Optimizing IUD Delivery for Adolescents and Young Adults

Mandy S. Coles • Aisha Mays

Editors

Optimizing IUD Delivery for Adolescents and Young Adults

Counseling, Placement, and Management

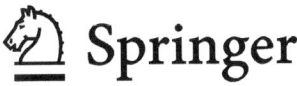 Springer

Editors
Mandy S. Coles, MD, MPH
Boston University Medical Center
Boston, MA, USA

Aisha Mays, MD
UC Berkley-UCSF Joint Medical Program
Berkeley, CA, USA

ISBN 978-3-030-17815-4   ISBN 978-3-030-17816-1   (eBook)
https://doi.org/10.1007/978-3-030-17816-1

This Springer imprint is published by the registered company Springer Nature Switzerland AG
The registered company address is: Gewerbestrasse 11, 6330 Cham, Switzerland

This text is dedicated to all of the amazing and resilient adolescents and young adults whom we serve.
May you always remember your strength and reach for your goals.

Acknowledgement

Style editing by Tricia J. Asklar

Introduction

Adolescents and young adults in the USA often experience barriers to IUD use, with unequal access to information, as well as service disparities. This book is designed to help support providers seeking to integrate, and/or expand IUD provision for adolescents and young adults in their practices. In recognizing the scope of experiences of our audience, we aim to provide a wide range of tools that may be useful. *Optimizing IUD Delivery for Adolescents and Young Adults: Counseling, Placement, and Management* is designed to serve as a working text that highlights the particular needs of adolescents and young adults surrounding IUD delivery; it is meant to act as a comprehensive IUD procedural text that is ideal for medical offices and teaching institutions alike.

We are lucky to have chapters written by experts in the fields of adolescent reproductive health and family planning from a variety of medical disciplines. Authors self-selected chapter topics based on their area of excellence and expertise. Many authors wrote collaboratively to add to the breadth and depth of the subject matter presented.

You will notice some similarities in each chapter of this book. Chapters all begin with **Learning Objectives** relevant to their topics, and all end with **Clinical Pearls** that are meant to be practical tips for the reader. Every chapter contains at least one case—to aid with integrating information and concepts presented in the text. As a reader, you will have the opportunity to think hypothetically about what you would do if you were put in these clinical case situations. Chapters are intended to be practical in nature. Each can be used as a stand-alone guide in clinical practice. Chapter 14 provides a list of additional resources organized by chapter, as well as full text or images of targeted materials for quick access.

Optimizing IUD Delivery for Adolescents and Young Adults: Counseling, Placement, and Management provides education and information to help providers incorporate developmentally appropriate counseling and IUD delivery approaches into their practice. Book chapters examine the history of IUDs, debunk commonly held IUD myths, and address IUD counseling, initiation, placement, and follow-up techniques unique to adolescent and young adult populations. The text closes with chapters on how to access IUD training, deliver IUD services in non-traditional settings, and how to utilize information on IUD billing and reimbursement. Clinical cases in each chapter provide both a clinical grounding and a context within which to apply the chapter material, in addition to integrating a variety of adolescent and young adult voices.

As editors and authors, we were very intentional about integrating reproductive justice and gender inclusivity into the text. The history of IUDs in the USA was not always a positive one—underserved communities and communities of color were often forced or coerced to adopt these methods. It is important for all IUD providers to be knowledgeable of these injustices in order to prevent them from recurring in their own practices; in the words of Loretta Ross, one of the leaders of the reproductive justice movement, "We can take advantage of this moment to advance reproductive justice for all...to advance and protect their full human rights." Aligned with reproductive justice principles—and discussed throughout this text—we support adolescents' and young adults' full autonomy regarding their reproductive life plans, access to the full range of contraceptive methods, and choice to have an IUD placed only if and when *they choose*—and to have it removed at any time as they request. Chapters on the history of IUDs (Chapter 1), counseling (Chapter 5), and when to insert IUDs (Chapter 6) all directly address the principles of reproductive justice in the context of IUD delivery.

Optimizing IUD Delivery for Adolescents and Young Adults: Counseling, Placement, and Management also fully supports gender diversity and inclusivity in clinical care and practice. We have been intentional in ensuring that all language in this text is gender neutral, except where citing research done with specific populations. You will notice that every case references the gender identity of the individual, and many cases include non-cisgender youth. Additionally, the chapters on adolescent-friendly clinical spaces (Chapter 2), consent (Chapter 7), and pain management (Chapter 9) specifically discuss strategies for working with individuals of all gender identities. Inclusion of and commitment to providing optimal reproductive health care for adolescents and young adults across the gender spectrum is one of the key tenets of reproductive justice.

We are grateful for the expert perspectives shared in this text. We hope that the richness of experience that is shared here will contribute to building access and equity in IUD counseling and provision, not only across socioeconomic, racial, cultural, geographic, and gender lines, but also within in our own communities. Dr. Jay Giedd reminds us that adolescence is "a time of enormous opportunity and of enormous risk." It is our intention that this book will help providers to support adolescents and young adults, empowering youth to take advantage of the opportunities that lie ahead.

Berkeley, CA, USA   Aisha Mays, MD
Boston, MA, USA   Mandy S. Coles, MD, MPH

Contents

Contributors

Aletha Y. Akers, MD, MPH The Craig Dalsimer Division of Adolescent Medicine, The Children's Hospital of Philadelphia, Philadelphia, PA, USA

Rebecca H. Allen, MD, MPH Department of Obstetrics and Gynecology, Women and Infants Hospital, Brown University, Providence, RI, USA

Lela R. Bachrach, MD, MS Department of Adolescent Medicine, UCSF Benioff Children's Hospital Oakland, Oakland, CA, USA

Yasmin Z. Bahar, DNP, RN, NP, FNP-BC Department of Pediatrics, New York Presbyterian Columbia University Medical Center, New York, NY, USA

Elise D. Berlan, MD, MPH Interim Chief, Adolescent Medicine, Associate Professor of Pediatrics, The Ohio State University College of Medicine, Division of Adolescent Medicine, Nationwide Children's Hospital, Columbus, OH, USA

Maria Brown, MD Division of Adolescent Medicine, Nationwide Children's Hospital, Columbus, OH, USA

Nicole Chaisson, MD, MPH Department of Family Medicine and Community Health, University of Minnesota, Minneapolis, MN, USA

Mandy S. Coles, MD, MPH Department of Pediatrics, Boston University Medical Center, Boston, MA, USA

Joy Friedman, MD Department of Pediatrics, Albert Einstein Medical Center, Philadelphia, PA, USA

Melanie A. Gold, DO, DMQ Department of Pediatrics, Division of Child and Adolescent Health, Columbia University Irving Medical Center/New York–Presbyterian Hospital, New York, NY, USA

Suzan Goodman, MD, MPH Bixby Center for Global Reproductive Health, Department of Family and Community Medicine, UCSF, San Francisco, CA, USA

Katherine Blumoff Greenberg, MD Departments of Pediatrics (Primary) and Obstetrics and Gynecology (Secondary), University of Rochester Medical Center, Rochester, NY, USA

Aisha Mays, MD UC Berkeley School of Public Health, UC Berkeley/UCSF Joint Medical Program, Berkeley, CA, USA

Rubiliatu A. Oluronbi, MD, MPH Department of Obstetrics and Gynecology, Albert Einstein Medical Center, Philadelphia, PA, USA

Rachel C. Passmore, MPH Department of Population and Family Health, Columbia University Mailman School of Public Health, New York, NY, USA

Amy Yoxthimer, PA-C, MPH Department of Women's Health, Open Door Family Medical Centers, Brewster, NY, USA

Chapter 1
The Intrauterine Device and Adolescents: History and Present

Maria Brown and Elise D. Berlan

Abbreviations

AAP	American Academy of Pediatrics
ACOG	American College of Obstetrics and Gynecology
AYA	Adolescent and Young Adult
CDC	Centers for Disease Control and Prevention
FDA	United States Food and Drug Administration
IUD	Intrauterine Device
LARC	Long-Acting Reversible Contraception
LNG	Levonorgestrel
MEC	Medical Eligibility Criteria
PID	Pelvic Inflammatory Disease
SAHM	Society of Adolescent Health and Medicine
SES	Socioeconomic Status
STI	Sexually Transmitted Infection
WHO	World Health Organization

Learning Objectives
Following completion of this chapter, you should be able to:

1. Discuss the history of intrauterine devices (IUDs) in the USA
2. Explain the history and commonly held misconceptions about adolescent IUD use.
3. Describe the history of reproductive coercion and injustice involving the IUD in the USA

M. Brown (✉)
Division of Adolescent Medicine, Nationwide Children's Hospital, Columbus, OH, USA
e-mail: maria.brown@nationwidechildrens.org

E. D. Berlan
Interim Chief, Adolescent Medicine, Associate Professor of Pediatrics,
The Ohio State University College of Medicine, Division of Adolescent Medicine,
Nationwide Children's Hospital, Columbus, OH, USA

© Springer Nature Switzerland AG 2019
M. S. Coles, A. Mays (eds.), *Optimizing IUD Delivery for Adolescents and Young Adults*, https://doi.org/10.1007/978-3-030-17816-1_1

Introduction

The modern IUD has existed in some shape or form since the beginning of the twentieth century [1]. Despite advances in this form of long-acting reversible contraception (LARC) and their demonstrated safety and efficacy for use in adolescents [2], there remain misconceptions among patients and providers regarding IUD safety and indications for use [3]. As adolescent and young adults (AYAs) are at especially high risk of unintended pregnancy, it is imperative that they are aware of all available forms of contraception, including IUDs, in order to make informed decisions that best fit their individual reproductive goals [4]. Approaches that support each patient and help them to choose a method that best meets their current and anticipated needs will be discussed in more detail in Chap. 5 [5].

Case

Callie is a 15-year-old cisgender female presenting for contraception options counseling with her mother. She was previously started on oral contraceptive pills for dysmenorrhea. However, despite many efforts to remember, she often forgets her pills. Her mother complains that her cramps have been worse recently because she is not consistent with her pills, and she has been missing more school. In private, Callie tells you that she is not currently having sex, but has a boyfriend of 6 months and they are talking about having sex soon. She has heard about IUDs from a friend and thinks that she would like to get one. With her mother back in the room, Callie voices interest in the hormonal IUD to help with her cramps. Her mother raises concerns that the IUD is too "new" and has not had enough time to be "proven safe."

IUD History

Reviewing the history of the IUD can help us to better understand some of the lingering misconceptions regarding current IUDs [1]. First-generation IUDs were made in Germany and consisted of silkworm gut, and later hard rubber or various metals [1, 6]. England and British overseas territories later adopted the "Gräfenberg Ring" a spirally coiled metal ring composed of copper, nickel, and zinc created by Ernest Gräfenberg of Berlin, in the mid-1900s [1]. Second-generation devices containing plastic components later emerged and included the Maizlin Spring, Incon Ring, and the Dalkon Shield [1]. The Dalkon Shield, produced by the A.H. Robins pharmaceutical company, was made available for use in the USA in 1971; approximately 3.6 million were sold worldwide. The Dalkon Shield IUD was a plastic, irregular oval shape device with "foot-like" projections to prevent expulsion, and was attached to a porous multifilament string. See Fig. 1.1 below.

Fig. 1.1 A number of
IUDs throughout history.
(Presented with permission
from the Dittrick Medical
History Center at Case
Western Reserve
University)

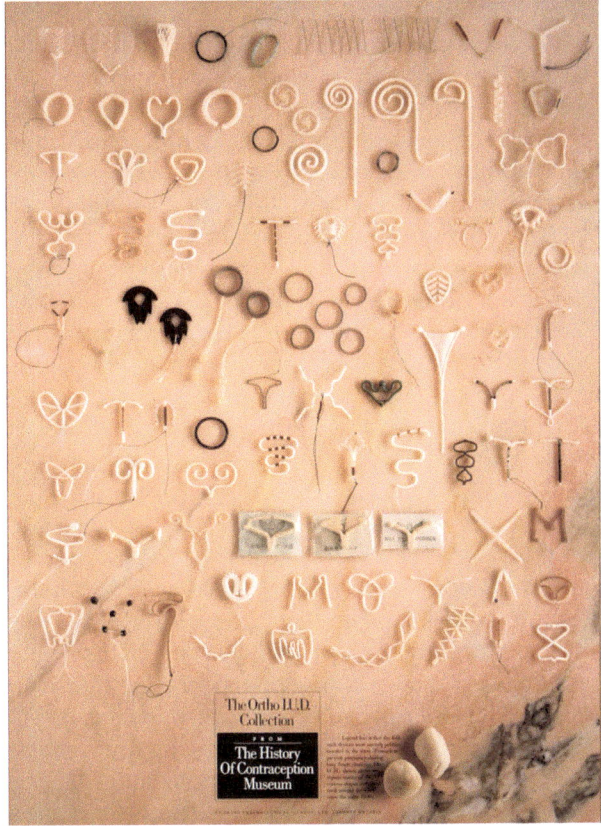

Concerns regarding IUD safety came to the forefront in 1968 with a published
report documenting critical IUD-associated complications and death [7]. Reports
of septic abortions among Dalkon shield users prompted the Centers for Disease
Control and Prevention (CDC) to conduct a physician survey in 1973 regarding
patients who had been hospitalized with or had died from complications related
to the use of an IUD in the previous 6 months [8]. This study estimated a device-
related hospitalization rate of 5 per 1000 IUD users. Five device-related fatalities
were noted, with four due to severe infection. There were additional reports around
that time of maternal morbidity and mortality associated with pregnancy and the
Dalkon shield in situ [9]. Use of the Dalkon shield was subsequently noted to be
associated with higher pregnancy rates than expected, and higher risk of complicated pregnancies including spontaneous and septic abortions [10]. Distribution
of the Dalkon Shield was halted after USA Food and Drug Administration (FDA)
hearings in 1974 [9]. More than 400,000 lawsuits were filed against A.H. Robins
and, in 1985, the company filed for bankruptcy.

There has been considerable controversy over the last several decades about IUD
use and the risk of pelvic inflammatory disease (PID), infection, and infertility, as
well as the role of the Dalkon Shield's multifilament tailstring in upper genital tract
infection among its users. While earlier retrospective case–control studies impli-

cated IUDs, and the Dalkon Shield in particular, with PID and tubal infertility [10, 11], researchers since have identified bias and methodologic flaws in these earlier studies [8, 12]. These included use of inappropriate comparison groups, ascertainment bias (over-diagnosing salpingitis among IUD users), and not controlling for confounding factors, such as number of sexual partners. When these biases were subsequently accounted for, the attributed increase in infection risk related to IUD use was greatly diminished [13]. However, some disagreement persists regarding the Dalkon Shield's multifilament tail strings and their possible role in ascending infection [14, 15].

With negative press about the Dalkon Shield and concerns about the safety of intrauterine contraception, use of IUDs plummeted in the USA from a peak of 9.6% of married women using contraception in 1973 [16] to a nadir of 0.8% of women 15–44 years of age using contraception in the mid-1990s [17]. Despite declines in IUD demand in the USA their use around the world remained strong, and investigators continued to actively work on IUD design. In 1969 gynecologists at the University of Santiago developed a third-generation copper-containing IUD [6]. Later, fourth- and fifth-generation IUDs – hormone-releasing devices – were developed in Finland, and led to the current levonorgestrel (LNG) IUDs [6]. These later-generation devices have not been associated with the complications of the earlier IUDs, resulting in their increased use. Worldwide use of IUDs varies across countries and regions for a variety of reasons, including geographic differences, government policies, and healthcare provider education [18]. The most recent analysis of IUD use among married or in-union women ages 15–49 from the United Nations found wide variation in IUD use, ranging from around 1% in Oceania to more than 17% in Asia. Among industrialized countries, IUD use in the USA falls behind other countries, with 5% of women married or in-union using an IUD compared to 11% across Europe [19]. Adolescents in the USA are even less likely to use IUDs compared to adult women [20].

Contemporary IUDs

IUDs have become more accepted in the USA in recent years. Between 2002 and 2012, the percentage of sexually active women aged 15–44 years using an IUD increased more than five-fold to 9.5% [21]. A solid body of evidence demonstrates that current FDA-approved IUDs (copper IUD and LNG IUDs) are very safe to use, including in AYAs [22]. Complications from IUDs are uncommon, and include expulsion, perforation, and infection [22]. Importantly, there is not an increased risk of PID or sexually transmitted infections (STIs) in adolescent IUD users compared to the general population [23]. As of 2019, there are five IUDs available in the USA (described in more detail in Chap. 3). The CuT380A copper IUD was FDA approved in 1984. There are four hormonal IUDs, including two LNG 52 mg devices (FDA approved in 2000 and 2015), one LNG 19.5 mg device (FDA approved in 2016), and one LNG 13.5 mg device (FDA approved in 2013).

Case

You explain that IUDs are known to be safe for adolescents – even those who have never had a baby, and that using an IUD would not affect Callie's future fertility. Her mom seems more comfortable knowing that the IUD would be safe for use in her daughter. However, she raises additional concerns. Why has she never heard of IUDs being used with adolescents before? What if Callie has it placed, but doesn't like it? Can it be removed early? How effective is this method compared to the pills Callie was on previously?

Adolescents and Reproductive Health

In 2017, an estimated 39.5% of USA high school students reported having had sexual intercourse at least once [24]. As adolescents age, they are more likely to become sexually active; in 2017, an estimated 20.4% of ninth graders reported having had intercourse and by twelfth grade, an estimated 57.3% reported having had intercourse [24]. While rates of adolescent sexual activity and pregnancy have declined over the past decades, the USA has the highest adolescent pregnancy rate among developed countries [25–27], and most adolescent pregnancies are unintended.

Younger adolescents are less likely to use contraception with first intercourse compared to older adolescents [28]. In those who use contraception, the most common methods among USA adolescents are condoms, withdrawal, and oral contraceptive pills [28]. IUDs and contraceptive implants are the least-used method in this population, as demonstrated by the 2017 Youth Risk Behavior Surveillance Study that found that 5.3% of female high school students in the USA used a form of LARC [24]. While rates of IUD use in recent years have increased in most cohorts of women of reproductive age, this growth has not been reflected among adolescents [29].

Provider Misconceptions Around IUDs

Despite established safety and benefits, many healthcare providers continue to have concerns about IUDs [3, 30]. For example, a 2015 study assessing IUD-related knowledge and experience among family medicine residents found that half of the respondents were unwilling to place an IUD in a woman with a history of STIs within the previous 6 months and more than a third would not place an IUD if there was a history of ectopic pregnancy. Many residents would also not insert an IUD if a Pap test had not been completed in the last year, if the patient was not in a monogamous relationship, or if there was a remote history of PID [30]. These misconceptions are not evidence-based and are not consistent with current guidelines [31].

Additionally, many pediatric providers remain uncomfortable with counseling on IUDs as an option for contraception. Misinformation, suspicion regarding recommendation reversals, and scientifically unsupported beliefs about adolescent IUD use are common themes in studies of pediatricians. In a 2013 study, only 11% of pediatricians would recommend the IUD as an appropriate form of contraception for their patients [32]. Pediatrician knowledge in this study was inconsistent with contemporaneous scientific evidence, which showed no increased risk of infections or infertility with IUD use. In a later study, primary care pediatricians perceived IUDs to pose significant risks for adverse reproductive health outcomes and to be poorly tolerated by adolescents [33]. Provider misconceptions regarding safety, efficacy and indications for an IUD impede adolescents' access to a full range of contraceptive options.

Adolescent Awareness and Misconceptions Around IUDs

Studies of AYAs have found that many are unfamiliar with IUDs [34, 35]. On a college campus, less than 25% of young women surveyed had heard of IUDs and most reported little or no knowledge of this method [36]. Among AYAs who knew about IUDs, the most common reasons for disinterest in the method included the "idea of something in my body," fear of pain with device insertion, and that a healthcare professional is required to insert and remove the device [35]. Interviews of female college students found mostly negative beliefs about IUDs as well, which were related to their fear of IUD-related infertility, hormonal side effects, and physical damage to their bodies [37]. AYAs may be influenced by friends' and family members' unfavorable opinions toward IUDs, as well as myths that IUDs are for women who have been pregnant before [37, 38], as further detailed in Chap. 5.

History of Reproductive Coercion and IUD Use

One cannot examine the history of IUDs in the USA without acknowledging how these methods have been used to control the fertility of particular communities over the past decades [39]. African American, Latinx, indigenous, and disabled persons in particular have experienced reproductive coercion around both LARC device placement and removal. In the 1990s, court judges from several states offered women the use of Norplant (a five-rod contraceptive implant) in exchange for lighter sentencing or to avoid federal prison terms [40, 41]. Similarly, during the same time period in California, additional financial public benefits were offered to women on government assistance if they agreed to have Norplant inserted. Evidence exists that healthcare providers are more likely to recommend the IUD to lower socioeconomic status (SES) Latinx and Black patients than to lower SES white patients [42]. Additionally, many young Black and Latinx women have reported feeling pressured in their experiences with contraceptive care and discussions with their providers, including IUDs, implants, and oral contraceptive pills [43]. Clinical practices continue to exist that promote same-day LARC insertion, but require multiple visits for LARC removal. It is our duty as healthcare providers to inform all of our patients of the full range of contraceptive options available to them, while keeping in line with a reproductive justice framework that patients have the ultimate say on whether or not to use contraception and on their method of choice. Our ultimate goal is "to enhance the health, social well-being, and bodily integrity of all our contraceptive clients," which includes honoring and respecting individuals "decisions not to use LARC, their ability to have LARC removed when they wish and their ability to have the children they want to have [44]."

Contemporary IUDs and Adolescents

In the story of IUDs, where are we now? The IUD is currently one of the most cost-effective methods of contraception in the USA [45, 46], and there has been a steady increase in use of IUDs over recent years [47]. Contemporary IUDs are safely used by adolescents and adults all over the world, without increased risk of STIs [48, 49]. In one large USA study, most adolescent IUD users were satisfied with their IUD, and only a minority opted for removal within the first year [50].

Case

Callie and her mother feel much better about an IUD as an acceptable option for Callie. Callie voices interest in the IUD because "I don't have to do anything!" Callie's only concern is that her cousin's best friend's sister-in-law posted on her social media account that there's a high infection rate. Is this true? You explain that using the IUD does not increase her risk of STIs. Callie and her mom decide that an IUD is the best option for her, and Callie is referred to an Adolescent Medicine provider for IUD placement. You advise Callie to continue her birth control pills for now, confidentially provide her counseling on condom use, and offer her condoms to take home.

Professional medical groups strongly support healthcare providers in recommending intrauterine contraception to adolescents. In 2004, the World Health Organization (WHO) released the Medical Eligibility Criteria for Contraceptive Use (MEC), which stated that the IUD was an acceptable contraceptive choice for this age group. For nulliparous women and women less than 20 years old, the WHO MEC indicates the advantages of using intrauterine contraception generally outweigh the theoretical or proven risks [51]. In 2007 and again in 2018, the American College of Obstetricians and Gynecologists (ACOG) released Committee Opinions supporting the use of IUD in nulliparous women and adolescents [23, 52]. Similarly, in 2013, the CDC released its Selected Practice Recommendations for Contraceptive Use, stating that IUDs can "be used by women of all ages, including adolescents, and both parous and nulliparous women" [53]. This statement was reconfirmed in the CDC's 2016 release [54]. The American Academy of Pediatrics (AAP) followed suit when it released a policy statement in 2014 declaring that pediatricians should educate adolescent patients about LARC and that LARC methods are "first line" contraceptives for adolescents [4]. The Society for Adolescent Health and Medicine (SAHM) went further in their 2017 position paper, specifically focused on AYA access to LARCs using a reproductive justice framework, in recommending that "LARCs are offered and are available as part of essential, comprehensive contraceptive options through education, counseling, and healthcare services [55]." Their website provides links to clinical care guidelines by the WHO, ACOG, CDC, and AAP to provide clinicians easy access to reproductive health clinical care guidelines and resources [56].

Clinical Pearls
- Despite prior safety outcomes, contemporary IUDs have been well studied and proven safe for use by all people, including AYAs.
- In contrast to historical IUDs, contemporary IUDs have a well-demonstrated safety record.
- Given past incidences of reproductive coercion and other attempts to control individuals' fertility, counseling around IUDs should incorporate the principles of reproductive justice.

References

1. Margulies L. History of intrauterine devices. Bull N Y Acad Med. 1975;51:662–7.
2. Allen S, Barlow E. Long-acting reversible contraception: an essential guide for pediatric primary care providers. Pediatr Clin North Am. 2017;64:359–69.
3. Stubbs E, Schamp A. The evidence is in. Why are IUDs still out?: family physicians' perceptions of risk and indications. Can Fam Physician. 2008;54:560–6.
4. Ott MA, Sucato GS. Committee on Adolescence. Contraception for adolescents. Pediatrics. 2014;134:e1257–81.
5. Gomez AM, Fuentes L, Allina A. Women or LARC first? Reproductive autonomy and the promotion of long-acting reversible contraceptive methods. Perspect Sex Reprod Health. 2014;46:171–5.
6. Thiery M. Intrauterine contraception: from silver ring to intrauterine contraceptive implant. Eur J Obstet Gynecol Reprod Biol. 2000;90:145–52.
7. Scott RB. Critical illnesses and deaths associated with intrauterine devices. Obstet Gynecol. 1968;31:322–7.
8. Sivin I. Another look at the Dalkon Shield: meta-analysis underscores its problems. Contraception. 1993;48:1–12.
9. Levinson CJ, Richardson DC. The Dalkon shield story. Adv Plan Parent. 1976;11:53–63.
10. Tietze C, Lewit S. Evaluation of intrauterine devices: ninth progress report of the cooperative statistical program. Stud Fam Plann. 1970;1:1.
11. Spellacy WN, Birk SA, Gordon L. Comparative randomized study of the Copper-T 200 and Dalkon Shield intrauterine devices. Contraception. 1975;12:453–63.
12. Grimes DA. Intrauterine device and upper-genital-tract infection. Lancet. 2000;356:1013–9.
13. Buchan H, Villard-Mackintosh L, Vessey M, Yeates D, McPherson K. Epidemiology of pelvic inflammatory disease in parous women with special reference to intrauterine device use. Br J Obstet Gynaecol. 1990;97:780–8.

14. Tennant C, Schreiber CA. Time to trim the loose ends of the tailstring debate. Contraception. 2011;84:108; author reply 108–9.
15. Lyus R, Lohr P, Prager S. The Dalkon Shield and pelvic infection. Contraception. 2011;84:108–9.
16. Mosher WD, Westoff CF. Trends in contraceptive practice: United States, 1965–76. Vital Health Stat. 1982;23:1–47.
17. Mosher WD, Martinez GM, Chandra A, Abma JC, Willson SJ. Use of contraception and use of family planning services in the United States: 1982–2002. Adv Data. 2004;(350):1–36.
18. Buhling KJ, Zite NB, Lotke P, Black K, INTRA Writing Group. Worldwide use of intrauterine contraception: a review. Contraception. 2014;89:162–73.
19. United Nations Department of Economic and Social Affairs, Division for the Advancement of Women Staff. Trends in contraceptive use worldwide 2015. New York: United Nations Department of Economic and Social Affairs, Division; 2015.
20. Daniels K, Daugherty J, Jones J, Mosher W. Current contraceptive use and variation by selected characteristics among women aged 15–44: United States, 2011–2013. Natl Health Stat Report. 2015;(86):1–14.
21. Mosher WD, Moreau C, Lantos H. Trends and determinants of IUD use in the USA, 2002–2012. Hum Reprod. 2016;31:1696–702.
22. Jatlaoui TC, Riley HEM, Curtis KM. The safety of intrauterine devices among young women: a systematic review. Contraception. 2017;95:17–39.
23. American College of Obstetricians and Gynecologists. ACOG Committee Opinion No. 392, December 2007. Intrauterine device and adolescents. Obstet Gynecol. 2007;110:1493–5.
24. Kann L, McManus T, Harris WA, Shanklin SL, Flint KH, Queen B, et al. Youth risk behavior surveillance - United States, 2017. MMWR Surveill Summ. 2018;67:1–114.
25. Kost K, Henshaw S. U.S. Teenage pregnancies births and abortions 2010- national and state trends by age race and ethnicity. New York: Guttmacher; 2014. [Internet]. [cited 28 Nov 2018]. Available: http://www.guttmacher.org/pubs/USTPtrends10.pdf.
26. Sedgh G, Finer LB, Bankole A, Eilers MA, Singh S. Adolescent pregnancy, birth, and abortion rates across countries: levels and recent trends. J Adolesc Health. 2015;56:223–30.
27. Abma JC, Martinez GM. Sexual activity and contraceptive use among teenagers in the United States, 2011–2015. Natl Health Stat Report. 2017;(104):1–23.
28. Martinez GM, Abma JC. Sexual activity, contraceptive use, and childbearing of teenagers aged 15–19 in the United States. NCHS Data Brief. 2015;(209):1–8.
29. Romero L, Pazol K, Warner L, Gavin L, Moskosky S, Besera G, et al. Vital signs: trends in use of long-acting reversible contraception among teens aged 15–19 years seeking contraceptive services—United States, 2005–2013. MMWR Morb Mortal Wkly Rep. 2015;64:363–9.
30. Schubert FD, Herbitter C, Fletcher J, Gold M. IUD knowledge and experience among family medicine residents. Fam Med. 2015;47:474–7.
31. Curtis KM, Tepper NK, Jatlaoui TC, Berry-Bibee E, Horton LG, Zapata LB, et al. U.S. medical eligibility criteria for contraceptive use, 2016. MMWR Recomm Rep. 2016;65:1–103.
32. Wilson SF, Strohsnitter W, Baecher-Lind L. Practices and perceptions among pediatricians regarding adolescent contraception with emphasis on intrauterine contraception. J Pediatr Adolesc Gynecol. 2013;26:281–4.
33. Berlan ED, Pritt NM, Norris AH. Pediatricians' attitudes and beliefs about long-acting reversible contraceptives influence counseling. J Pediatr Adolesc Gynecol. 2017;30:47–52.
34. Barrett M, Soon R, Whitaker AK, Takekawa S, Kaneshiro B. Awareness and knowledge of the intrauterine device in adolescents. J Pediatr Adolesc Gynecol. 2012;25:39–42.
35. Fleming KL, Sokoloff A, Raine TR. Attitudes and beliefs about the intrauterine device among teenagers and young women. Contraception. 2010;82:178–82.
36. Hall KS, Ela E, Zochowski MK, Caldwell A, Moniz M, McAndrew L, et al. "I don't know enough to feel comfortable using them:" women's knowledge of and perceived barriers to long-acting reversible contraceptives on a college campus. Contraception. 2016;93:556–64.
37. Payne JB, Sundstrom B, DeMaria AL. A qualitative study of young women's beliefs about intrauterine devices: fear of infertility. J Midwifery Womens Health. 2016;61:482–8.

38. Hoopes AJ, Teal SB, Akers AY, Sheeder J. Low acceptability of certain contraceptive methods among young women. J Pediatr Adolesc Gynecol. 2018;31:274–80.
39. Roberts D. Killing the black body: race, reproduction, and the meaning of liberty. New York: Vintage Books; 2014.
40. The Norplant Sentence. In: Washington Post [Internet]. The Washington Post; 24 Jan 1991 [cited 28 Nov 2018]. Available: https://www.washingtonpost.com/archive/opinions/1991/01/24/the-norplant-sentence/aa7453d8-639f-4fa8-bacb-b96e77dc6c0f/.
41. Walker KM. Judicial control of reproductive freedom: the use of norplant as a condition of probation. Iowa L Rev. 1992–1993;78:779.
42. Dehlendorf C, Ruskin R, Grumbach K, Vittinghoff E, Bibbins-Domingo K, Schillinger D, et al. Recommendations for intrauterine contraception: a randomized trial of the effects of patients' race/ethnicity and socioeconomic status. Am J Obstet Gynecol. 2010;203:319.e1–8.
43. Gomez AM, Wapman M. Under (implicit) pressure: young Black and Latina women's perceptions of contraceptive care. Contraception. 2017;96:221–6.
44. Higgins JA. Celebration meets caution: LARC's boons, potential busts, and the benefits of a reproductive justice approach. Contraception. 2014;89:237–41.
45. Trussell J, Lalla AM, Doan QV, Reyes E, Pinto L, Gricar J. Cost effectiveness of contraceptives in the United States. Contraception. 2009;79:5–14.
46. Trussell J. Update on and correction to the cost-effectiveness of contraceptives in the United States. Contraception. 2012;85:611.
47. Kavanaugh ML, Jerman J, Finer LB. Changes in use of long-acting reversible contraceptive methods among U.S. women, 2009–2012. Obstet Gynecol. 2015;126:917–27.
48. Alton TM, Brock GN, Yang D, Wilking DA, Hertweck SP, Loveless MB. Retrospective review of intrauterine device in adolescent and young women. J Pediatr Adolesc Gynecol. 2012;25:195–200.
49. Paterson H, Ashton J, Harrison-Woolrych M. A nationwide cohort study of the use of the levo-norgestrel intrauterine device in New Zealand adolescents. Contraception. 2009;79:433–8.
50. Grunloh DS, Casner T, Secura GM, Peipert JF, Madden T. Characteristics associated with discontinuation of long-acting reversible contraception within the first 6 months of use. Obstet Gynecol. 2013;122:1214–21.
51. World Health Organization. Medical eligibility criteria for contraceptive use. 3rd ed. Geneva: World Health Organization; 2010. p. 1–17.
52. ACOG Committee Opinion No. 735: adolescents and long-acting reversible contraception: implants and intrauterine devices. Obstet Gynecol. 2018;131:e130–e139.
53. Curtis KM, Tepper NK, Jamieson DJ, Marchbanks PA. Adaptation of the World Health Organization's selected practice recommendations for contraceptive use for the United States. Contraception. 2013;87:513–6.
54. Curtis KM, Jatlaoui TC, Tepper NK, Zapata LB, Horton LG, Jamieson DJ, et al. U.S. selected practice recommendations for contraceptive use, 2016. MMWR Recomm Rep. 2016;65:1–66.
55. Society for Adolescent Health and Medicine. Improving knowledge about, access to, and utilization of long-acting reversible contraception among adolescents and young adults. J Adolesc Health Care. 2017;60:472–4.
56. Pregnancy – Society for Adolescent Health and Medicine [Internet]. [cited 28 Nov 2018]. Available: https://www.adolescenthealth.org/Resources/Clinical-Care-Resources/Sexual-Reproductive-Health/Clinical-Care-Guidelines/Pregnancy.aspx#Contraception.

Chapter 2
Making Your Office Accessible for Adolescent and Young Adult IUD Services

Suzan Goodman and Lela R. Bachrach

Abbreviations

AYA	Adolescent and young adult
EC	Emergency contraception
EHR	Electronic health records
IUD	Intrauterine device
LARC	Long-acting reversible contraception
LGBTQIA	Lesbian, gay, bisexual, transgender, queer or questioning, intersex, asexual, agender or allied
STI	Sexually transmitted infection

Learning Objectives

Following completion of this chapter, you should be able to:

1. Consider key barriers and solutions tailored for adolescent-friendly contraceptive care.
2. Plan specific improvements to assure privacy, confidentiality, and patient autonomy in contraceptive services for adolescent and young adult (AYAs).
3. Learn best practices to meet adolescent clients' needs across the cultural and gender spectrum.

S. Goodman (✉)
Bixby Center for Global Reproductive Health, Department of Family and Community Medicine, UCSF, San Francisco, CA, USA

L. R. Bachrach
Department of Adolescent Medicine, UCSF Benioff Children's Hospital Oakland, Oakland, CA, USA

© Springer Nature Switzerland AG 2019
M. S. Coles, A. Mays (eds.), *Optimizing IUD Delivery for Adolescents and Young Adults*, https://doi.org/10.1007/978-3-030-17816-1_2

11

4. Discuss key modifications to assure rapid-access scheduling, clinic flow, and/or timely referral for contraception, including quick-start of all methods including Long-acting reversible contraception (LARC).
5. Apply key principles, evidence, and cost considerations for equitable contraceptive services.

Introduction

Many of the barriers that AYAs face in accessing health services are unique to young people, due to their stage in life and associated needs, perceptions, and abilities. Adolescent-friendly services are those effectively able to attract young people, responsively meet AYA needs, and go on serving those needs through continuing care. This chapter discusses key obstacles faced by AYAs, important elements of adolescent-friendly health service provision and patient-centered contraceptive care, as well as best practices and real-world examples for successful integration of same-day intrauterinee device (IUD) provision for both emergency and ongoing contraception.

Case

Dillon, a 16-year-old transgender male (assigned female at birth) high school student, drops in to clinic asking for an appointment for "a cough, and um… (under his breath) the morning after pill." He usually has sex with cis-women, but twice in the last week he had receptive vaginal penile intercourse without condoms. The busy front desk staff person asks impatiently: "Have we seen you before? Have your parents given consent for you to be seen?" and states, "For birth control, there are condoms in the jar." The staff person is confused about Dillon's gender and thinks emergency contraception (EC) is for Dillon's partner. Dillon nearly leaves out of embarrassment and fear of parental disclosure, but cannot afford over-the-counter EC pills, so decides to wait. After waiting idly for an hour, Dillon texts a friend who recommends that he goes to a "better clinic that really listens and will see you today." Dillon leaves to head across town to the other clinic.

How might this clinic have better accommodated Dillon's needs?

The Importance of Clinical Services Tailored to Adolescents

Healthcare providers can best approach the developmental, sexual, and reproductive health needs of AYAs if they appreciate the particular obstacles patients may face negotiating the healthcare system. Barriers frequently faced by trans or cis adolescents include insensitive attitudes by care providers and a perceived (or real) lack of confidentiality [1, 2]—for example, via inadvertent lapses due to insurance billing (detailed explanation of benefits to policyholders) or electronic health record (EHR) glitches, such as after-visit summaries that include sensitive diagnoses [3]. Limited hours and services offered, combined with transportation challenges, which many adolescents face, create another barrier.

Providers can take an active role in increasing awareness of LARC among young people, rather than relying on patient requests for methods of which they have little knowledge [4]. Clinic policies should address a variety of system- and provider-level updates to facilitate same-day provision and meet patient needs. A recent survey of USA publicly funded family planning facilities found most ensured confidential services for young clients, however 36% lacked flexible hours, 33% required appointments for contraceptive refills, and 30% lacked outreach and/or education focusing on adolescents [5]. When clinical services are specially tailored to the needs of AYAs, providers have greater opportunities to offer timely services and improve adolescent health outcomes [6].

Case continuation

Dillon arrives at a colorful, busy, adolescent medicine clinic near his school during evening hours. He feels at home seeing a rainbow placard in the window, contraceptive pamphlets, and privacy dividers between the front desk and the waiting area. The staff person is friendly and uses gender-neutral language to avoid assumptions based on appearance. A poster reads: "Our Policy on Confidentiality: Our discussions with you are private. We hope that you feel free to talk openly with us about yourself and your health..." Dillon gets help applying for state health insurance coverage that will protect his confidentiality regarding sensitive services, receives a pamphlet on the pros and cons of EC methods, and watches a video on contraceptive options for AYAs. Dillon learns that oral EC medications are less effective at higher body weights, and thinks about his two recent episodes of unprotected sex, which have put him at risk of pregnancy (because he still has a uterus and testosterone is not effective contraception). Dillon desires ongoing contraception and decides to choose a copper IUD. A medical assistant prepares placement materials and consents, and a clinician places the IUD and collects Sexually transmitted infection (STI) screening tests. Dillon is very grateful that he is able to receive EC and have an IUD placed for ongoing pregnancy prevention on the same day.

Best Practices and Real-World Applications

There have been increasing USA and global efforts to design services aimed to overcome barriers faced by AYAs and to improve the quality of care to specifically meet their healthcare needs. Below we outline overarching principles, best practices, and real-world applications for providing adolescent-friendly health services, with a specific focus on contraceptive services, including IUDs. These principles from Advocates for Youth [7], the Adolescent Sexual and Reproductive Health

Education Program (Physicians for Reproductive Health) [8], the Society for Adolescent Health and Medicine [9, 10], the American College of Gynecology and Obstetrics [11], and the World Health Organization [12, 13] are adapted throughout this chapter, unless otherwise noted.

Principle #1—Create a visually appealing atmosphere and material Providing a youth-friendly setting will help to attract and allow AYAs to feel more comfortable in clinical spaces. Figure 2.1 shows an open and colorful reception area. Consider both the space and clinic flow to allow for optimal ways to reach patients before and throughout their visit. Use multimedia educational materials (print, video, audio, web-based) that are eye-catching, up-to-date, evidence-based, at appropriate reading and comprehension levels, in the languages and cultures reflective of your patient community (see Figs. 2.2 and 2.3). Consider using technology to facilitate engagement while maintaining confidentiality, such as social media to engage and communicate with AYAs [37]. A study in an urban pediatric emergency department offered AYAs the opportunity to watch a tablet-based contraceptive education video, and found it feasible, acceptable, and successful in building interest in highly effective methods [38].

Other examples of how to make clinic atmosphere and materials appealing to AYAs:

- Incorporate technology when feasible—including access to educational materials with high-yield websites bookmarked on tablets or kiosks—and text health education pearls or appointment reminders.
- Encourage apps and websites that provide evidence-based sexual health information. Some examples include: bedsider.org, reproductiveaccess.org, teensouce. org, and plannedparenthood.org, as well as myriad period-tracking apps.
- Explore social media opportunities to engage AYAs and provide information about the clinic and services, as well as health education [14].

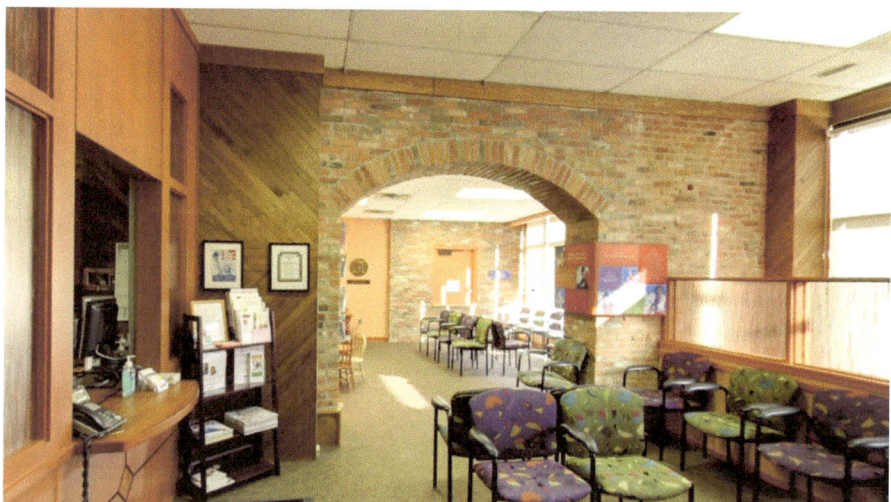

Fig. 2.1 AYAs welcomed by a light-filled, colorful waiting area. Image source: (The Corner Health Center)

Fig. 2.2 Playful dots and ample materials make a space more welcoming. (Image source: Michigan Medical – Saline Health Center)

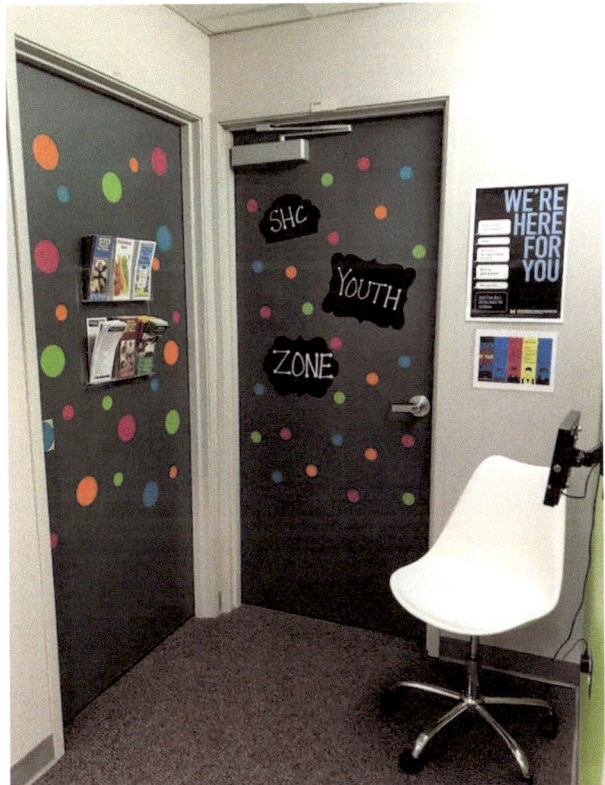

Fig. 2.3 Colorful exam room with informative posters and comfortable chair. (Image source: Dream Youth Clinic)

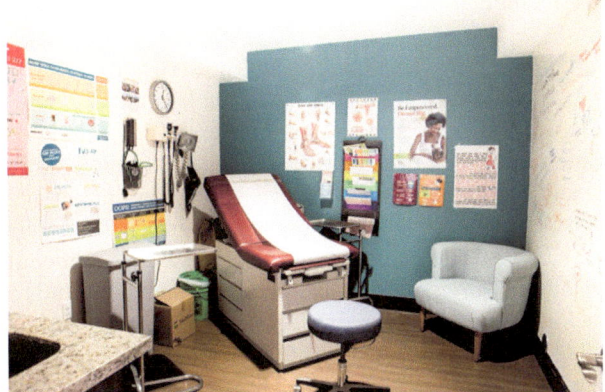

- Provide AYA-focused magazines, videos, educational materials, and posters on topics to discuss with a clinician.
- Consider creating infographics and other visual aids to improve patients' understanding of health risks and intervention outcomes [15, 16]. See Fig. 2.4 for some examples.
- Use anatomical posters of individuals from varied ethnic backgrounds and gender identities.

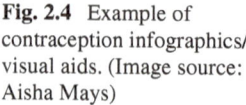

Fig. 2.4 Example of contraception infographics/ visual aids. (Image source: Aisha Mays)

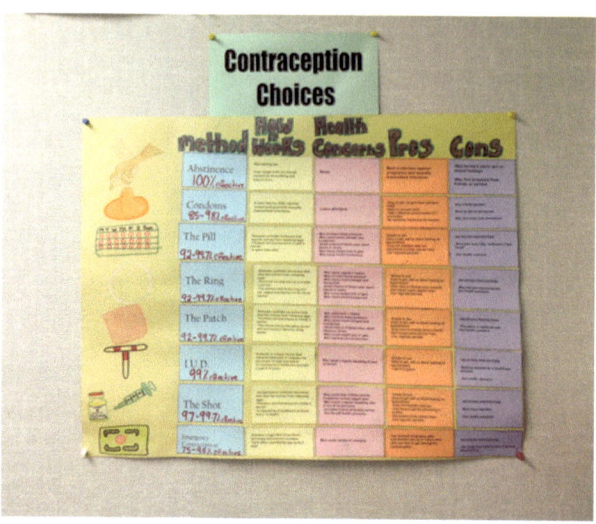

- Create clinic environments that are bright, clean, gender inclusive, and relevant to the different cultural groups of AYAs you serve. Consider reviewing "Drawing a Picture: Adolescent-Centered Medical Homes" video created by the Adolescent Health Initiative [17].
- Utilize peer education support methods by showing videos that highlight peer experiences about birth control and side effects (see www.bedsider.org).
- Display anatomic models and contraceptive devices in patient rooms to allow opportunities for patients to ask questions, and to provide modalities for visual learning.

Principle #2—Ensure privacy and confidentiality AYAs have their own cultures, which often include a distinct language, a particular attire, a focus on peers and pop culture, and an ongoing search for individual identity [18]. To best serve adolescents, clinical services should foster the culture, relationships, and environment in which they will engage. Adolescents are more likely to seek health services, disclose health risk behaviors, and return for follow-up care when confidentiality is assured [19]. Young people greatly value confidentiality while receiving family planning services [20]. Requiring parental consent is a significant barrier for many adolescents who may not feel safe discussing birth control, pregnancy testing, or STI screening and treatment with parents. Many AYAs may forgo care if confidentiality is not guaranteed [7, 21, 22]. The following strategies focus on improving privacy before, during, and after the visit.

- Post signs about the importance of provider-patient confidentiality to alert both adolescents and parents/guardians that patients will be seen alone at every visit. These can be posted in waiting and exam rooms. Figure 2.5 shows a sample posting.

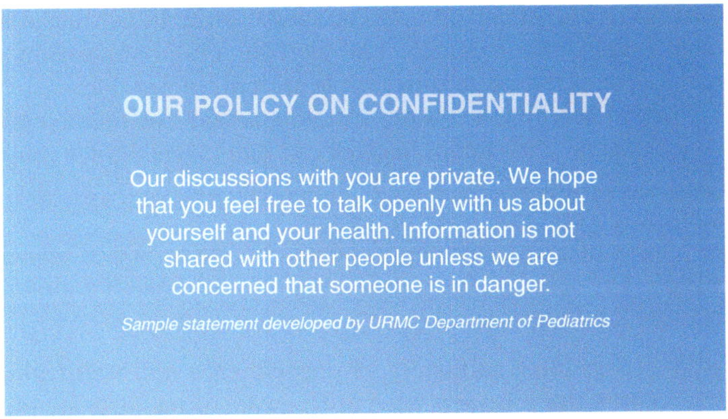

OUR POLICY ON CONFIDENTIALITY

Our discussions with you are private. We hope that you feel free to talk openly with us about yourself and your health. Information is not shared with other people unless we are concerned that someone is in danger.

Sample statement developed by URMC Department of Pediatrics

Fig. 2.5 A sample confidentiality policy that can be posted in waiting rooms and exam rooms: [18]. (Image source: PRH ARSHEP Adolescent Friendly Health Services Slide Set)

- Discuss confidentiality (and its limits) with patients and families during early adolescence to set expectations about the transition from childhood to adolescence. Educate about the need for AYAs to develop autonomy and assume more responsibility for their own health and health care. An example of this may be:
  - "Everything we discuss in this visit is confidential, which means that I don't discuss any information that you share with me with anyone else unless you tell me that you're going to hurt yourself, hurt someone else, or if someone is hurting you."
- Ensure time alone with patients during every clinic history, even when AYAs are accompanied by a parent, partner, or peer.
- Know the laws and policies around minor access for contraception, STI and HIV testing, and abortion in the state in which you practice. While all states and D.C. allow minors to consent to STI services, only 26 states allow all minors to consent to contraceptive services (and another 20 only allow consent to certain categories of minors) [23]. Go to the American Civil Liberties Union website (www.aclu.org) or the Guttmacher Institute (https://www.guttmacher.org/state-policy/laws-policies) to find minor consent laws for each state.
- List the sexual and reproductive services the clinic offers in public spaces, exam rooms, and online and via social media so patients need not ask about them.
- Utilize privacy screens, white noise makers, and/or music in the front office to allow for private conversations with front desk staff and/or communicate via a quick written form regarding chief concern.
- Design screening forms to elicit a client's needs, method eligibility, and coverage.
- Assure privacy and security of all medical records. Tell clients when the clinic cannot guarantee third-party privacy, and seek avenues that will enhance privacy [24–26]. For example, individuals in California can submit a Confidential Communication Request via the Confidential Care Act [27].

- Create relevant policies and optimize processes for EHR use that assure adolescent confidentiality. For example, have the option to print a patient's after-visit summary that does not list sensitive lab tests or diagnoses.
- Disclose sensitive information only with the patient's permission and in accordance with state laws to parents, teachers, or employers. Foster youth and other dependent minors are entitled to confidential reproductive health care, and not all child welfare workers may be aware of this.
- Make a plan to communicate confidentially via phone or text according to client's wishes. For example, use a code name for the clinic if a message must be left, and note this in the chart.

Principle #3—Guarantee culturally responsive care and well-trained diverse staff Adolescent health providers need to be aware of the diversity of AYAs who they serve, and understand the ways in which race, ethnicity, sexual orientation, gender identity, culture, and socioeconomic status interact with health behaviors and outcomes. Implicit biases (thoughts existing outside of conscious awareness) are as common among healthcare providers as they are among the general population [24] and significantly influence patient-provider interactions, treatment decisions, treatment adherence, and patient health outcomes [28]. "As more health care organizations work toward achieving health equity, it is not enough to focus on avoiding intentional discrimination; we must also acknowledge implicit bias and address it [29]." One way to do this, is to prioritize cultural diversity in clinic leadership and clinical program decision making. In New Mexico, strategic work to increase LARC access statewide was led by a young women's reproductive justice organization, with the goal of leveraging resources to increase access to all forms of contraception, while preventing coercion [30].

The following strategies focus on improving cultural awareness, diversifying staff, mitigating discrimination, and managing implicit biases affecting care in order to provide equitable healthcare services for all AYAs:

- Ensure cultural and ethnic diversity, with particular inclusion of underrepresented groups and people of color, in all clinical staffing, including clinic leadership, medical providers, medical support staff, and other direct service staff.
- Establish clear, unambiguous, universal policies against discrimination.
- Ensure the same level of care to all patients regardless of age, social status, gender, sexual orientation, cultural background, ethnicity, disability, or other areas of differences.
- Provide regular trainings on cultural complexity, humility, and culturally responsive care that encompasses cultural diversity and inclusivity, sexual orientation, gender identity, and the cultures you serve.
- Encourage staff to be friendly, inclusive, non-judgmental, and open-minded. They should try not to assert their personal views on patients.
- Offer opportunities for staff to evaluate their biases by learning about personal history and the contexts that bring patients in for care.
- Hire medical staff at all levels of clinical care that represent the diversity of cultures, ethnicities, gender identities, and languages of your clinical population.

- Put the onus on staff and providers to equalize power imbalances in patient-physician interactions. For example, during a contraceptive visit, first ask patients what is most important to them in their contraception method, rather than assuming a shared framework of efficacy as the most important factor in contraceptive decision making.
- Train your team to help destigmatize the biopsychosocial needs of vulnerable youth (e.g., youth impacted by foster care, unstable housing, human trafficking, the juvenile justice system, etc.).
- Involve AYAs in design, feedback, quality, and provision of services [31]:

  - Recruit and support AYAs to be active on your clinical advisory board, in focus groups, as outreach workers, and as media spokespeople.
  - Brainstorm with AYAs about their ideas to create adolescent-friendly services.
  - Provide formats for patient feedback (in writing, in person, or online), to be reviewed and incorporated as part of your clinic's quality improvement process.
  - Incorporate patient-facing quality measures assessing counseling, autonomy, and satisfaction.

- Involve community stakeholders, such as youth-serving agencies, in advocating for AYA services and providing preventive education.

Principle #4—Affirm the gender spectrum and sexual preferences of clients Many lesbian, gay, bisexual, transgender, queer or questioning, intersex, asexual, agender or allied (LGTBQIA) individuals have faced stigmatizing medical care in the past and then avoided further healthcare interactions, fearing reactions from staff or providers [32, 33]. Such stigma can create a significant barrier to care, as can a provider's appearance-based assumptions. For example, studies show that sexual minority women are less likely than heterosexual women to use highly or moderately effective contraceptive methods, putting them at increased risk for unintended pregnancy [34–36]. Creating a safe, welcoming, and gender-inclusive clinic environment will help ensure LGBTQIA AYAs not only seek care, but also return for follow-up. There are many aspects of care that can affirm the gender spectrum and sexual preferences of your clients [37]:

- Uphold values of patient centered, non-judgmental care for all clients.
- Understand your patient population and tailor services that are sensitive to gender, gender identity, gender expression, and sexual orientation.
- Ask about and track patients' used name and pronouns, current gender identity, and sex assigned at birth. This is important in keeping track of individual organs and corresponding preventive health needs, improving visibility in research and policy, and increasing patient satisfaction.
- Introduce yourself with your used pronouns and ask patients' pronouns if not shared. For example: "My name is [name] and I use they/them pronouns. What name and pronouns do you use?" Be honest and apologize if you get a pronoun wrong or forget.

- Provide patient intake forms and EHR templates that use gender-neutral language.
- Offer services based not on patients' gender expression but on their sex assigned at birth, hormonal status, and surgical status (i.e., organs present). For example, address the pregnancy prevention needs of sexual minority and gender noncon-forming AYAs who may be less likely than heterosexual women to use highly or moderately effective contraceptive methods [34].
- Make all available contraceptive, prenatal, and abortion care services available to all, including LGBTQIA youth. Utilize educational resources, like Birth Control Across the Gender Spectrum (available at: https://www.reproductiveaccess.org), which address contraceptive options for all individuals regardless of sexual ori-entation or gender identity [38].
- Check in about terms used for body parts, to assess for terms the patient would like you to use.
- Allow self-collection of test samples when possible (such as swabs or urine for STI testing), to help increase comfort in those individuals who experience dys-phoria about their current anatomy.

Principle #5—Improve scheduling access to optimize contraception deliv-ery Barriers including restrictive eligibility criteria, scheduling issues, and out-dated screening protocols have long stood in the way of patient access to IUDs [39]. We know that many patients do not return for follow-up visits for IUD placement if they are unable to have an IUD placed at their initial visit. Various studies have shown that access can be greatly improved through staff training and relatively sim-ple, low-cost, and administrative changes [40]. In a pilot study in nine family plan-ning clinics, efforts to accommodate patients desiring IUDs as EC showed that the clinics were able to accommodate more than 75% of patients as same-day place-ments, while the remaining patients returned for placement within the 5-day win-dow after unprotected intercourse [41].

- Scheduling and front desk tips:
  - Provide patient forms online (with smartphone compatibility), ensuring that your practice has processes in place to maintain patient confidentiality.
  - Offer visits after school, in the evening, and on weekends.
  - Consider phone hold messages that provide contraceptive education and high-light new service availability, such as IUDs.
- Call Center/Scheduling Staff Tips and Scripts. Ask patients that are calling in
  - "Are you wanting to become pregnant now?" [if no, continue] "Are you using anything to prevent becoming pregnant?" [if yes or no] "At your visit, would you like to talk to your provider about birth control?"
  - "Did you know that you can get any birth control method, including the IUD, right here in clinic!"
  - Schedulers need to be aware of contraceptive services. Assure ability for walk in visits.
  - Staff can mention that bedsider.org has great information.

- For patients that are in clinic, give them this brief questionnaire. If privacy is an issue, these questions can be provided on paper.

  - "Are you interested in discussing birth control today?" If yes:
  - Offer patient education materials, including paper handouts, videos on tablet, or access to online resources if feasible.
  - Alert staff/medical provider of patient with contraceptive need.

- Verify insurance (pre-authorization or patient assistance plans as needed)

  - Make changes necessary to adapt same-day screening and IUD insertion protocols at your clinic. For example, modify clinic template to include both scheduled and drop-in appointment slots, or make all appointment slots 20 minutes to accommodate procedures at any visit.
  - Convert no-show appointments swiftly, by calling or texting patients immediately when they are late to see if they will be using their appointment slot. Offer slots that become available to walk-in patients.
  - Give patients who are waiting a choice: "Do you prefer to wait (range) minutes or to be seen later this afternoon?" and keep them updated about wait times.
  - Make confidential reminder calls (or send texts) to all patients, preferably on the same day as the appointment.
  - Build walk-in slots into the clinic templates in order to accommodate LARC and EC visits.
  - Prioritize contraceptive needs that arise during a visit, even if the appointment was scheduled for other reasons.
  - Triage EC clients to see a clinician if interested, to ensure all EC options are presented, including the option of using an IUD as EC.
  - Work toward availability of IUD-trained providers in clinic at all times and refer if you cannot accommodate patients' needs.

- Rapid-access referral

  - Become familiar with and improve lines of communication with referral sites.
  - Assist adolescents in making appointments for time-sensitive issues or situations in which they fear stigmatization.
  - Offer patients help with transportation and notes for school or work as needed.

Principle #6—Offer free or low-cost services (front desk/billing issues) Although LARC methods are cost-effective for patients over time, up-front costs of devices are significantly higher than other contraceptives and may be a barrier for AYAs [42]. The LARC Quick Coding Guide (excerpted below in Fig. 2.6) presents one resource to manage billing issues [43]. The following strategies focus on cost and reimbursement mechanisms:

- Verify patient's insurance benefits, help with enrollment for available coverage options, and get pre-authorization, if needed, ahead of the visit.
- Utilize all available coverages for services (i.e., city or state LARC access programs, school-based health centers, patient assistance plans covering LARCs; state family planning expansion programs, etc.) to reduce patient costs.

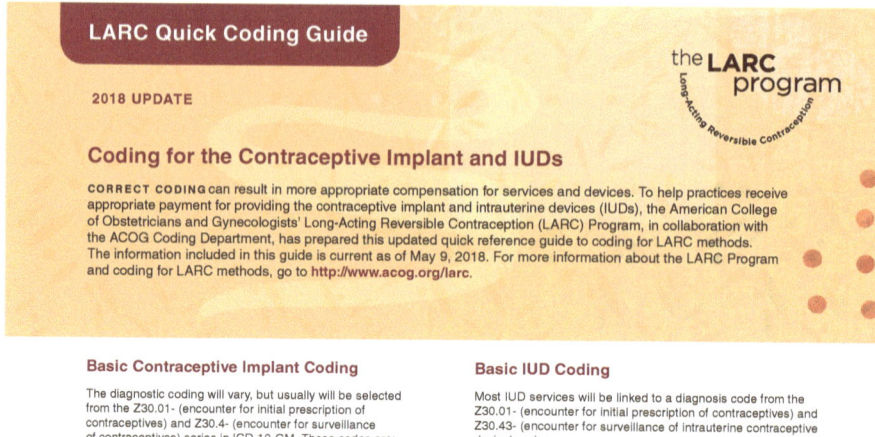

Fig. 2.6 The LARC Quick Coding Guide. (Image source: American College of Obstetrics and Gynecology)

- Do background research necessary to ensure that LARC devices are acquired in the most cost-effective manner (i.e., 340B pricing for federally qualified health centers or group purchasing plans, Title X).
- Create and post job aids so staff are aware of what common insurance payers cover for contraception.
- Offer sliding scale payment plans if a patient's insurance does not fully cover contraception.
- Use manufacturer assistance plans to help self-pay patients who do not qualify for state- or grant-based programs.
- Build two-way communications between the clinic and billing services around denials and to get feedback to improve coding and reimbursement.

Principle #7—Ensure *appropriate* **services, with autonomy and choice for AYAs** Reproductive health services have not always been patient-centered; in fact, there is a long history of contraceptive services that have incentivized or coerced in the USA and beyond (see Chap. 1). With increasing interest in highly effective methods by medical and public health organizations, it is critical that our programs are intentional about providing services in a manner that honors every client as the expert in their own life and decisions about contraception [44–46]. We must strive to ensure patient choice, at the same time as we work to broaden access. Although this chapter focuses on improving access to IUDs, it seeks to level the playing field, rather than endorsing IUDs over other methods. The following strategies focus on ensuring appropriate contraceptive services:

- Assure enthusiasm for LARC methods does not inadvertently compromise patient choice.
- Affirm LARC methods can be removed at any time.

- Improve quality of rapport and interpersonal care that are associated with critical contraceptive outcomes, including better method satisfaction and continuation [47]. Newly validated measures for interpersonal quality of family planning care include [48]:
  - Respect individuals as people.
  - Let patients say what matters about their method.
  - Take client preferences seriously.
  - Offer enough information for patients to make a decision.
- Adopt a patient-centered, noncoercive contraceptive counseling approach to support AYAs in making their contraceptive choice. The approach includes accurate, comprehensive information that takes into account AYAs individual needs, developmental level, and preferences for pregnancy planning and prevention through the following strategies:
  - Explain why you will be asking sensitive questions.
  - Build open and trusting relationships with patients [49, 50].
  - Ask open-ended questions, prioritizing information delivery based on a patient's preferences [51].
  - Parse problems into smaller pieces and consider multiple visits for younger adolescents.
  - Use role playing and shared decision-making to assist with contraceptive counseling for older AYAs.
  - Learn to read patient cues and respond with active listening—by restating and using reflective and summary statements [52, 53].
  - Use the OARS acronym (Open-ended questions, Affirmations, Reflections, and Summaries) [54] to engage AYAs in their contraceptive decision-making.
  - Conduct a full psychosocial assessment using the HEADSS acronym and making sure to additionally assess for strength and goals, after reviewing ground rules of confidentiality [18, 55].
- Inquire directly about partner involvement, safety, and reproductive coercion or contraceptive sabotage [56]. At no time should any patient be forced to use a method chosen by someone other than themself, including a partner, parent, guardian, or provider [53, 57].
- Schedule appointments of appropriate length, since AYAs may require more time to build rapport in discussing sensitive services.
- Ensure visits are frequent enough, as AYAs may need timely check ins to reinforce healthy decision making, and to assess method satisfaction, adherence, side effects, and condom use.
- Assure patients that they have a right to have an IUD or implant removed at any time without undue provider resistance or multiple clinic visit requirements.
- Encourage continuity of care by arranging follow-up visits, welcoming future visits and helping AYA patients transition smoothly to adult healthcare services when appropriate.

Principle #8—Make services *effective* in fulfilling the needs of young people While AYAs may receive both sexual and reproductive healthcare and primary care services in the same medical setting, they are less likely to consider health professionals as a primary source of information around sexual health [58]. Providers may also be less likely to discuss these topics during routine health maintenance visits [59]. It is essential that health professionals offer sexual and reproductive healthcare services in ways that provide accessibility to AYAs, and make a positive contribution to AYA health. The following strategies focus on ensuring effective reproductive health services for this population:

• Provide a comprehensive package of information, counseling, diagnosis, and treatment services to meet the needs of all your patients at the clinic or by referral.
• Follow professional guidelines when conducting a comprehensive sexual health history, examination, counseling and education, testing and treatment [9].
• Ensure LARCs are offered and are available as part of essential, comprehensive contraceptive options through education, counseling, and healthcare services [10].
• Offer STI prevention, testing, treatment, and counseling on all forms of contraception; offer options counseling for unintended pregnancy, and referral information for abortion or pregnancy care [9].
• Train staff and providers in up-to-date knowledge and skills to provide AYAs with the most comprehensive health services.
• Make changes that improve capacity to provide same-day contraception, which promotes quick-starting all methods including LARC.
• Provide contraceptive counseling for patients who come in for other sexual and reproductive health services, including STI or pregnancy testing, if they want to avoid future pregnancy.

Principle #9—Engage your entire clinical team (healthcare providers, managers, and support staff) in making your office friendly for adolescent IUD delivery It is integral to include the entire medical team in providing efficient contraceptive care. One study showed that a half-day evidence-based training for clinic staff on counseling and LARC placement skills was associated with twice as many patients being counseled about all contraceptive methods [60]. Another study showed that tailored, on-site technical assistance and LARC proctoring was useful for increasing LARC proficiency at the clinic, staff, and provider level [61]. The following strategies focus on clinic flow, as well as specific efforts that can be made by the entire healthcare team to optimize adolescent IUD delivery:

• Avoid duplicate efforts (i.e., repeat counseling provided by more than one person), as this is a time loss and may be interpreted as coercive by patients.
• Empower staff to work at the top of their training and licensure, including counseling, consenting, and setting up for LARC procedures, so clinicians can focus on answering questions and doing procedures.

- Allow office staff and managers to make decisions about adding on clients, rather than requiring clinician approval. Consider a flow facilitator role.
- Ensure enough support staff, as well as IUD-trained clinicians.
- Use staff meetings and huddles for training, daily needs, stocking, anticipating challenges, and tracking progress.
- Improve efforts to shorten cycle time (patient entry to exit), via time studies and data, to help support change.
- Make CDC medical eligibility criteria charts [62] or apps available to clinicians and staff.
- Help arrange proctoring for clinicians new to IUD placements and removals (see Chap. 8).
- Develop a network of specialists for challenging case referrals.
- Mobilize experienced clinicians to train other clinicians at your site on new skills (such as paracervical block, dilation for difficult placements, IUD localization, and difficult removal).
- Have fact sheets and consents easily available in every room, and via the EHR.
- Keep adequate supplies, including IUD insertion kits, ready in every room.
- Pre-stock rooms to avoid accidental method disclosure (IUD carried into room after patient).

Summary/Take Home Messages

AYAs face many barriers in obtaining contraception. Healthcare providers remain their most trusted source for information. Working toward more accessible and same-day services is important in the provision of IUDs. A coordinated effort to make clinics adolescent-friendly can enhance quality of care, and timely access to the full range of contraceptive options.

Clinical Pearls
- Create a visually appealing atmosphere and materials that are informed by AYAs to help improve patient comfort.
- Ensure patient privacy and confidentiality with staff members who are culturally responsive and gender-affirming to allow clinics to provide care to a diverse group of AYAs.
- Consider office practices including easy scheduling for contraceptive access and follow-up, and options for free or low-cost services in order to reduce barriers to care.

References

1. Harris SK, Aalsma MC, Weitzman ER, Garcia-Huidobro D, Wong C, Hadland SE, et al. Research on clinical preventive services for adolescents and young adults: where are we and where do we need to go? J Adolesc Health. 2017;60:249–60.
2. Brittain AW, Williams JR, Zapata LB, Pazol K, Romero LM, Weik TS. Youth-friendly family planning services for young people: a systematic review. Am J Prev Med. 2015;49:S73–84.
3. Society for Adolescent Health and Medicine, Gray SH, Pasternak RH, Gooding HC, Woodward K, Hawkins K, et al. Recommendations for electronic health record use for delivery of adolescent health care. J Adolesc Health. 2014;54:487–90.
4. Teal SB, Elizabeth Romer S. Awareness of long-acting reversible contraception among teens and young adults. J Adolesc Health Care. 2013;52:S35–9.
5. Kavanaugh ML, Jerman J, Ethier K, Moskosky S. Meeting the contraceptive needs of teens and young adults: youth-friendly and long-acting reversible contraceptive services in U.S. family planning facilities. J Adolesc Health Care. 2013;52:284–92.
6. Moriarty Daley A, Sadler LS, Dawn Reynolds H. Tailoring clinical services to address the unique needs of adolescents from the pregnancy test to parenthood. Curr Probl Pediatr Adolesc Health Care. 2013;43:71–95.
7. Best practices for youth-friendly sexual and reproductive health services in schools – advocates for youth. In: Advocates for Youth [Internet]. [cited 28 Nov 2018]. Available: https://advocatesforyouth.org/resources/health-information/bp-youth-friendly-services/.
8. Medical education – Physicians for reproductive health [Internet]. [cited 28 Nov 2018]. Available: https://prh.org/medical-education/.
9. Society for Adolescent Health and Medicine, Burke PJ, Coles MS, Di Meglio G, Gibson EJ, Handschin SM, et al. Sexual and reproductive health care: a position paper of the Society for Adolescent Health and Medicine. J Adolesc Health. 2014;54:491–6.
10. Society for Adolescent Health and Medicine. Improving knowledge about, access to, and utilization of long-acting reversible contraception among adolescents and young adults. J Adolesc Health Care. 2017;60:472–4.
11. ACOG Committee Opinion No. 735. Obstet Gynecol. 2018;131:e130–e139.
12. World Health Organization, UNAIDS. Global standards for quality health-care services for adolescents: a guide to implement a standards-driven approach to improve the quality of health care services for adolescents. Geneva: World Health Organization; 2015.
13. Shafii T, Serrano J. Adolescent-friendly services key criteria and assessment tool. Adapted from 2009 WHO quality assessment guidebook [Internet]. [cited 28 Nov 2018]. Available: http://www.k12.wa.us/HIVSexualhealth/pubdocs/AdolescentFriendlyServices_OSPI.pdf.
14. Yonker LM, Zan S, Scirica CV, Jethwani K, Bernard Kinane T. "Friending" teens: systematic review of social media in adolescent and young adult health care. J Med Internet Res. 2015;17:e4.
15. Zipkin DA, Umscheid CA, Keating NL, Allen E, Aung K, Beyth R, et al. Evidence-based risk communication: a systematic review. Ann Intern Med. 2014;161:270–80.
16. Garcia-Retamero R, Cokely ET. Designing visual aids that promote risk literacy: a systematic review of health research and evidence-based design heuristics. Hum Factors. 2017;59:582–627.
17. Drawing a picture: adolescent centered medical homes [Internet]. 2015. Available: https://www.youtube.com/watch?v=vAu5ad827I8.
18. ARSHEP presentations & case videos – Physicians for reproductive health [Internet]. [cited 28 Nov 2018]. Available: https://prh.org/arshep-ppts/#best-practices.
19. Ford CA, Millstein SG, Halpern-Felsher BL, Irwin CE Jr. Influence of physician confidentiality assurances on adolescents' willingness to disclose information and seek future health care. A randomized controlled trial. JAMA. 1997;278:1029–34.
20. Brittain AW, Briceno ACL, Pazol K, Zapata LB, Decker E, Rollison JM, et al. Youth-friendly family planning services for young people: a systematic review update. Am J Prev Med. 2018;55:725–35.

21. Fuentes L, Ingerick M, Jones R, Lindberg L. Adolescents' and young adults' reports of barriers to confidential health care and receipt of contraceptive services. J Adolesc Health. 2018;62:36–43.
22. Jones RK, Boonstra H. Confidential reproductive health services for minors: the potential impact of mandated parental involvement for contraception. Perspect Sex Reprod Health. 2004;36:182–91.
23. An overview of minors' consent law. In: Guttmacher Institute [Internet]. 14 Mar 2016 [cited 28 Nov 2018]. Available: https://www.guttmacher.org/state-policy/explore/overview-minors-consent-law.
24. Bayer R, Santelli J, Klitzman R. New challenges for electronic health records: confidentiality and access to sensitive health information about parents and adolescents. JAMA. 2015;313:29–30.
25. American Academy of Pediatrics. Confidentiality protections for adolescents and young adults in the health care billing and insurance claims process. Pediatrics. 2016;137:e20160593.
26. Anoshiravani A, Gaskin GL, Groshek MR, Kuelbs C, Longhurst CA. Special requirements for electronic medical records in adolescent medicine. J Adolesc Health. 2012;51:409–14.
27. Keep It Confidential. | My Health My Info [Internet]. [cited 28 Nov 2018]. Available: https://myhealthmyinfo.org/.
28. Hall WJ, Chapman MV, Lee KM, Merino YM, Thomas TW, Payne BK, et al. Implicit racial/ethnic bias among health care professionals and its influence on health care outcomes: a systematic review. Am J Public Health. 2015;105:e60–76.
29. How to reduce implicit bias [Internet]. [cited 28 Nov 2018]. Available: http://www.ihi.org/communities/blogs/how-to-reduce-implicit-bias.
30. Young Women United – Young Women United – Albuquerque, NM – By and For Young Women of Color [Internet]. [cited 28 Nov 2018]. Available: https://youngwomenunited.org/.
31. Ambresin A-E, Bennett K, Patton GC, Sanci LA, Sawyer SM. Assessment of youth-friendly health care: a systematic review of indicators drawn from young people's perspectives. J Adolesc Health. 2013;52:670–81.
32. Dean MA, Victor E, Guidry-Grimes L. Inhospitable healthcare spaces: why diversity training on LGBTQIA issues is not enough. J Bioeth Inq. 2016;13:557–70.
33. Nadal KL, Whitman CN, Davis LS, Erazo T, Davidoff KC. Microaggressions toward lesbian, gay, bisexual, transgender, queer, and genderqueer people: a review of the literature. J Sex Res. 2016;53:488–508.
34. Blunt-Vinti HD, Thompson EL, Griner SB. Contraceptive use effectiveness and pregnancy prevention information preferences among heterosexual and sexual minority college women. Womens Health Issues. 2018;28:342–9.
35. Light AD, Obedin-Maliver J, Sevelius JM, Kerns JL. Transgender men who experienced pregnancy after female-to-male gender transitioning. Obstet Gynecol. 2014;124:1120–7.
36. Richards C, Seal L. Trans people's reproductive options and outcomes. J Fam Plann Reprod Health Care. 2014;40:245–7.
37. Guidelines for the primary and gender-affirming care of transgender and gender nonbinary people [Internet]. [cited 28 Nov 2018]. Available: http://transhealth.ucsf.edu/protocols.
38. Birth control access the gender spectrum. In: Reproductive health access project [Internet]. Aug 2018 [cited 28 Nov 2018]. Available: https://www.reproductiveaccess.org/wp-content/uploads/2018/06/bc-across-gender-spectrum.pdf.
39. Biggs MA, Kaller S, Harper CC, Freedman L, Mays AR. "Birth control can easily take a back seat": challenges providing IUDs in community health care settings. J Health Care Poor Underserved. 2018;29:228–44.
40. Thompson KMJ, Rocca CH, Stern L, Morfesis J, Goodman S, Steinauer J, et al. Training contraceptive providers to offer intrauterine devices and implants in contraceptive care: a cluster randomized trial. Am J Obstet Gynecol. 2018;218:597.e1–7.
41. Kohn JE, Nucatola DL. EC4U: results from a pilot project integrating the copper IUC into emergency contraceptive care. Contraception. 2016;94:48–51.
42. Eisenberg D, McNicholas C, Peipert JF. Cost as a barrier to long-acting reversible contraceptive (LARC) use in adolescents. J Adolesc Health. 2013;52:S59–63.

43. LARC quick coding guide. In: ACOG [Internet]. [cited 28 Nov 2018]. Available: https://www. acog.org/-/media/Departments/LARC/Coding-Guide-2018FINAL.pdf.
44. Gomez AM, Fuentes L, Allina A. Women or LARC first? Reproductive autonomy and the promotion of long-acting reversible contraceptive methods. Perspect Sex Reprod Health. 2014;46:171–5.
45. Higgins JA. Celebration meets caution: LARC's boons, potential busts, and the benefits of a reproductive justice approach. Contraception. 2014;89:237–41.
46. Gubrium AC, Mann ES, Borrero S, Dehlendorf C, Fields J, Geronimus AT, et al. Realizing reproductive health equity needs more than long-acting reversible contraception (LARC). Am J Public Health. 2016;106:18–9.
47. Dehlendorf C, Anderson N, Vittinghoff E, Grumbach K, Levy K, Steinauer J. Quality and content of patient-provider communication about contraception: differences by race/ethnicity and socioeconomic status. Womens Health Issues. 2017;27:530–8.
48. Dehlendorf C, Henderson JT, Vittinghoff E, Steinauer J, Hessler D. Development of a patient-reported measure of the interpersonal quality of family planning care. Contraception. 2018;97:34–40.
49. Dehlendorf C, Krajewski C, Borrero S. Contraceptive counseling: best practices to ensure quality communication and enable effective contraceptive use. Clin Obstet Gynecol. 2014;57:659–73.
50. Jaccard J, Levitz N. Counseling adolescents about contraception: towards the development of an evidence-based protocol for contraceptive counselors. J Adolesc Health. 2013;52:S6–13.
51. Callegari LS, Aiken ARA, Dehlendorf C, Cason P, Borrero S. Addressing potential pitfalls of reproductive life planning with patient-centered counseling. Am J Obstet Gynecol. 2017;216:129–34.
52. Tomescu O, Ginsburg KR. Interviewing the adolescent: strategies that promote communication and foster resilience. In: Obgyn key [Internet]. 13 Jun 2016 [cited 28 Nov 2018]. Available: https://obgynkey.com/interviewing-the-adolescent-strategies-that-promote-communication-and-foster-resilience/.
53. Committee on Adolescent Health Care. Committee Opinion No. 710: counseling adolescents about contraception. Obstet Gynecol. 2017;130:e74–80.
54. Miller WR, Rollnick S. Motivational interviewing: preparing people for change. New York: Guilford Press; 2002.
55. HEEADSSS 3.0: The psychosocial interview for adolescents updated for a new century fueled by media. In: Contemporary pediatrics [Internet]. [cited 28 Nov 2018]. Available: http://www.contemporarypediatrics.com/article/heeadsss-30-psychosocial-interview-adolescents-updated-new-century-fueled-media.
56. Grace KT, Anderson JC. Reproductive coercion: a systematic review. Trauma Violence Abuse. 2018;19:371–90.
57. Committee on Adolescent Health Care. Committee Opinion No 699: adolescent pregnancy, contraception, and sexual activity. Obstet Gynecol. 2017;129:e142–9.
58. Marcell AV, Halpern-Felsher BL. Adolescents' beliefs about preferred resources for help vary depending on the health issue. J Adolesc Health. 2007;41:61–8.
59. Alexander SC, Fortenberry JD, Pollak KI, Bravender T, Davis JK, Ostbye T, et al. Sexuality talk during adolescent health maintenance visits. JAMA Pediatr. 2014;168:163–9.
60. Harper CC, Rocca CH, Thompson KM, Morfesis J, Goodman S, Darney PD, et al. Reductions in pregnancy rates in the USA with long-acting reversible contraception: a cluster randomised trial. Lancet. 2015;386:562–8.
61. Mays A, Harper C, Freeman L, Biggs MA. The role of proctoring to increase LARC access in Community Health Centers. 2016 American Public Health Conference; 2016.
62. Summary chart of U.S. medical eligibility criteria for contraceptive use. In: CDC [Internet]. 2016 [cited 28 Nov 2018]. Available: https://www.cdc.gov/reproductivehealth/unintended-pregnancy/pdf/legal_summary-chart_english_final_tag508.pdf.

Chapter 3
Types of IUDs and Mechanism of Action

Joy Friedman and Rubiliatu A. Oluronbi

Abbreviations

ACOG	The American College of Obstetrics and Gynecology
AYA	Adolescent and Young Adult
EC	Emergency Contraception
FDA	United States Federal Drug Administration
IUD	Intrauterine Device
LARC	Long-Acting Reversible Contraception
LNG	Levonorgestrel
UPIC	Unprotected Intercourse

Learning Objectives
Following completion of this chapter, you should be able to:

1. Present the different forms of intrauterine devices (IUDs) that USA Federal Drug Administration (FDA) approved for use in the USA
2. Describe the differences between the current IUDs used in the USA
3. Outline the mechanism of action of the various forms of IUDs used in the USA

J. Friedman (✉)
Department of Pediatrics, Albert Einstein Medical Center, Philadelphia, PA, USA
e-mail: friedmjo@einstein.edu

R. A. Oluronbi
Department of Obstetrics and Gynecology, Albert Einstein Medical Center, Philadelphia, PA, USA

© Springer Nature Switzerland AG 2019
M. S. Coles, A. Mays (eds.), *Optimizing IUD Delivery for Adolescents and Young Adults*, https://doi.org/10.1007/978-3-030-17816-1_3

Background

IUDs vary in composition and shape (see Fig. 3.1). Modern IUDs are categorized as copper-releasing, progestin-releasing, and inert or unmedicated. This chapter will focus on the intrauterine contraceptives currently available in the USA as of 2018, which includes four levonorgestrel (LNG) IUDs and the Copper T 380A (brand name ParaGard) IUD, and their mechanisms of action.

While the percentage of adolescents selecting this highly effective and long-acting method has been increasing in recent years, the IUD remains underutilized among adolescent and young adults (AYAs) compared to other contraceptive options [7]. Barriers to use of IUDs in AYAs include lack of method knowledge and under-standing, misconceptions about safety, fears of insertion pain and post-insertion infertility, low parental acceptance, and lack of health care providers' knowledge and recommendation regarding use [8, 9]. Discussion regarding IUD types should be tailored to patient preferences (see Chap. 5: Contraceptive Counseling), address confidentiality, and be cognizant of state laws regarding privacy and consent practices for contraception (see Chap. 7). Addressing common misconceptions and myths regarding IUDs, explaining reproductive anatomy, addressing safety concerns, and reviewing the mechanism of action of the IUD provides the space for adolescents to consider this highly effective contraceptive method [8, 10].

Case

Erin is a 16-year-old cisgender female who presents for contraception management. She is in a new relationship and is currently using condoms for contraception. After you provide information regarding contraceptive options, she is interested in an IUD, but is also hesitant because she heard that IUDs cause abortion, and she does not believe in abortion. She had menarche at age 13, and her menstrual cycle occurs every 28 days and lasts for 5 days. She reports heavy menstrual bleeding with associated menstrual cramping that bothers her. Her LMP was 2 weeks ago. She has never been tested for STIs and is interested in testing today. She denies any medical problems and reports no known drug allergies. Her urine pregnancy test is negative. She last had sex a few days before her most recent period began. How would you address Erin's concerns before placing her IUD?

IUD Mechanisms of Action

All types of IUDs have both primary and secondary mechanisms of action. **The primary mechanism of action** for all IUDs is **prevention of fertilization** [11], though different types of IUDs do this differently, as discussed in the method-specific sections below. Secondary mechanisms of actions are also well studied.

"Intrauterine devices and the contraceptive implant should be offered routinely as safe and effective contraceptive options for nulliparous women and adolescents."
" The American Academy of Pediatrics and The American College of Obstetricians and Gynecologists endorse the use of LARC, including IUDs, for adolescents."

	Intrauterine Devices (IUD)				
	Levonorgestrel IUD				Copper IUD
	Mirena	Liletta	Skyla	Kyleena	Paragard
FDA Approval Date	2000	2015	2013	2016	1988
Approved for (Acceptable duration of use)	5 years (7 years)	5 years (7 years)	3 years	5 years	10 years (12 years)
Total Hormone	52 mg	52 mg	13.5 mg	19.5 mg	N/A
Changes in menses	Irregular bleeding initially, decreases over time				Heavier period, longer duration, more cramps
Notable characteristics	▪ String color: Brown ▪ FDA-approved for treatment of heavy menstrual bleeding	▪ String color: Blue ▪ Reloadable	▪ String color: Brown ▪ Silver ring visible on ultrasound	▪ String color: Blue ▪ Silver ring visible on ultrasound ▪ Smallest 5-year IUD	▪ String color: White ▪ Can be used as emergency contraceptive
Cumulative efficacy over approved period of use	99.3%	99.27%	99.1%	98.6%	>99%
Quick Resources:	www.bedsider.org https://www.acog.org/-/media/Departments/Government-Relations-and-Outreach/FactsAreImportantEC.pdf				

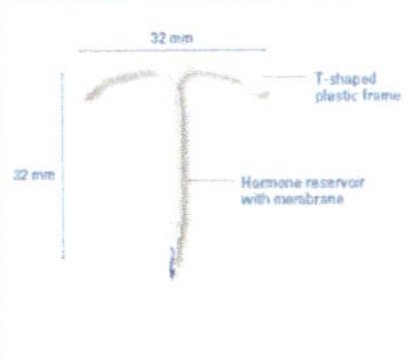

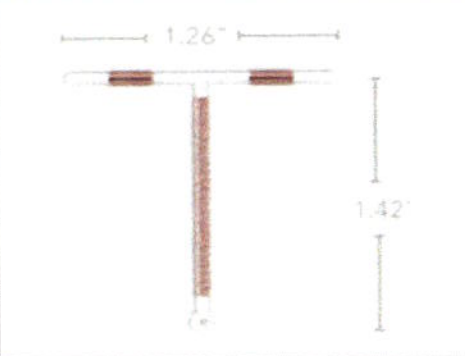

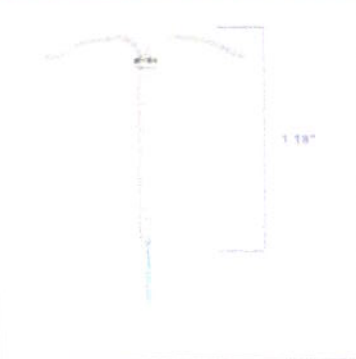

Fig. 3.1 IUD information by type. (Source: [1–6]) Safety and efficacy of Mirena, Kyleena, and Skyla has been established in women of reproductive age. Efficacy is expected to be the same for postpubertal females under the age of 18 as for users 18 years and older. Use of these products before menarche is not indicated

Fig. 3.2 IUDs from Around the World. (Image source: Case Western Reserve University: College of Arts and Sciences. Dittrick Medical History Center [16])

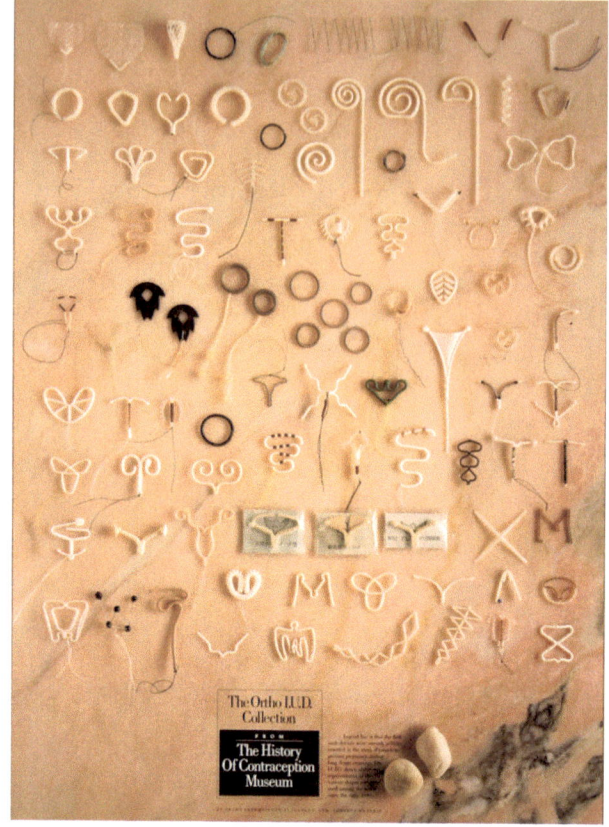

IUDs induce a sterile local inflammatory reaction that affects the viability of gametes and reduces the likelihood of fertilization [12], likely due to increased concentrations of inflammatory cytokines in the uterus [13] and macrophage engulfment of sperm [14]. While these mechanisms are very effective at preventing fertilization in IUD users, unintended pregnancies including ectopics can rarely occur. The precise evaluation of the secondary mechanisms of action is not complete due to difficulties in carrying out relevant investigations in humans [15].

Types of IUDs

While there are many types of IUDs available worldwide, there are currently five IUDs marketed in the USA **four LNG-releasing IUDs (LNG IUDs)** and **one copper-containing IUD**. After insertion, these IUDs can be differentiated by the *color of their threads* (see Fig. 3.2).

Levonorgestrel IUDs The LNG-IUDs are T-shaped polyethylene structures with steroid reservoirs that contain polydimethylsiloxane with varying amounts of LNG and are >99% effective in preventing pregnancy. Barium sulfate is also found in the

T-frame of all the LNG IUDs, *permitting their visualization on X-ray* [1–3, 5, 6]. The LNG IUDs are formulated such that LNG is released continuously from the vertical stem of the T-shaped device. The amount of hormone declines steadily over time. Most people who have an LNG IUD in place will continue to ovulate, but many experience a reduced menstrual flow or amenorrhea due to the atrophic effect of LNG on the endometrium. The Mirena branded LNG 52 mg IUD is also FDA approved for treatment of heavy menstrual bleeding [2]. The other LNG IUDs likely cause a similar effect. One of the most common effects of LNG IUDs is vaginal bleeding pattern alterations, especially in the first few months of use; therefore, it is imperative that providers explain this possible change to patients prior to placement of the IUDs as described in Chap. 7 (Consenting for IUDs).

LNG-containing IUDs prevent fertilization by thickening the cervical mucus, such that the mucus prevents sperm passage through the cervical canal [17]. This effect has been shown to occur within 5 days of insertion of the LNG 52 mg IUD [18], and is the primary mechanism of action of all hormonal IUDs in order to prevent fertilization. The higher dose LNG IUDs may suppress ovulation in approximately 20% of users [19], whereas greater than 90% of users of the LNG 19.5 mg IUD and LNG 13.5 mg IUD continued to ovulate [17]. In the rare event that sperm penetrates the viscous cervical mucus in individuals using hormonal IUDs, the secondary mechanisms of action, as discussed above, may prevent fertilization.

It takes seven days for the LNG IUDs to start working reliably. Patients using the contraceptive pill, patch, ring, or the etonogestrel subdermal implant should be instructed to continue use for seven days after insertion and/or use condoms for back up contraception during that time frame [17, 20]. Patients using the hormonal contraceptive injection at 14 weeks or greater from their last shot, should also use condoms as a seven-day backup method. While LNG IUDs are not currently recommended for emergency contraception (EC), preliminary research suggests that they may be effective [21].

LNG 52 mg IUD: There are currently **two FDA-approved LNG 52 mg IUD devices**, Mirena and Liletta (see Fig. 3.3), which are bioequivalent devices with equal amounts and release rates of LNG. Mirena (FDA approved in 2000) and Liletta (FDA approved in 2015) IUDs both contain a total of 52 mg of LNG and measure 32 mm × 32 mm. The inserter diameter measures 4.4 mm and 4.8 mm, respectively [22]. Both devices are FDA approved for up to 5 years, although evidence supports their use for up to 7 years [23, 24]. These IUDs initially release approximately 20 mcg/day LNG, with a five year average release rate of 14 mcg/day. The rate decreases gradually to approximately 10 mcg/day by 5 years of use [25]. As noted above, Mirena was also FDA approved in 2009 for the management of heavy menstrual bleeding with approximately 20% of users experiencing amenorrhea after 1 year of use [2].

Mirena has **brown polyethylene** monofilament strings that are attached to a loop at the end of the vertical stem of the T-frame. Liletta can be distinguished by its **blue polypropylene** monofilament strings, which are attached to an eyelet at the end of the vertical stem of the T-frame. Unlike Mirena, the Liletta IUD inserter is reloadable, meaning that if the IUD is loaded incorrectly in the insertion device or prematurely released, it may be repositioned and reloaded [6].

Levonorgestrel 52 mg: Mirena and Liletta

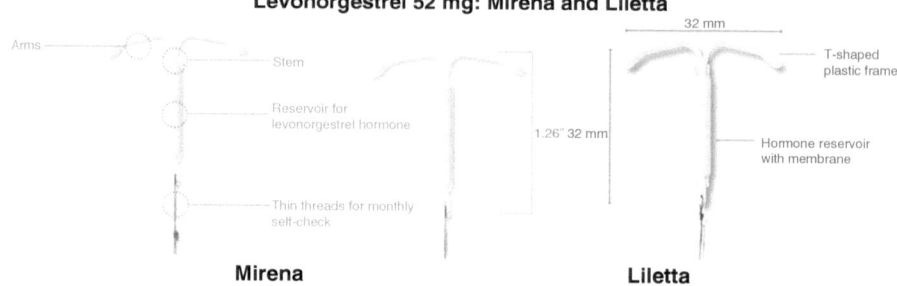

Mirena **Liletta**

Fig. 3.3 Image of the LNG 52 mg IUD devices available in the USA (Image sources: Bayer (Mirena) and Allergan (Liletta))

LNG 19.5 mg IUD: The LNG 19.5 mg IUD (see Fig. 3.4) measures 28 mm × 30 mm and was FDA approved in 2016 for pregnancy prevention for up to 5 years. It initially releases 17.5 mcg/day with a five-year average release rate of 9 mcg/day. This rate decreases gradually to 7.4 mcg/day by 5 years of use [3]. The LNG 19.5 mg IUD has an inserter diameter of 3.8 mm, slightly smaller than the LNG 52 mg IUDs. The LNG 19.5 mg IUD shares the same non-reloadable applicator for insertion as the Mirena IUD (above) and the LNG 13.5 mg IUD (below) [4]. Approximately 12% of LNG 19.5 mg IUD users developed amenorrhea after 1 year of use. The LNG 19.5 mg IUD can be distinguished from other IUDs by **the combination of the visibility of the silver ring on ultrasound and the *blue color* of the removal strings** [3].

Fig. 3.4 Image of the LNG 19.5 mg IUD device Kyleena available in the USA (Image source: Bayer. Safety and efficacy of Kyleena have been established in women of reproductive age. Efficacy is expected to be the same for postpubertal females under the age of 18 as for users 18 years and older. Use of this product before menarche is not indicated.)

Levonorgestrel 19.5 mg: Kyleena

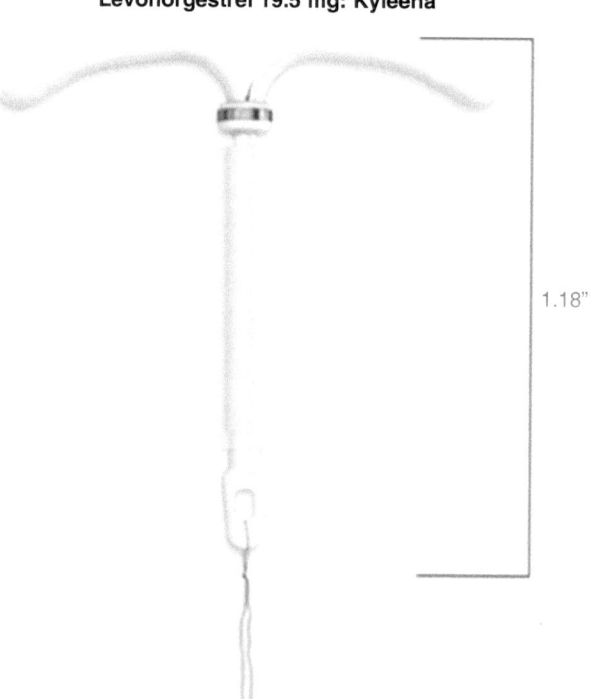

LNG 13.5 mg IUD: The LNG 13.5 mg IUD (see Fig. 3.5) is the same size as the LNG 19.5 mg IUD, measuring 28 mm × 30 mm, and was FDA approved in 2013 for the prevention of pregnancy for up to 3 years. The LNG 13.5 mg IUD initially releases 14 mcg/day with a 6 mcg/day over the course of 3 years. This rate decreases to 5 mcg/day after 3 years of use. It uses the same non-reloadable applicator and has the same inserter diameter (3.8 mm) as the LNG 19.5 mg IUD (above) [5]. Patients using LNG 13.5 mg IUD may experience more irregular bleeding on average than those using IUDs with higher doses of LNG [4] due to lower endometrial hormone levels. Approximately 6% of 13.5 mg LNG IUD users experience amenorrhea by the end of the first year of use [5]. This IUD can be distinguished from others by the **combination of the visibility of the silver ring on ultrasound (similar to the Kyleena) and the *brown color* of the removal** strings [5].

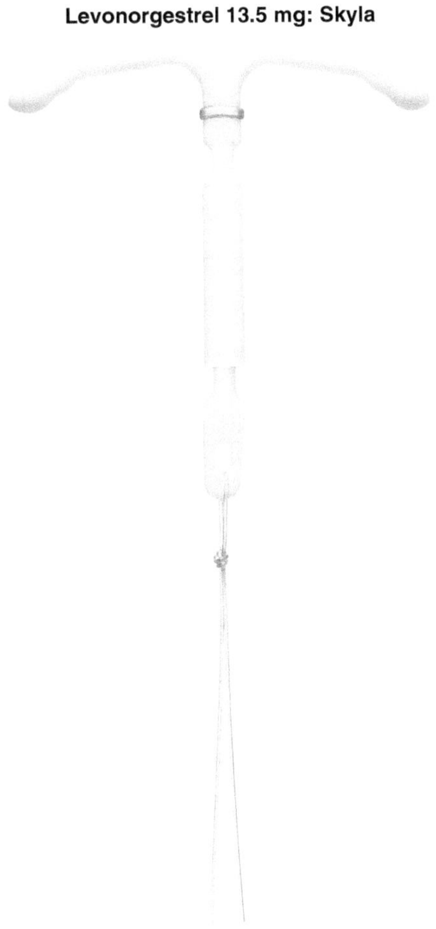

Fig. 3.5 Image of the LNG 13.5 mg IUD device Skyla available in the USA (Image source: Bayer. Safety and efficacy of Skyla have been established in women of reproductive age. Efficacy is expected to be the same for postpubertal females under the age of 18 as for users 18 years and older. Use of this product before menarche is not indicated.)

Levonorgestrel 13.5 mg: Skyla

Copper IUD The CuT380A IUD, brand name ParaGard (see image in Fig. 3.6 below), is a T-shaped polyethylene structure that is wrapped with copper wire around the stem and arms. The CuT380A IUD works by releasing copper ions into the cervical mucus and endometrial cavity, which act to impair sperm migration and prevents sperm from reaching ova [26]. In addition, and as described above, all IUDs induce a sterile local inflammatory reaction that affects sperm motility and prevents fertilization. This effect is more pronounced in individuals using copper IUDs [27]. As the copper IUD does not contain any hormones, it has no effect on ovulation. It may, however, have effects on both fertilized oocytes, and on the endometrium that contribute to its high efficacy and pregnancy prevention [28].

The CuT380A IUD is the only copper-containing IUD available in the USA and was FDA approved for use in 1988 for pregnancy prevention lasting up to 10 years [1]; there is strong evidence to support use for up to 12 years [24]. In typical use, the CuT380A is 99.2% effective for prevention of pregnancy in the first year of use [1] and is effective as soon as it has been placed [29].

In addition to preventing pregnancy, copper IUDs are also **the most effective form of EC**, working in part to disrupt the normal development of a fertilized oocyte and prevent implantation. AYAs should be fully educated regarding all of their options for EC. AYAs can be assured that they can use the CuT380A for EC up to seven days after unprotected intercourse (UPIC), with efficacy for pregnancy prevention of 99% [30]. Please note that the American College of Obstetrics and Gynecology (ACOG) recommends the CuT380A be used for EC only up to 5 days after UPIC [31], though it is recommended by the Canadian Contraception Consensus group for use as EC up to 7 days after UPIC based on current evidence [32, 33].

There are approximately 176 mg of copper wire coiled along the vertical stem and a 68.7 mg collar on each side of the horizontal arm of the CuT380A IUD, with the total exposed copper surface area measuring approximately 380mm^2. The IUD stem contains a 3 mm ball at the base, which is designed to decrease the risk of cervical perforation [1]. It has an inserter tube diameter that measures 4.01 mm [34] and a monofilament polyethylene thread that is tied through the tip, resulting in **two white strings**, which distinguish it from other IUDs. Barium sulfate in the T frame aids in detecting the device under X-ray [35].

Fig. 3.6 Image of the CuT380A IUD device ParaGard available in the USA (Image source: Cooper Surgical)

CuT380A IU: ParaGard

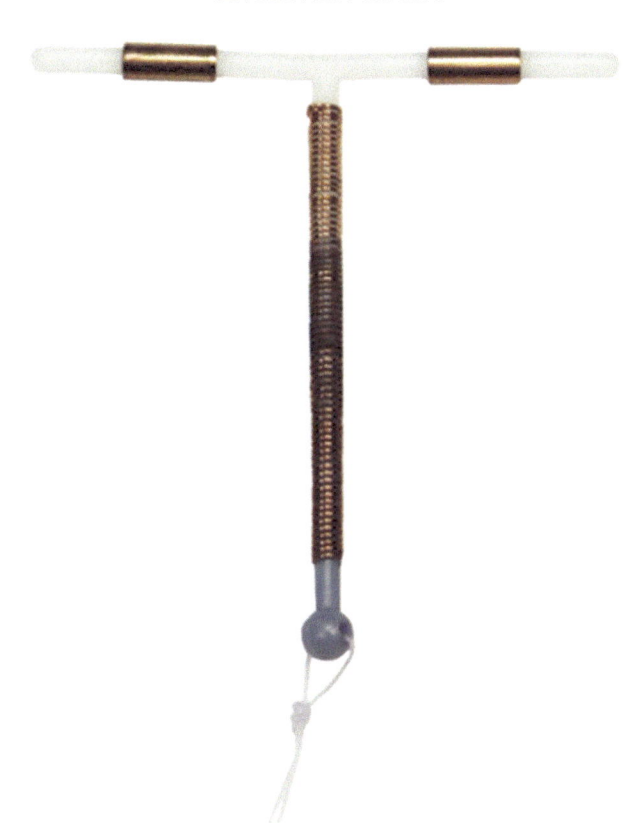

Case

Erin chose the LNG 19.5 mg IUD because she wanted the reliability of a long-acting method, and preferred to have a more regular period. She opted not to get the copper IUD because she was worried it would make her period heavier. The IUD was placed without difficulty. A few days later, her STI screening test resulted positive for chlamydia, and she was appropriately treated with azithromycin with her IUD left in place. Erin returned to clinic 4 weeks later for an IUD follow-up. Repeat STI testing was done, and the results were negative. She shares with you that her best friend Jessie is also interested in contraception, and Erin can't remember the specific details about each method that you had talked about last month. You refer her to www.bedsider.org and www.reproductiveaccess.org for fact sheets about each method.

A few days later, Erin returns to clinic with her mother, who demands that her daughter's IUD be removed. She is concerned that IUDs can cause infertility, and also believes that IUDs cause abortion—which the family does not believe in. You meet with Erin privately, who shares that she had some irregular bleeding, and when her mother questioned why she was using more pads, she told her mother that she had an IUD. Erin would like to continue using her IUD. You offer support, and ask Erin's permission to speak with her mother about the IUD's mechanisms of action, safety profile, and efficacy. Erin agrees.

In summary, in order to optimally counsel AYA's about IUDs it is important to be aware of the composition and mechanism of action of the various types of IUDs available in your community. Addressing important concepts that IUDs work prior to fertilization to prevent pregnancy, and do not impact an ongoing pregnancy, may be important for some individuals. Certain types of IUDs may also be good options for patients seeking EC, and research in ongoing in this field. Further information on addressing IUD myths, fears, and misinformation can be found in Chap. 4.

Clinical Pearls
- There are currently 5 types of IUDs FDA approved for use in the USA all of which are appropriate for use in AYAs.
- IUDs primary mechanism of action, to prevent fertilization, has been well studied and confirmed.
- The copper IUD is the most effective form of EC and can be used safely for up to 7 days after UPIC.
- Promising research is underway investigating the LNG IUDs for EC.

References

1. ParaGard T 380A intrauterine copper contraceptive [Internet]. [cited 28 Nov 2018]. Available: https://www.accessdata.fda.gov/drugsatfda_docs/label/2005/018680s060lbl.pdf.
2. Mirena (levonorgestrel-releasing intrauterine system). Highlights of prescribing information [Internet]. [cited 28 Nov 2018]. Available: https://www.accessdata.fda.gov/drugsatfda_docs/label/2009/021225s027lbl.pdf.
3. Kyleena (levonorgestrel-releasing intrauterine system). Highlights of prescribing information [Internet]. [cited 28 Nov 2018]. Available: https://labeling.bayerhealthcare.com/html/products/pi/Kyleena_PI.pdf.
4. Nelson AL. LNG-IUS 12: a 19.5 levonorgestrel-releasing intrauterine system for prevention of pregnancy for up to five years. Expert Opin Drug Deliv. 2017;14:1131–40.
5. Skyla (levonorgestrel-releasing intrauterine system). Highlights of prescribing information [Internet]. [cited 28 Nov 2018]. Available: http://labeling.bayerhealthcare.com/html/products/pi/Skyla_PI.pdf.
6. Liletta (levonorgestrel-releasing intrauterine system). Highlights of prescribing information [Internet]. [cited 28 Nov 2018]. Available: https://www.allergan.com/assets/pdf/lilettashi_pi.
7. Secura GM, Madden T, McNicholas C, Mullersman J, Buckel CM, Zhao Q, et al. Provision of no-cost, long-acting contraception and teenage pregnancy. N Engl J Med. 2014;371:1316–23.
8. Potter J, Rubin SE, Sherman P. Fear of intrauterine contraception among adolescents in New York City. Contraception. 2014;89:446–50.
9. Pritt NM, Norris AH, Berlan ED. Barriers and facilitators to adolescents' use of long-acting reversible contraceptives. J Pediatr Adolesc Gynecol. 2017;30:18–22.
10. Committee on Adolescent Health Care. Committee Opinion No. 710: counseling adolescents about contraception. Obstet Gynecol. 2017;130:e74–80.
11. Speroff L, Darney PD. A clinical guide for contraception. Philadelphia: Lippincott Williams & Wilkins; 2010.

12. Ortiz ME, Croxatto HB, Bardin CW. Mechanisms of action of intrauterine devices. Obstet Gynecol Surv. 1996;51:S42–51.
13. Ammälä M, Nyman T, Strengell L, Rutanen EM. Effect of intrauterine contraceptive devices on cytokine messenger ribonucleic acid expression in the human endometrium. Fertil Steril. 1995;63:773–8.
14. Sağiroğlu N. Phagocytosis of spermatozoa in the uterine cavity of woman using intrauterine device. Int J Fertil. 1971;16:1–14.
15. Rivera R, Yacobson I, Grimes D. The mechanism of action of hormonal contraceptives and intrauterine contraceptive devices. Am J Obstet Gynecol. 1999;181:1263–9.
16. IUD Poster – Dittrick Medical History Center. In: Dittrick Medical History Center [Internet]. [cited 28 Nov 2018]. Available: http://artsci.case.edu/dittrick/shop/iud-poster/.
17. Apter D, Gemzell-Danielsson K, Hauck B, Rosen K, Zurth C. Pharmacokinetics of two low-dose levonorgestrel-releasing intrauterine systems and effects on ovulation rate and cervical function: pooled analyses of phase II and III studies. Fertil Steril. 2014;101:1656–62.e1–4.
18. Natavio MF, Taylor D, Lewis RA, Blumenthal P, Felix JC, Melamed A, et al. Temporal changes in cervical mucus after insertion of the levonorgestrel-releasing intrauterine system. Contraception. 2013;87:426–31.
19. Sonalkar S, Schreiber CS, Barnhart KT. Contraception. In: Degroot LJ, Chrousos G, Dungan K, et al, editors. Endotext [Internet]. South Dartmouth: MDText.com, Inc.; 2000–2017. Last updated 2014 Nov 11.
20. CDC - Intrauterine contraception - US SPR - Reproductive health [Internet]. 25 Dec 2017 [cited 28 Nov 2018]. Available: https://www.cdc.gov/reproductivehealth/contraception/mmwr/spr/intrauterine.html.
21. Turok DK, Sanders JN, Thompson IS, Royer PA, Eggebroten J, Gawron LM. Preference for and efficacy of oral levonorgestrel for emergency contraception with concomitant placement of a levonorgestrel IUD: a prospective cohort study. Contraception. 2016;93:526–32.
22. Costescu DJ. Levonorgestrel-releasing intrauterine systems for long-acting contraception: current perspectives, safety, and patient counseling. Int J Womens Health. 2016;8:589–98.
23. McNicholas C, Swor E, Wan L, Peipert JF. Prolonged use of the etonogestrel implant and levonorgestrel intrauterine device: 2 years beyond Food and Drug Administration-approved duration. Am J Obstet Gynecol. 2017;216:586.e1–6.
24. Wu JP, Pickle S. Extended use of the intrauterine device: a literature review and recommendations for clinical practice. Contraception. 2014;89:495–503.
25. Creinin MD, Jansen R, Starr RM, Gobburu J, Gopalakrishnan M, Olariu A. Levonorgestrel release rates over 5 years with the Liletta® 52-mg intrauterine system. Contraception. 2016;94:353–6.
26. Ortiz ME, Croxatto HB. Copper-T intrauterine device and levonorgestrel intrauterine system: biological bases of their mechanism of action. Contraception. 2007;75:S16–30.
27. Stanford JB, Mikolajczyk RT. Mechanisms of action of intrauterine devices: update and estimation of postfertilization effects. Am J Obstet Gynecol. 2002;187:1699–708.
28. Gemzell-Danielsson K, Berger C, Lalitkumar PGL. Emergency contraception — mechanisms of action. Contraception. 2013;87:300–8.
29. Shen J, Che Y, Showell E, Chen K, Cheng L. Interventions for emergency contraception. Cochrane Database Syst Rev. 2017;(8):CD001324.
30. IUD most effective post-coital contraception. Contracept Technol Update. 1995;16:78–80.
31. Practice Bulletin No. 152: emergency contraception. Obstet Gynecol. 2015;126:e1–11.
32. Black A, Guilbert E; Co-Authors, Costescu D, Dunn S, Fisher W, et al. Canadian contraception consensus (Part 2 of 4). J Obstet Gynaecol Can. 2015;37:1033–1039.
33. Goldstuck ND, Wildemeersch D. Practical advice for emergency IUD contraception in young women. Obstet Gynecol Int. 2015;2015:986439.
34. LARC clinical training opportunities. In: ACOG [Internet]. [cited 28 Nov 2018]. Available: https://www.acog.org/-/media/Departments/LARC/LARC-Clinical-Training-Opportunities-Replaceable.pdf?dmc=1&ts=20180618T0337178645.
35. Hoffman B, Schorge J, Bradshaw K, Halvorson L, Schaffer J, Corton MM. Williams gynecology. 3rd ed. New York: McGraw Hill Professional; 2016.

Chapter 4
Addressing IUD Efficacy, Eligibility, Myths, and Satisfaction with Adolescents and Young Adults

Mandy S. Coles and Aisha Mays

Abbreviations

ACOG	American College of Obstetrics and Gynecology
AYA	Adolescents and Young Adults
CDC	Centers for Disease Control and Prevention
IUD	Intrauterine Device
LARC	Long-Acting Reversible Contraception
LNG	Levonorgestrel
MEC	Medical Eligibility Criteria
PID	Pelvic Inflammatory Disease
SBHC	School-Based Health Center
SPR	Selected Practice Recommendations for Contraceptive Use
STI	Sexually Transmitted Infection

Learning Objectives

Following completion of this chapter, you should be able to:

1. Review the evidence-based guidelines for safe intrauterine device (IUD) delivery, continuation, and management.
2. Discuss and dispel common myths associated with IUD use among adolescents and young adults (AYAs).
3. Illustrate how AYAs can provide peer education regarding IUDs.

M. S. Coles (✉)
Department of Pediatrics, Boston University Medical Center, Boston, MA, USA
e-mail: mcoles@bu.edu

A. Mays
UC Berkeley School of Public Health, UC Berkeley/UCSF Joint Medical Program, Berkeley, CA, USA

© Springer Nature Switzerland AG 2019
M. S. Coles, A. Mays (eds.), *Optimizing IUD Delivery for Adolescents and Young Adults*, https://doi.org/10.1007/978-3-030-17816-1_4

Background

The American Academy of Pediatrics, the Americal College of Obstetrics and Gynecology (ACOG), and the Society for Adolescent Medicine and Health have all published recommendations for long-acting reversible contraception (LARC) to be included in the contraceptive methods offered to AYAs [1–3]. Despite these recommendations, use of LARC in the USA remains low in women ages 15–44 years, with just 6.4% using IUDs and 0.8% using the contraceptive implant in 2012 [4]. Studies examining this age disparity have found that many medical providers still believe that LARC methods are inappropriate for use with AYA patients [5–9]. This chapter will address some of the potential gaps in knowledge noted above, including a review of IUD efficacy and eligibility in AYAs, a list of resources for evidence-based guidelines, and a discussion of common IUD myths.

Case

Tamira is a 15-year-old cisgender female in tenth grade. She had an IUD placed at her school-based health center (SBHC) last month, and is surprised how much she likes it. One day, in the school cafeteria, Tamira is talking with her friends about the lecture they just had in health class about sex, birth control, and pregnancy. One of her friends was happy to hear that condoms will prevent both pregnancy and sexually transmitted infections (STIs), because she knows that this is the best and safest form of birth control. Another friend, who uses the contraceptive patch, thinks this is the best birth control for teenagers because the sticker makes it easy to use. Tamira tells her friends that she just had an IUD placed and really likes it. Her friends look at her strangely, with one saying that her mother told her that, "IUDs cause you not to be able to have children in the future." Another friend agrees, and said that she heard that people their age shouldn't get IUDs because their bodies aren't fully developed. Tamira's friends say that they're worried that the IUD will "mess up" her body and that she should get it taken out. Tamira is so confused because her medical provider said that IUDs are safe, and that she will be able to have babies in the future. Now she's not sure what to believe.

Efficacy

IUDs are among the most effective contraceptive method for preventing pregnancy. When discussing efficacy, it is important to be aware of the distinction between *typical* use failure rates and *perfect* use failure rates [10]. Perfect use failure rates refer to the number of pregnancies occurring when the contraceptive is used consistently and correctly. Typical use failure rates reflect pregnancy risk due to inconsistent or incorrect use of their contraceptive method. Failure rates for AYAs under are significantly higher than typically quoted efficacy data across most contraceptive methods [11]. One study, which looked at data worldwide, did show a difference in typical use failure rates for AYA IUD users under 25 years (3.2%) compared to adults ages 25 years and older (1.1%). Another study systematically reviewed all published research on IUDs and young adults and found a similar failure rate at less than one percent, regardless of age [12]. Although the aforementioned studies presented inconsistent results, IUDs remain among the most effective contraceptive methods for AYAs.

Safety and IUD Use in Adolescents and Young Adults

AYAs can safely use IUDs. Complications such as pelvic inflammatory disease (PID), uterine perforation, and heavy bleeding are rare [12]. The risk of PID with IUD placement is very low, even in the event of a positive STI screening test performed at the time of insertion of the IUD [13, 14]. It is prudent to screen for infection when placing IUDs, and a speculum exam revealing mucopurulent cervicitis is a contraindication placement [15]. Other serious complications such as uterine perforation, which occurs in 1 out of 1,000 IUD placements, and infertility are not related to patient age at time of placement [12]. We know that infertility rates after IUD removal are very low, and are similar to those after discontinuation of other types of reversible contraceptives [14]. IUD expulsion was slightly more common among AYAs compared to adults who used the copper IUD [12].

Medical Eligibility Criteria (MEC)

The Centers for Disease Control and Prevention (CDC) publishes the USA Medical Eligibility Criteria (MEC), a series of recommendations for using specific USA Food and Drug Administration-approved contraceptive methods by patients who have certain characteristics or medical conditions [16]. These recommendations, **formulated from evidence-based research** and adapted from the World Health Organization [17], are intended to assist health care providers when they counsel patients about contraceptive method choice. The USA MEC was most recently updated in 2016. It provides guidelines on the *safe* **initiation** and **continuation** of all contraceptive methods. The MEC gives recommendations on contraceptive use for conditions including STIs, migraines with and without aura, PID, postpartum conditions, and systemic lupus erythematosus. These guidelines can be

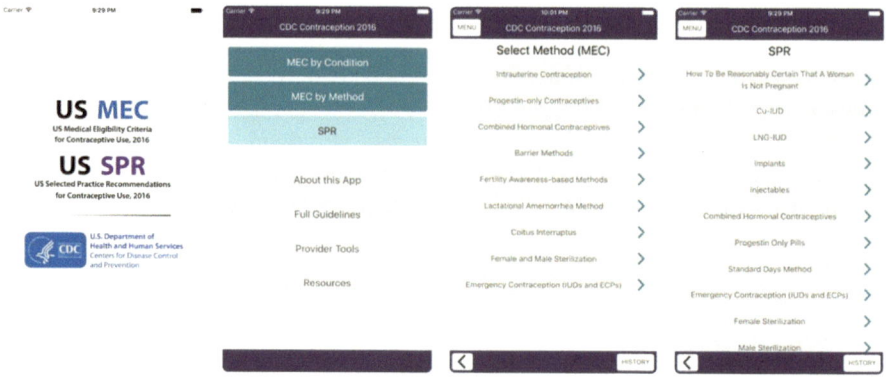

Fig. 4.1 Screenshots of the CDC MEC mobile app. (Image source: [18])

used to dispel myths about contraception suitability and safety. Medical providers can use the MEC guidelines to ensure that they are practicing unbiased, evidenced-based contraceptive care.

The CDC MEC has a mobile **app for download** and use on a smartphone (as seen here in Fig. 4.1):

The MEC recommendations also come in **printable table** format (Fig. 4.2), which can be posted in office work areas and clinic exam rooms [19].

Selected Practice Recommendations

The CDC publishes the USA Selected Practice Recommendations for Contraceptive Use (SPR), which address a select group of common, yet sometimes controversial or complex, issues regarding use of specific contraceptive methods [20]. The SPR recommendations were created from a review of scientific evidence-based research and national expert opinion and were most recently updated in 2016. The SPR helps to guide clinicians through management of contraceptive care including, how to **initiate contraception, provide contraception with co-occurring medical conditions, and switch between methods**. In the SPR, you will find up-to-date information on initiation and management of IUDs. The SPR can be referenced as an initial source to aid in IUD management.

The CDC SPR is provided in combination with the CDC MEC mobile app. This combination app provides integrated information about management and eligibility that helps to optimize contraceptive care (Fig. 4.3).

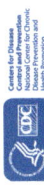

Fig. 4.2 The summary chart of USA MEC guidelines is available to print. (Image source: [181])

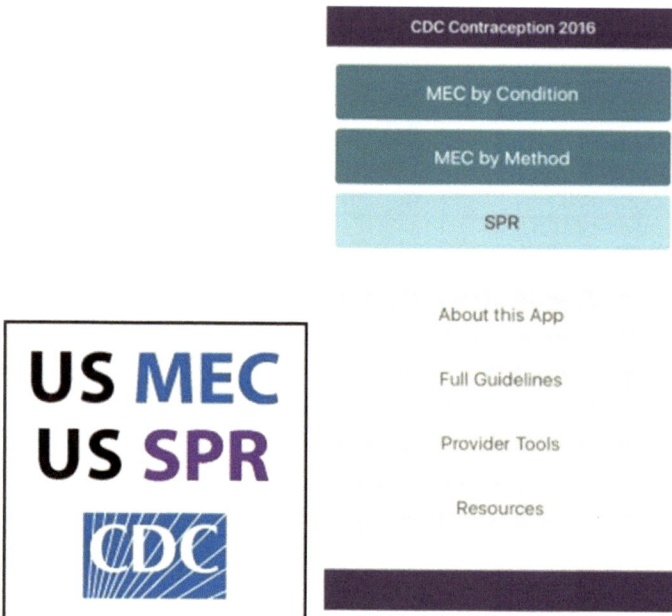

Fig. 4.3 The CDC provides a combination mobile application. (Image source: [18])

Case

Tamira goes back for her IUD follow-up visit at her SBHC and tells her provider that she wants her IUD removed. When her provider asks why, Tamira tells her about the conversation that she had with her friends. Tamira reports she didn't know that the IUD wasn't good for someone her age, and is afraid because her friends said that she wouldn't be able to have children in the future. She is scared and wants it out. Her SBHC provider is sympathetic and says that she can definitely remove Tamira's IUD if she wants but tells her that the information that her friends gave her is not true. She tells Tamira that she used research-proven guidelines to make sure that the IUD was safe for Tamira. Her medical provider also tells Tamira that the fear of not being able to have a baby in the future is a common myth, and it is simply not true. She tells Tamira that many people use the IUD as birth control between their pregnancies. Tamira feels relieved and is happy that she had this follow-up visit to speak with her provider.

Addressing IUD Myths, Fears, and Misinformation

The CDC MEC and SPR, along with current additional evidence-based recommendations, are debunking myths related to AYA eligibility for and safety of IUDs. While knowledge about IUDs has improved among AYAs, myths and misconceptions still exist and, "several myths must be dispelled before IUDs are more widely utilized by AYAs or recommended by more clinicians" [21]. Listed below are some concerns that we have heard from patients, and the data that can be used to reassure our patients (as well as ourselves). Common myths include:

Myth 1 *"I didn't think I could get an IUD if I hadn't been pregnant."* Many parents tell us, and tell their children, that they didn't think adolescents could get an IUD. And young people themselves may have seen or heard an advertisement for Mirena that was directly marketed to women who had a child. However, clear data on both safety and efficacy guided the CDC's MEC to categorize both age (menarche to <20 years) and nulliparity as Category 2 (benefits outweigh risks) conditions for both copper and levonorgestrel (LNG) type IUDs [15]. Past concerns about fertility issues stemming from IUD use may also be tied into the idea that IUDs should/could not be used in younger people. However, as covered in Chap. 1, a large body of evidence now ties issues of infertility to untreated STIs (as discussed below) and to a type of IUD that is no longer available. Despite this evidence, many providers rarely (or never) provide IUDs to nulliparous patients [6], despite research that shows those who have never had children (including AYAs) can successfully use IUDs.

Myth 2 *"I heard that IUDs cause infection."* As noted above, concerns about infection continue to be a barrier to IUD use. We now know that flaws in early research exaggerated the risk of infection, and that PID was associated with chlamydia infection and not with IUDs. A large number of newer randomized controlled studies have demonstrated that the risk of PID in IUD users is low [13, 14, 22, 23]—and, in fact, LNG IUDs may decrease the long-term risk of PID, due to a thickening of cervical mucus [24]. The IUD insertion process itself does pose a transient increased risk of ascending infection for up to 3 weeks post-insertion only if an STI is present, though overall PID risks are similar for those with and without IUDs [13, 22]. As AYAs are at higher risk of STIs in general, we do recommend screening for infections either at the time of, or prior to, IUD insertion. There is no data to support the misconception that IUDs increase the rate of infection among AYAs or persons of any age.

Myth 3 *"Isn't the IUD going to fall out of me?"* Concerns that IUD expulsion is more likely in AYAs compared to adults may be based on older studies that raised concerns of higher expulsion rates (5–22%) with younger and nulliparous individuals compared to adults (3–5%). However, current data supports similar (and *low*) rates of IUD expulsion compared for AYAs compared to adult patients [22, 25, 26].

Myth 4 *"Don't IUDs increase the risk of ectopic pregnancies?"* It is well documented that IUDs are highly effective at reducing the risk of pregnancy, and this is especially true for intrauterine pregnancies. While the overall risk of ectopic pregnancy is lower for individuals with IUDs than for those not using contraception, if a pregnancy occurs with an IUD in place, there is a higher likelihood of it being ectopic [27].

Myth 5 *"Do IUDs cause abortion?"* An abortifacient is defined as an agent that disturbs an embryo that is fertilized and has implanted in the uterine lining. In contrast to abortifacients, LNG and copper IUDs work to prevent fertilization of an egg by sperm [28]. Copper IUDs also work by reducing sperm motility and viability, and produce an inflammatory endometrial environment that may also impact implantation of a fertilized egg [29]. Neither type of IUD has an effect after implantation [30]. ACOG provides a fact sheet that can also help explain the differences to patients and families [31].

Myth 6 *"I would like to get an IUD, but I'm afraid it's going to hurt."* Fear of pain has been reported as a primary reason younger patients were not interested in using IUDs [32, 33]. However, it is clear that AYAs are able to successfully tolerate IUD insertions, and manage whatever sensations they experience based on the numbers who get IUDs placed; research informs us of this as well [34, 35]. Individual experiences of pain can be impacted both positively and negatively by knowledge, prior learning, emotions, and expectations, among a number of factors [36]. While many people report discomfort with their IUD insertion and overall pain scores tend to be low, the severity of these sensations can range widely. We know that the language we use to discuss what an IUD insertion feels like with individual patients during the counseling process can impact their expectation and future experiences of pain, and help either allay or worsen their fear [37]. Please see Chaps. 9 and 10 for further information on both pharmacologic and nonpharmacologic pain-management strategies.

Case: A moment for peer education

Tamira and her friends are having lunch again after health education class and Tamira's friends ask her if she got her IUD taken out yet. Tamira told them that she spoke with the SBHC medical provider about the issues that her friends talked about. She shared that the provider told her that the IUD was safe for her at her age, and that it does not cause problems with having children in the future. Tamira told her friends that IUD guidelines are based on research. Tamira added that the SBHC medical provider even showed her the guidelines on her medical websites. Tamira said that she was relieved because she really likes her IUD and wants to keep it. She told her friends that the SBHC provider also talked about lots of myths about the IUD, and that these medical guidelines really tell the truth. Tamira encouraged her friends to go to the SBHC to get more information about the IUD. Suddenly the bell rang and it was time to go to the next class. As they were walking to class, Tamira's friend Mirella thanked her for what she said during lunch. Mirella wants an IUD but has been scared. Now Mirella's going to go to the SBHC after school to discuss it further.

Contraindications to IUD Use

IUDs are a completely safe form of contraception for AYAs, if they choose this method. However, there are a **few contraindications** to IUD use for which clinicians should be familiar. Below see a list of absolute contraindications to IUD use, with those pertinent to AYAs in **bold**.

Absolute contraindications to the IUD:

- **Current purulent cervicitis or known gonorrhea or chlamydia infection (up to one week after treatment)**
- **Current PID (up to three months after treatment)**
- **Pregnancy**
- Postpartum sepsis
- **Immediate post-septic abortion**
- Unexplained vaginal bleeding, suspicious for a serious condition and not yet evaluated
- Gestational trophoblastic disease, with persistent elevation in beta hCG levels and evidence or suspicion of intrauterine disease
- Lupus with positive or unknown antiphospholipid antibodies
- Cervical cancer (awaiting treatment) (initiation)
- Endometrial cancer (initiation)
- Current breast cancer
- Distortion of the uterine cavity that is incompatible with IUD placement
- Pelvic tuberculosis (initiation)

Relative contraindications to the IUD (conditions most pertinent to AYAs in bold):

- Pelvic tuberculosis (continuation)
- Complicated solid organ transplantation with graft failure, rejection, or cardiac allograft vasculopathy (initiation)
- Hepatic disease including hepatocellular tumors (LNG IUD)
- Severe thrombocytopenia (Copper IUD)

Satisfaction and Continuation

Despite recent increases in IUD use (7.7–10.3%) from 2009 to 2012 among 15-44 year olds, the use of IUDs among those aged 15–19 years old in the USA has been relatively stable (4.5–4.3%) [38], with no significant differences in type of IUD use by age. Researchers have theorized that these low and stable rates of IUD use among AYAs may be related to a number of factors, including healthcare provider beliefs of patient preferences against the IUD, pelvic examination avoidance, and a higher likelihood of early removal as a result of dissatisfaction [33]. However, data show us that AYAs who choose IUDs tend to be both satisfied with, and likely to continue this method.

The largest body of research on LARC satisfaction and continuation comes from the Contraceptive CHOICE Project, which offered a wide variety of contraceptive methods to women in the St. Louis area seeking to avoid pregnancy for at least one year, who were interested in starting a new form of contraception [39]. The CHOICE Project, which used a tiered contraceptive counseling model that prioritized effectiveness [40]—and offered all reversible contraceptive options, free of charge to participants—found reasonably high levels of IUD acceptance among both adolescents (26% of 14–17-year-olds (n = 214)) and young adults (43% of 18–20-year-olds (n = 840) [41]). Some family planning advocates have raised concerns that the efficacy-prioritized contraceptive counseling model used in the CHOICE project may have guided women toward choosing LARC methods [42] over other methods. Contraceptive choice is a personal decision, and based on many factors including not only contraceptive effectiveness (as in the CHOICE project), but also the experiences of friends and family [43], relationship context [44], preferences for bleeding patterns, and control over method, to name a few [45].

After 3 years, the CHOICE Project reported that more than half of young people who initially chose a LARC method continued their method, compared to only about 20% of AYAs who chose a non-LARC method [46]. The findings of two review articles supported these findings of high continuation and satisfaction rates among AYAs who used IUDs. One systematic review that evaluated research done between 1946–2015 found statistically higher 12-month continuation rates for the AYAs who used IUDs (86.5%)—compared to users of the pill, patch, ring, or progesterone injection [47]. The other systematic review and meta-analysis of study that included AYA IUD users reported a 74% continuation rate at 12 months, with slightly higher continuation rates among post-partum individuals (84%) [48].

Few studies assess AYA user satisfaction with IUDs. One study of youth (n = 79) who received IUDs in an urban adolescent center reported similar satisfaction rates (75.4%) at three and six months, and did not identify consistent patient characteristics (parity, prior contraceptive use, device choice) that predicted higher method satisfaction over time [49]. The CHOICE Project conducted focus groups with adolescent IUD users and identified **effectiveness, duration of use, convenience, and potential bleeding changes** as themes for both choosing and continuing IUDs. Copper IUD users also reported desires for a **non-hormonal method**, and for **continued menses** as influencing their choice. For those who chose to **discontinue** their method, LNG-IUD users reported **bleeding changes and not liking "how it made me feel"** as important decision-making points, while the most common reported reasons for discontinuation of copper IUDs were **bleeding changes and cramping** [50]. IUD users also noted an adjustment period where side effects were present, which is clearly important to discuss during method counseling. A separate study at a family medicine clinic found that adolescents were more likely to make follow-up appointments to discuss concerns after an IUD insertion but reported similar concerns as adult women (bleeding changes and abdominal or pelvic pain) and had similar rates of IUD removals [25].

Clinical Pearls
- Evidence-based **eligibility** criteria have expanded AYAs access to IUDs. IUDs should be among the first-line methods for teens.
- LARC methods including IUDs have the highest **efficacy** at preventing pregnancy over short-acting, reversible contraceptives in all individuals including AYAs.
- IUDs are **safe** and are without increased complications or adverse outcomes in AYAs.
- Among adolescents, LARCs including IUDs have the highest rates of **satisfaction** and **continuation** rates, versus non-LARC methods.
- Accurate patient education around efficacy, safety, and reversibility is core to informed consent and reproductive justice.

Conclusion

Access to the full spectrum of contraceptive options, including IUDs, is recommended for AYA service providers [1, 3, 51]. However, a focus on LARC methods above others may actually limit young people's reproductive autonomy if providers do not respect individual decisions to not use these methods, or to have them removed if/when patients wish [52]. IUDs are incredibly safe and highly effective forms of birth control, with higher continuation rates compared to non-LARC methods. While IUDs are safe for the vast majority of youth, the CDC's MEC and SPR should be used as evidenced-based guides for determining their appropriateness for each individual patient. Myths of previous decades, fueled by complications from previous devices no longer available, still exist, but can be dispelled. Clinicians play a pivotal role in addressing common misperceptions around the use of IUDs, as well as responding to fears and misinformation with compassion, understanding, and patience. Understanding patients' motivating factors for IUD use is equally as important as understanding and alleviating potential barriers.

References

1. Ott MA, Sucato GS. Committee on adolescence. Contraception for adolescents. Pediatrics. 2014;134:e1257–81.
2. Society for Adolescent Health and Medicine, Burke PJ, Coles MS, Di Meglio G, Gibson EJ, Handschin SM, et al. Sexual and reproductive health care: a position paper of the society for adolescent health and medicine. J Adolesc Health. 2014;54:491–6.
3. ACOG Committee Opinion No. 735: adolescents and long-acting reversible contraception: implants and intrauterine devices. Obstet Gynecol. 2018;131:e130–e139.
4. Contraceptive use in the United States. In: Guttmacher Institute [Internet]. Jul 2018 [cited 29 Nov 2018]. Available: https://www.guttmacher.org/fact-sheet/contraceptive-use-united-states.

5. Luchowski AT, Anderson BL, Power ML, Raglan GB, Espey E, Schulkin J. Obstetrician-gynecologists and contraception: practice and opinions about the use of IUDs in nulliparous women, adolescents and other patient populations. Contraception. 2014;89:572–7.

6. Tyler CP, Whiteman MK, Zapata LB, Curtis KM, Hillis SD, Marchbanks PA. Health care provider attitudes and practices related to intrauterine devices for nulliparous women. Obstet Gynecol. 2012;119:762–71.

7. Rubin SE, Davis K, McKee MD. New York city physicians' views of providing long-acting reversible contraception to adolescents. Ann Fam Med. 2013;11:130–6.

8. Whitaker AK, Sisco KM, Tomlinson AN, Dude AM, Martins SL. Use of the intrauterine device among adolescent and young adult women in the United States from 2002 to 2010. J Adolesc Health. 2013;53:401–6.

9. Biggs MA, Kaller S, Harper CC, Freedman L, Mays AR. "Birth Control can Easily Take a Back Seat": challenges providing IUDs in community health care settings. J Health Care Poor Underserved. 2018;29:228–44.

10. Schreiber CA, Barnhart K. In: Strauss JF, Jerome F, Strauss III, Barbieri RL, editors. Yen and Jaffe's reproductive endocrinology. Philadelphia, PA. Elsevier Health Sciences; 2013.

11. Polis CB, Bradley SEK, Bankole A, Onda T, Croft T, Singh S. Typical-use contraceptive failure rates in 43 countries with Demographic and Health Survey data: summary of a detailed report. Contraception. 2016;94:11–7.

12. Jatlaoui TC, Riley HEM, Curtis KM. The safety of intrauterine devices among young women: a systematic review. Contraception. 2017;95:17–39.

13. Mohllajee AP, Curtis KM, Peterson HB. Does insertion and use of an intrauterine device increase the risk of pelvic inflammatory disease among women with sexually transmitted infection? A systematic review. Contraception. 2006;73:145–53.

14. Grimes DA. Intrauterine device and upper-genital-tract infection. Lancet. 2000;356:1013–9.

15. Curtis KM, Tepper NK, Jatlaoui TC, Berry-Bibee E, Horton LG, Zapata LB, et al. U.S. medical eligibility criteria for contraceptive use, 2016. MMWR Recomm Rep. 2016;65:1–103.

16. CDC – Summary – USMEC – Reproductive Health [Internet]. 28 Sep 2017 [cited 30 Nov 2018]. Available: https://www.cdc.gov/reproductivehealth/contraception/mmwr/mec/summary.html.

17. World Health Organization, Reproductive Health and Research, World Health Organization, World Health Organization, Family and Community Health. Selected practice recommendations for contraceptive use. Geneva: World Health Organization; 2005.

18. CDC – Summary – USMEC – Reproductive Health [Internet]. 2 Nov 2018 [cited 6 Jan 2019]. Available: https://www.cdc.gov/reproductivehealth/contraception/mmwr/mec/summary.html.

19. Summary chart of U.S. medical eligibility criteria for contraceptive use. In: CDC [Internet]. [cited 1 Dec 2018]. Available: https://www.cdc.gov/reproductivehealth/contraception/pdf/summary-chart-us-medical-eligibility-criteria_508tagged.pdf.

20. CDC – Summary – US SPR – Reproductive Health [Internet]. 27 Sep 2017 [cited 30 Nov 2018]. Available: https://www.cdc.gov/reproductivehealth/contraception/mmwr/spr/summary.html.

21. Yen S, Saah T, Hillard PJA. IUDs and adolescents--an under-utilized opportunity for pregnancy prevention. J Pediatr Adolesc Gynecol. 2010;23:123–8.

22. Alton TM, Brock GN, Yang D, Wilking DA, Hertweck SP, Loveless MB. Retrospective review of intrauterine device in adolescent and young women. J Pediatr Adolesc Gynecol. 2012;25:195–200.

23. Hubacher D, Lara-Ricalde R, Taylor DJ, Guerra-Infante F, Guzmán-Rodríguez R. Use of copper intrauterine devices and the risk of tubal infertility among nulligravid women. N Engl J Med. 2001;345:561–7.

24. Toivonen J, Luukkainen T, Allonen H. Protective effect of intrauterine release of levonorgestrel on pelvic infection: three years' comparative experience of levonorgestrel- and copper-releasing intrauterine devices. Obstet Gynecol. 1991;77:261–4.

25. Ravi A, Prine L, Waltermaurer E, Miller N, Rubin SE. Intrauterine devices at six months: does patient age matter? Results from an urban family medicine federally qualified health center (FQHC) network. J Am Board Fam Med. 2014;27:822–30.
26. Aoun J, Dines VA, Stovall DW, Mete M, Nelson CB, Gomez-Lobo V. Effects of age, parity, and device type on complications and discontinuation of intrauterine devices. Obstet Gynecol. 2014;123:585–92.
27. Heinemann K, Reed S, Moehner S, Minh TD. Comparative contraceptive effectiveness of levonorgestrel-releasing and copper intrauterine devices: the European Active Surveillance Study for Intrauterine Devices. Contraception. 2015;91:280–3.
28. Ortiz ME, Croxatto HB. Copper-T intrauterine device and levonorgestrel intrauterine system: biological bases of their mechanism of action. Contraception. 2007;75:S16–30.
29. Stanford JB, Mikolajczyk RT. Mechanisms of action of intrauterine devices: update and estimation of postfertilization effects. Am J Obstet Gynecol. 2002;187:1699–708.
30. Videla-Rivero L, Etchepareborda JJ, Kesseru E. Early chorionic activity in women bearing inert IUD, copper IUD and levonorgestrel-releasing IUD. Contraception. 1987;36:217–26.
31. Facts are important emergency contraception (EC) and intrauterine devices (IUDs) are not abortifacients. The American College of Obstetricians and Gynecologists [Internet]. Jun 2014 [cited 6 Jan 2019]. Available: www.acog.org/-/media/Departments/Government-Relations-and-Outreach/FactsAreImportantEC.pdf.
32. Fleming KL, Sokoloff A, Raine TR. Attitudes and beliefs about the intrauterine device among teenagers and young women. Contraception. 2010;82:178–82.
33. Kavanaugh ML, Frohwirth L, Jerman J, Popkin R, Ethier K. Long-acting reversible contraception for adolescents and young adults: patient and provider perspectives. J Pediatr Adolesc Gynecol. 2013;26:86–95.
34. Allen RH, Carey MS, Raker C, Goyal V, Matteson K. A prospective cohort study of pain with intrauterine device insertion among women with and without vaginal deliveries. J Obstet Gynaecol. 2014;34:263–7.
35. Akers AY, Harding J, Perriera LK, Schreiber C, Garcia-Espana JF, Sonalkar S. Satisfaction with the intrauterine device insertion procedure among adolescent and young adult women. Obstet Gynecol. 2018;131:1130–6.
36. Tracey I. Getting the pain you expect: mechanisms of placebo, nocebo and reappraisal effects in humans. Nat Med. 2010;16:1277–83.
37. Krauss BS. "This may hurt": predictions in procedural disclosure may do harm. BMJ. 2015;350:h649.
38. Kavanaugh ML, Jerman J, Finer LB. Changes in use of long-acting reversible contraceptive methods among U.S. women, 2009–2012. Obstet Gynecol. 2015;126:917–27.
39. Secura GM, Allsworth JE, Madden T, Mullersman JL, Peipert JF. The Contraceptive CHOICE Project: reducing barriers to long-acting reversible contraception. Am J Obstet Gynecol. 2010;203:115.e1–7.
40. Madden T, Mullersman JL, Omvig KJ, Secura GM, Peipert JF. Structured contraceptive counseling provided by the Contraceptive CHOICE Project. Contraception. 2013;88:243–9.
41. Mestad R, Secura G, Allsworth JE, Madden T, Zhao Q, Peipert JF. Acceptance of long-acting reversible contraceptive methods by adolescent participants in the Contraceptive CHOICE Project. Contraception. 2011;84:493–8.
42. Stanback J, Steiner M, Dorflinger L, Solo J, Cates W Jr. WHO tiered-effectiveness counseling is rights-based family planning. Glob Health Sci Pract. 2015;3:352–7.
43. Gilliam ML, Neustadt A, Whitaker A, Kozloski M. Familial, cultural and psychosocial influences of use of effective methods of contraception among Mexican-American adolescents and young adults. J Pediatr Adolesc Gynecol. 2011;24:79–84.
44. Kusunoki Y, Upchurch DM. Contraceptive method choice among youth in the United States: the importance of relationship context. Demography. 2011;48:1451–72.
45. Gomez AM, Fuentes L, Allina A. Women or LARC first? Reproductive autonomy and the promotion of long-acting reversible contraceptive methods. Perspect Sex Reprod Health. 2014;46:171–5.

46. Diedrich JT, Zhao Q, Madden T, Secura GM, Peipert JF. Three-year continuation of reversible contraception. Am J Obstet Gynecol. 2015;213:662.e1–8.
47. Usinger KM, Gola SB, Weis M, Smaldone A. Intrauterine contraception continuation in adolescents and young women: a systematic review. J Pediatr Adolesc Gynecol. 2016;29:659–67.
48. Diedrich JT, Klein DA, Peipert JF. Long-acting reversible contraception in adolescents: a systematic review and meta-analysis. Am J Obstet Gynecol. 2017;216:364.e1–364.e12.
49. Friedman JO. Factors associated with contraceptive satisfaction in adolescent women using the IUD. J Pediatr Adolesc Gynecol. 2015;28:38–42.
50. Schmidt EO, James A, Curran KM, Peipert JF, Madden T. Adolescent experiences with intrauterine devices: a qualitative study. J Adolesc Health. 2015;57:381–6.
51. Society for Adolescent Health and Medicine. Improving knowledge about, access to, and utilization of long-acting reversible contraception among adolescents and young adults. J Adolesc Health. 2017;60:472–4.
52. Gubrium AC, Mann ES, Borrero S, Dehlendorf C, Fields J, Geronimus AT, et al. Realizing reproductive health equity needs more than long-acting reversible contraception (LARC). Am J Public Health. 2016;106:18–9.

Chapter 5
IUD Counseling: What's Choice Got to Do With It?

Aisha Mays

Abbreviations

AAP	American Academy of Pediatrics
ACOG	The American College of Obstetrics and Gynecology
HEADSS	Home, Education/Employment, Activities, Drugs/Depression, Suicidality, Sex
LARC	Long-acting reversible contraception
RJ	Reproductive justice
SAHM	Society of Adolescent Health and Medicine
SDM	Shared decision-making

Learning Objectives
Following completion of this chapter, you should be better able to:

- Discuss the history of reproductive abuse in the USA, and understand how the medical community has contributed.
- Describe the common models of contraceptive counseling.
- Describe and apply the shared decision-making model (SDM) for contraceptive counseling.
- Address additional points to consider with intrauterine device (IUD) counseling for adolescents and young adults (AYAs).

A. Mays (✉)
UC Berkeley School of Public Health, UC Berkeley/UCSF Joint Medical Program, Berkeley, CA, USA
e-mail: amays@berkeley.edu

© Springer Nature Switzerland AG 2019
M. S. Coles, A. Mays (eds.), *Optimizing IUD Delivery for Adolescents and Young Adults*, https://doi.org/10.1007/978-3-030-17816-1_5

Introduction

Since 2009, several USA medical organizations have supported the use of IUDs as safe and "forgettable" [1] contraceptive methods for AYAs [2, 3]. In addition to citing safety and ease of use of these methods, these organizations highlighted their *effectiveness* as a primary driver for recommending that providers counsel AYAs on IUDs and implants as the *first-line method* of contraception [2, 3]. This recommendation, primarily centered on the outcomes of reducing unintended pregnancy and achieving *perfect contraceptive use* for AYAs, has been criticized by medical providers, family planning researchers, and reproductive justice organizations as a threat to reproductive autonomy—those original 2009 and 2014 recommendations put AYAs at risk for reproductive coercion [4–8]. In 2018, The American College of Obstetrics and Gynecology (ACOG) revised their recommendations to mirror those in the position statement released by Society of Adolescent Health and Medicine (SAHM) in 2017 [9]. This updated committee opinion supported patient choice as the principal factor driving choice of method of contraception, respected the adolescent's right to choose or decline any method of reversible contraception as critical, and recommended that providers not prefer any one contraceptive method over another [10].

Current best practices in contraceptive counseling reflect reproductive justice principles that *access to reproductive health care is a human right* [10, 11]—that individuals should have autonomous choice of when, and if, they choose to parent, irrespective of age, socioeconomic status, gender identity, or social vulnerabilities [8, 12]. Adopting counseling techniques that avoid all forms of reproductive coercion and promote ultimate patient choice ensures that providers follow these tenets. This chapter will describe best-practice models for providing contraceptive counseling, and methods for integrating these counseling models around IUD placement, continuation, and removal for AYAs.

Case

Rohan is a 15-year-old, cisgender female who has received her care at your adolescent clinic for the past 2 years. Rohan is seen frequently in clinic because of challenges with school attendance, volatile relationships with friends, and a lack of parental support. She comes in today, and is seen by the second-year family medicine resident who is working with you. The resident reports that Rohan has a new boyfriend who she is excited about, especially because she always felt that boys were, "just not that into her." Rohan and her boyfriend have now been dating for about 3 months, and he has been hinting around about wanting to have sex with her. When asked by the resident how she felt about sex, Rohan replied that she isn't really sure if she's ready now, but, "maybe when I'm sixteen…" Rohan told the resident that she thinks her boyfriend has lots of experience with sex because he has a child, so he could probably show her what to do. Rohan is sure that she doesn't want to get pregnant, and asks if you can give her some birth control today.

Your resident shares that she feels concerned Rohan is going to have sex when she's not really ready, but is relieved that Rohan wants birth control. The resident wants to talk to Rohan about choosing a long-acting reversible contraception (LARC) method, so that Rohan "definitely doesn't get pregnant."

Sexual Readiness

Before delving into contraceptive counseling with AYAs, it is important that patients are able to have conversations with their providers about sexual empowerment, including discussions about sexual readiness and consent [13]. A 2017 systematic review of adolescents' understanding of sexual readiness found that adolescents are often unsure of how to assert sexual decisions outside of models presented through dominant (and often repressive) gender norms. Therefore, as part of AYA sexual and reproductive health care, it is critical to engage adolescents in critiquing ideas about gender equality, sexual rights, and sexual readiness [14]. Conversations about sexual readiness and consent should be part of the routine Home, Education/Employment, Activities, Drugs/Depression, Suicidality, Sex (HEADSS) assessment with AYAs, and are especially important to include in all family planning and contraceptive visits. Below are some examples of how to begin discussions about sexual readiness and sexual consent.

Sexual readiness:

1. How do you feel about beginning to have sex?
2. How did you all decide to begin to have sex?
3. When you think about having sex with [insert how patient describes the individual], and how does that make you feel?

Sexual consent:

1. How do you know if you've said "yes" (or "no") to having sex?

Regardless of whether an AYA has had sex in the past, **it is important that they feel ready to have sex, and that that sex be consensual, on every occasion**. For more information on how to support AYA sexual empowerment, sexual readiness, and sexual consent, please see the following resources from Advocates for Youth and Futures Without Violence [15, 16].

Case (continued)

You look a little perplexed at your resident and share that from what she's told you, it seems like Rohan is not sure if she's ready to have sex. You ask your resident if they talked about sexual readiness, and she responds eagerly that she asked some of the follow-up questions that she learned during your Adolescent Sexual Empowerment presentation. Rohan answered very positively to questions about sexual readiness and sexual consent. Your resident informs you that she also spent a significant amount of time counseling Rohan about birth control methods using a tiered effectiveness counseling approach, and encouraged Rohan to get an IUD, as it is one of the most effective methods.

Contraceptive Counseling

Medical providers are given a unique and privileged opportunity to support AYAs in their contraceptive decision-making. Alongside personal social networks, providers are highly influential in guiding the contraceptive choices of AYAs [17, 18]. One study of low-income young women showed that AYAs were more likely to choose a new contraceptive method that was recommended by their provider [19, 20]. Because of this significant power, it is crucial that providers are both aware of how contraception has been used to negatively impact individuals and families and, conversely, how it can be used to support individuals in their overall life goals.

History of Contraception Abuse and Reproductive Coercion

To truly understand why it is *so important to be mindful of how we discuss and counsel* AYAs on contraception, medical providers **must be knowledgeable about the history of contraception abuse** in the USA and how healthcare providers have contributed to these injustices (also discussed in Chap. 1). The USA has a history of reproductive control dating back to colonialism, slavery, and the eugenics movement when Native American, African slave, and other vulnerable women of color were forcibly sterilized [5, 21–23]. This level of control and abuse continues throughout USA history, most recently in the 1990s, wherein California women on public benefits were provided increased financial incentives if they agreed to use Norplant, a five-rod, 5-year contraceptive device [24]. During this same time, in the judicial system, women were offered reduced sentences in exchange for using LARC methods [25]. Coercion, bias, and reproductive control of low-income women, vulnerable women, and women of color also continue within the medical community [26–28]. In a study of women's experiences of reproductive health care, Black and Latina participants were more likely to describe being discouraged by their providers from having future children, than middle-class white women participants [27]. These findings are further supported by a 2011 study that found providers were more likely to recommend IUD use for low-income Black and Latina women, than for low-income white women [29].

These experiences and studies highlight how medicine has been used—and the medical community has been complicit—to harm women of color and vulnerable populations. Given this, medical providers must make particular efforts to ensure that patients are able to freely choose contraceptive methods of their own choice.

Medical providers must take steps to make certain that use of these methods is driven by patients' own expressed desires for them and not by population-level goals of reducing unintended or "teenage" pregnancy rates [7]. Medical providers have the potential to shift the tides and positively support patient's contraceptive use by optimizing patient-centered, patient-first contraceptive counseling.

Common Types of Contraceptive Counseling

Studies have shown that while patients want control over the ultimate selection of their birth control, most also want their provider to participate in the decision-making process in a way that emphasizes the patients' values and preferences [7, 18, 30, 31]. When counseling AYAs about contraception, it is paramount to ensure that they are able to make informed decisions, free from coercion [32]. There are several common styles of contraception counseling; three styles are discussed: consumerist counseling, directive counseling, and SDM counseling.

Consumerist Counseling Consumerist Counseling, also termed the "informed choice" model [33, 34], focuses on being objective and non-judgmental—**providing *only information*** and **not participating in the selection** of the method itself—so as to ensure that patients are not inappropriately influenced [19, 20].

One example of consumerist counseling is A medical provider, without discussion, continues to refill an AYA's birth control pills because they say that they like the pill and want to stay on it, although they consistently miss pills and lose pill packs. This provider continues to provide the patient with the method that they want (*good*), without providing any assessment or guidance that may assist the patient in contracepting effectively (*bad*).

• **We do not recommend the Consumerist Counseling Model**.

Directive Counseling Another popular counseling model, Directive Counseling [35, 36], implores a more directive approach, where providers directly recommend methods that are associated with a predetermined "best outcome," such as population-based data (reduction in unintended or teen pregnancy) or scientific data (the most effective contraceptive method) [36]. One well-known form of directive counseling is **Tiered Effectiveness Counseling** [37], in which methods are presented in order of **effectiveness,** so as to emphasize and draw attention to these methods. **Motivational interviewing** [38] is an approach developed initially in the context of working with patients with substance-use disorder [39], and designed to promote **certain behavior choices**. Using motivational interviewing techniques, patients are encouraged by providers on method choice.

An example of directive counseling is A sexually active adolescent whose maturity and behavior history strongly suggest that she would struggle managing the daily requirements of oral contraceptives or consistent use of a barrier method is steered by a medical provider to use a LARC method [40]. This counseling approach is criticized as being "disease centered and not patient centered and supports techniques that place patients **at risk of reproductive coercion** at the hand of providers" [40].

- **We do not recommend the Directive Counseling Model.**

Shared Decision-Making Counseling SDM counseling is a *collaborative process* that allows patients and their providers to make healthcare decisions together, taking into account the best scientific evidence available, as well as the ***patient's values and preferences*** [41]. This process provides patients with the **support** they need to make the best **individualized care** decisions [42]. In the SDM model, each party is recognized as having relevant expertise, with the **healthcare provider having superior knowledge of the medical information** and **the patient being the expert regarding their own values and preferences** [43]. SDM counseling uses principles designed to partner with, and empower, patients in their health care [44]. SDM counseling focuses on patient-centered, rather than provider-driven approaches. The model is associated with improved satisfaction with contraceptive counseling, contraceptive choice, and method continuation [44, 45]. The SDM model can be thought of as an overlap between portions of the consumerist and directive counseling models with an emphasis on patient-centeredness [42] (see Fig. 5.1).

Qualitative research suggests that AYAs prefer contraceptive counseling that uses SDM principles [46], leading to its recommendation as the preferred method of contraceptive counseling for AYAs [47]. In SDM counseling, both the provider and the patient play important roles in facilitating the patient's contraceptive choices, while recognizing that the ultimate decision always lies with the patient.

- **We *recommended* the SDM counseling model for contraceptive counseling.**

Medical providers' roles in the SDM model include [18, 42–44]**:**

- Providing clear and accurate contraceptive information
- Facilitating the identification of patient preferences
- Ensuring that preferences are not based on misinformation

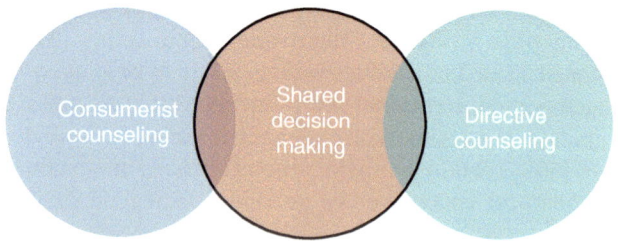

Fig. 5.1 The SDM model can be thought of as an overlap between portions of the consumerist and directive counseling models with an emphasis on patient-centeredness. (Source: Dehlendorf [42])

Consumerist counseling

Shared decision making

Directive counseling

- Helping patients to think about how their preferences relate to the available contraceptive options
- Supporting the patient to be successful using their chosen contraceptive method

Patient's role in the SDM model includes:

- Sharing what they know about birth control with their provider
- Informing the provider what they tried in the past and what they did (or did not) like about the method
- Informing the provider of what they are looking for in their birth control method (preferences)
- Asking clarifying questions of the provider to assist themselves in making the best contraceptive choice

SDM Counseling *DOES*:

- Elicit the patient's preferences for what they would like in their birth control method.
  - "What are important features that your birth control should have?"
- Use open, non-judgmental language in discussing contraception with patients.
- Provide decision support, without pressure.

SDM Counseling *DOES NOT:*:

- Make general recommendations for the patient.
  - "You should choose an IUD. Most of my patients like them!"
- Use social information to lead (coerce) patients to choose a particular method.
  - "Well, since homeless youth are at high risk of forgetting about their birth control, you should get an IUD."
- Even if *seemingly* well intentioned.
  - "It's probably best for you to have an IUD because I know you have to conceal your birth control."
- Use fear tactics to lead (coerce) patients to choose a particular method.
  - "If you really don't want to get pregnant, it's probably best that you choose something like the IUD."

How to Discuss Preferences with AYAs

One of the key aspects of the SDM model is eliciting patients' preferences. Understanding what an individual may value or prefer, in regard to specific contraceptive options, can help clinicians tailor their counseling and support informed contraception choice [48]. Patient preferences are defined contraceptive features that patients may desire, or wish to avoid, in choosing their birth control method [18, 49]. Examples of commonly stated contraceptive preferences among AYAs include [46, 50]:

- Desire to have or stop periods
- Desire for regular periods

- Contraceptive effectiveness
- Frequency of method use (daily, weekly, monthly, yearly)
- How to take/use method
- "Forgetability"
- Desire to not depend on refills
- Duration of use

Because the concept of discussing preferences may be new for AYAs, it is important to explain to your AYA patients what you mean by *preferences*. Questions such as the ones below can help you to determine what is most important to your patients. The features outlined in the above preferences should be drawn upon in supporting your patients to choose their contraceptive method. Here are examples of how to begin a discussion to elicit AYAs' preferences in a birth control method:

1. "Tell me what is important to you about your birth control?"
2. "What are important features that your birth control should have?" (You can give examples, as below).
   (a) Shorter, absent, or no change in your period.
   (b) A method that cannot be seen.
   (c) A method that you manage outside of clinic, or one that you manage in the clinic with your provider.
3. "We offer birth control that you manage every day, once a week, a few times a month, yearly? Which do you think would be best for you?"
4. "What did you like/dislike about the birth control methods that you have used in the past?"

Applying the SDM Model in Contraceptive Counseling and IUD Choice

The SDM model can be a new way for providers to discuss birth control with AYAs. As such, it may be helpful to practice some common steps of applying SDM principles to your contraceptive counseling visits. Additionally, AYAs consider their medical provider to play a significant role in their adoption of (and adjustment to) an IUD [31, 48]. Therefore, it is important that providers are able to also apply SDM principles to help support patients in choosing between IUD types. Figures 5.2 and 5.3 detail typical steps in applying SDM principles to contraceptive counseling visits, along with examples of how to apply SDM principles when providing counseling on the different IUD types.

Applying Shared Decision-Making Principles to Contraceptive Counseling Visits (Steps 1–3)

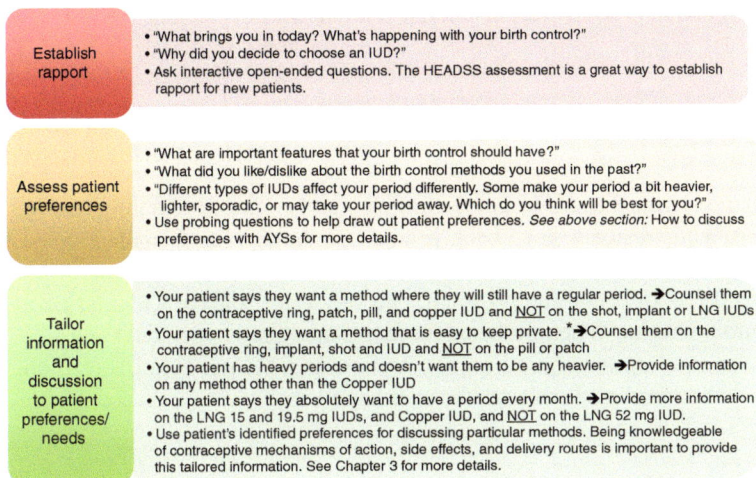

Fig. 5.2 Steps 1–3 in applying SDM principles to contraceptive counseling visits, along with examples of how to apply the principles when addressing different IUD types. It is important to identify why a patient may want or require a private form of birth control. This can include an assessment for sexual readiness, consent, and reproductive coercion. For more information on this, see the Sexual Readiness section at the beginning of this chapter, and resources from Futures Without Violence [16]

Applying Shared Decision-Making Principles to Contraceptive Counseling Visits (Steps 4–6)

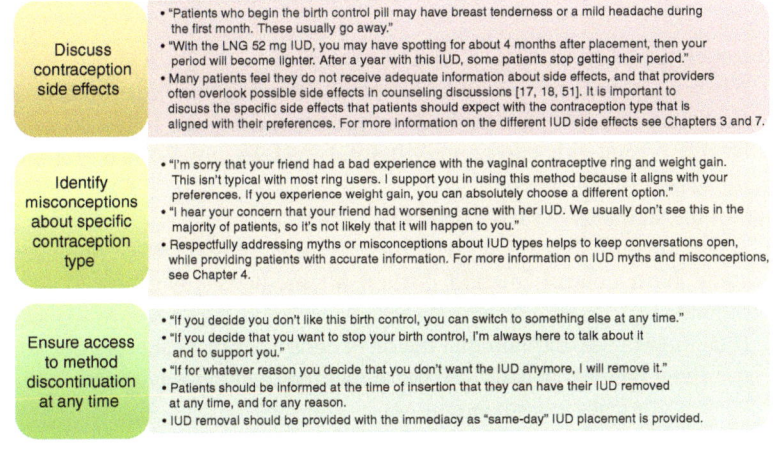

Fig. 5.3 Steps 4–6 in applying SDM principles to contraceptive counseling visits, along with examples of how to apply the principles when addressing different IUD types

Remember that even with scripts and language to facilitate SDM counseling (as shown in Figs. 5.2 and 5.3), the medical provider is only the facilitator of information and support. The patient is the ultimate driver of their contraceptive decision, and may or may not decide to choose a method.

Case (continued)

After reviewing the SDM counseling principles and practicing some of the techniques, your resident goes back in and has another birth control discussion with Rohan. Rohan informs the resident that she wants to be on a method where she has the least risk of becoming pregnant, and she wants to have a regular period because her mom checks. When the resident mentioned the copper IUD and LNG 19.5 mg IUD as good options based on her preferences, Rohan is not sure if she wants to have something inside of her "for so many years."

Special Points to Consider

Discussing effectiveness in contraceptive counseling Effectiveness of a contraceptive method is often very important to AYAs [46, 50, 51], and has been identified as a leading reason why AYAs choose IUDs [51]. With the knowledge that AYAs value this information on effectiveness, **contraceptive effectiveness should be included when discussing the patient's preferred method using SDM practices.** However, if contraceptive effectiveness is NOT important to a specific AYA, this information should not be used to lead the contraceptive counseling visit. When discussing the effectiveness of contraception, it's important to:

1. Use understandable statistics [52]. For example:
   (a) Nine in 100 patients may become pregnant using the birth control patch.
   (b) Less than 1 in 100 patients become pregnant using the IUD.
   (c) NOTE: Visual aids can be very helpful [53]. Figure 5.4 is a great image to illustrate effectiveness:
2. Explain the statistics—**VERY IMPORTANT**
   (a) AYAs may not understand why there is an increased rate of pregnancy with some birth control methods, when all methods are designed to prevent pregnancy.
   (b) It is important to explain that the birth control failure rates are due to *typical* use (how patients usually use these methods), and not *perfect* use (based on perfect clinical recommendations).
3. Explain to AYA what *typical* use is: "The birth control pill is designed to be taken every day to prevent pregnancy. However, some patients may forget to take their

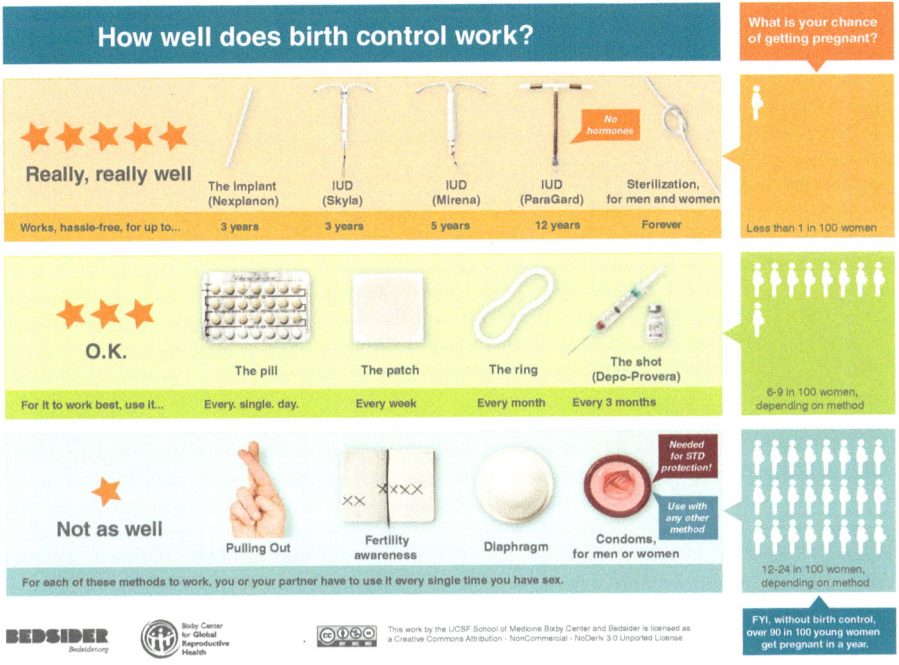

Fig. 5.4 A visual aid can be helpful in discussing method effectiveness in contraceptive counseling. (Source: UCSF School of Medicine Bixby Center and Bedsider.org: [54])

pill for one or several days, or may begin their next pill pack too late, AND THIS is what increases their risk of pregnancy while on the pill."

4. Partner with patients to help them facilitate correct and consistent contraception use. Examples: setting a reminder on their cell phone, adding text message reminders, recommending reminder apps, scheduling frequent clinic visits.

SDM Principles and IUD Removal

Some AYAs have reported that fear of not being able to have their IUD removed when they want leads them to not choose the IUD as their birth control method [55–57]. As stated above in the SDM counseling process, it is *absolutely imperative* that AYAs know that they can have their IUD **removed at any time,** and **for any reason.** Requiring AYAs to continue a newly placed IUD for a specified amount of time, to try side effect temporizing measures, or to have multiple medical visits for counseling before IUD removal are *coercive practices* and should be avoided; these are not in line with the recommended reproductive justice framework for providing IUDs to AYAs [10].

Table 5.1 It is vital to inform patients of common bleeding patterns by IUD type in supporting patients in choosing an IUD

Common bleeding patterns by IUD type			
IUD type	Bleeding pattern post-placement	Menstrual pattern	Chance of amenorrhea
LNG 52 mg	Spotting for 4–6 months after placement	90% have lighter and/or shorter periods	**Yes**. Can happen in up to 50% of patients after 1 year of use
LNG 19.5 mg	Spotting for 3–6 months after placement	Lighter and/or shorter periods	**Less likely**
LNG 13.5 mg	Spotting for 3–6 months after placement	**Likely lighter and irregular periods**	No
Copper IUD	Spotting for 1–2 days	**Often heavier and longer periods**	No

Bleeding Patterns

One of the most common reasons that AYAs discontinue the IUD is due to intolerable bleeding patterns and/or menstrual irregularities [51, 55, 57]. Clearly informing patients about common bleeding patterns with the different IUDs is vital when supporting patients in choosing their IUD type. Below is a summary of expected bleeding patterns by IUD type (Table 5.1). Please refer to Chaps. 3, 7, and 11 for additional information on IUD bleeding patterns.

Case (wrap up)

Your resident makes sure that Rohan knows that if she chooses an IUD, she can have it removed at any time and does not need to keep it for multiple years. Rohan feels relieved by this and decides to give the LNG 19.5 mg IUD a try. In reviewing Rohan's visit with you, your resident admits that she was surprised to hear that patients can have their IUDs removed at any time, as this seems to be a wasteful use of medical resources, "especially for patients who are at such a high risk of becoming pregnant." You remind the resident of the principles of patient-centered, unbiased medical care, which include providing contraceptive care within a reproductive justice framework.

Conclusion

Medical providers have a unique opportunity to provide supportive patient-centered contraceptive counseling to AYAs for all methods, including IUDs. Best practices of contraceptive counseling are in line with reproductive justice principles, both respecting patient autonomy and ensuring health equity. A paradigm shift must take place in healthcare delivery and medical education, so that providers are knowledgeable of reproductive injustices in the USA and aware of the historical role medical providers have played, in both direct and indirect reproductive coercion. SDM counseling techniques are the best-practice model for providing non-coercive and patient-centered contraceptive counseling around IUDs for AYAs.

References

1. Hillard PJA. What is LARC? And why does it matter for adolescents and young adults? J Adolesc Health. 2013;52:S1–5.
2. American College of Obstetricians and Gynecologists Committee on Gynecologic Practice, Long-Acting Reversible Contraception Working Group. ACOG Committee Opinion no. 450: increasing use of contraceptive implants and intrauterine devices to reduce unintended pregnancy. Obstet Gynecol. 2009;114:1434–8.
3. Ott MA, Sucato GS. Committee on adolescence. Contraception for adolescents. Pediatrics. 2014;134:e1257–81.
4. Dehlendorf C, Rodriguez MI, Levy K, Borrero S, Steinauer J. Disparities in family planning. Am J Obstet Gynecol. 2010;202:214–20.
5. Roberts D. Killing the black body: race, reproduction, and the meaning of liberty. New York: Vintage Books; 2014.
6. Christopherson S. NWHN-SisterSong joint statement of principles on LARCs – NWHN. In: NWHN [Internet]. 14 Nov 2016 [cited 9 Jan 2019]. Available: https://www.nwhn.org/nwhn-joins-statement-principles-larcs/.
7. Gomez AM, Fuentes L, Allina A. Women or LARC first? Reproductive autonomy and the promotion of long-acting reversible contraceptive methods. Perspect Sex Reprod Health. 2014;46:171–5.
8. Gubrium AC, Mann ES, Borrero S, Dehlendorf C, Fields J, Geronimus AT, et al. Realizing reproductive health equity needs more than Long-Acting Reversible Contraception (LARC). Am J Public Health. 2016;106:18–9.
9. Society for Adolescent Health and Medicine. Improving knowledge about, access to, and utilization of long-acting reversible contraception among adolescents and young *adults*. J Adolesc Health. 2017;60:472–4.
10. ACOG Committee Opinion No. 735. Adolescents and long-acting reversible contraception: implants and intrauterine devices. Obstet Gynecol. 2018;131:e130–9.
11. Ross L, Solinger R. Reproductive justice: an Introduction. Oakland: University of California Press; 2017.
12. Gilliam ML, Neustadt A, Gordon R. A call to incorporate a reproductive justice agenda into reproductive health clinical practice and policy. Contraception. 2009;79:243–6.
13. Higgins JA, Hirsch JS. Pleasure, power, and inequality: incorporating sexuality into research on contraceptive use. Am J Public Health. 2008;98:1803–13.
14. Templeton M, Lohan M, Kelly C, Lundy L. A systematic review and qualitative synthesis of adolescents' views of sexual readiness. J Adv Nurs. 2017;73:1288–301.
15. Rights, respect, responsibility: don't have sex without them a lesson plan from rights, respect, responsibility: A K-12 curriculum [Internet]. [cited 18 Jan 2019]. Available: https://advocatesforyouth.org/wp-content/uploads/3rscurric/documents/10-Lesson-1-3Rs-RightsRespectResponsibility.pdf.
16. Hanging out or hooking up: a train the trainers curriculum on responding to adolescent relationship abuse – futures without violence. In: Futures without violence [Internet].

2 Feb 2015 [cited 18 Jan 2019]. Available: https://www.futureswithoutviolence.org/hanging-hooking-train-trainers-curriculum-responding-adolescent-relationship-abuse/.

17. Yee L, Simon M. The role of the social network in contraceptive decision-making among young, African American and Latina women. J Adolesc Health. 2010;47:374–80.

18. Dehlendorf C, Levy K, Kelley A, Grumbach K, Steinauer J. Women's preferences for contraceptive counseling and decision making. Contraception. 2013;88:250–6.

19. Harper CC, Brown BA, Foster-Rosales A, Raine TR. Hormonal contraceptive method choice among young, low-income women: how important is the provider? Patient Educ Couns. 2010;81:349–54.

20. Bitzer J, Cupanik V, Fait T, Gemzell-Danielsson K, Grob P, Oddens BJ, et al. Factors influencing women's selection of combined hormonal contraceptive methods after counselling in 11 countries: results from a subanalysis of the CHOICE study. Eur J Contracept Reprod Health Care. 2013;18:372–80.

21. Gold RB. Guarding against coercion while ensuring access: a delicate balance. Guttmacher Policy Rev. 2014;17:8–14.

22. Geronimus AT. Damned if you do: culture, identity, privilege, and teenage childbearing in the United States. Soc Sci Med. 2003;57:881–93.

23. Collins PH. From black power to hip hop: racism, nationalism, and feminism. Philadelphia: Temple University Press; 2006.

24. Burrell DE. The Norplant solution: Norplant and the control of African-American motherhood. UCLA Womens Law J. 1995;5. Available: https://cloudfront.escholarship.org/dist/prd/content/qt9861n279/qt9861n279.pdf?t=mlr84z.

25. Walker KM. Judicial control of reproductive freedom: the use of Norplant as a condition of probation. Iowa L Rev. 1993;78:779.

26. Borrero S, Schwarz EB, Creinin M, Ibrahim S. The impact of race and ethnicity on receipt of family planning services in the United States. J Women's Health. 2009;18:91–6.

27. Downing RA, LaVeist TA, Bullock HE. Intersections of ethnicity and social class in provider advice regarding reproductive health. Am J Public Health. 2007;97:1803–7.

28. Spain JE, Peipert JF, Madden T, Allsworth JE, Secura GM. The Contraceptive CHOICE Project: recruiting women at highest risk for unintended pregnancy and sexually transmitted infection. J Women's Health. 2010;19:2233–8.

29. Dehlendorf C, Ruskin R, Grumbach K, Vittinghoff E, Bibbins-Domingo K, Schillinger D, et al. Recommendations for intrauterine contraception: a randomized trial of the effects of patients' race/ethnicity and socioeconomic status. Am J Obstet Gynecol. 2010;203:319.e1–8.

30. Wyatt KD, Anderson RT, Creedon D, Montori VM, Bachman J, Erwin P, et al. Women's values in contraceptive choice: a systematic review of relevant attributes included in decision aids. BMC Womens Health. 2014;14. https://doi.org/10.1186/1472-6874-14-28.

31. Brown MK, Auerswald C, Eyre SL, Deardorff J, Dehlendorf C. Identifying counseling needs of nulliparous adolescent intrauterine contraceptive users: a qualitative approach. J Adolesc Health. 2013;52:293–300.

32. Raidoo S, Kaneshiro B. Contraception counseling for adolescents. Curr Opin Obstet Gynecol. 2017;29:310–5.

33. Upadhyay UD. Informed choice in family planning. Helping people decide. Popul Rep J. 2001:1–39.

34. Kim YM, Kols A, Mucheke S. Informed choice and decision-making in family planning counseling in Kenya. Int Fam Plann Persp. 1998;24:4–11, 42.

35. Nathanson CA, Becker MH. The influence of client-provider relationships on teenage women's subsequent use of contraception. Am J Public Health. 1985;75:33–8.

36. Verme CS, Harper PB, Misra G, Neamatalla GS. Family planning counseling: an evolving process. Int Fam Plan Perspect. 1993;19:67.

37. Stanback J, Steiner M, Dorflinger L, Solo J, Jr Cates W. WHO tiered-effectiveness counseling is rights-based family planning. Glob Health Sci Pract. 2015;3:352–7.

38. Stevens J, Lutz R, Osuagwu N, Rotz D, Goesling B. A randomized trial of motivational interviewing and facilitated contraceptive access to prevent rapid repeat pregnancy among adolescent mothers. Am J Obstet Gynecol. 2017;217:423.e1–9.

39. DiClemente CC, Corno CM, Graydon MM, Wiprovnick AE, Knoblach DJ. Motivational interviewing, enhancement, and brief interventions over the last decade: a review of reviews of efficacy and effectiveness. Psychol Addict Behav. 2017;31:862–87.

40. Moskowitz E, Jennings B. Directive counseling on long-acting contraception. Am J Public Health. 1996;86:787–90.

41. Charles C, Gafni A, Whelan T. Shared decision-making in the medical encounter: what does it mean? (or it takes at least two to tango). Soc Sci Med. 1997;44:681–92.

42. Dehlendorf C. Contraceptive counseling and LARC uptake. October 2014 [slides].

43. Makoul G, Clayman ML. An integrative model of shared decision making in medical encounters. Patient Educ Couns. 2006;60:301–12.

44. Chen M, Lindley A, Kimport K, Dehlendorf C. An in-depth analysis of the use of shared decision making in contraceptive counseling. Contraception. 2018; https://doi.org/10.1016/j.contraception.2018.11.009.

45. Abdel-Tawab N, Roter D. The relevance of client-centered communication to family planning settings in developing countries: lessons from the Egyptian experience. Soc Sci Med. 2002;54:1357–68.

46. Melo J, Peters M, Teal S, Guiahi M. Adolescent and young women's contraceptive decision-making processes: choosing "The Best Method for Her". J Pediatr Adolesc Gynecol. 2015;28:224–8.

47. Curtis KM, Tepper NK, Jatlaoui TC, Berry-Bibee E, Horton LG, Zapata LB, et al. U.S. medical eligibility criteria for contraceptive use, 2016. MMWR Recomm Rep. 2016;65:1–103.

48. Rubin SE, Felsher M, Korich F, Jacobs AM. Urban adolescents' and young adults' decision-making process around selection of intrauterine contraception. J Pediatr Adolesc Gynecol. 2016;29:234–9.

49. Jackson AV, Karasek D, Dehlendorf C, Foster DG. Racial and ethnic differences in women's preferences for features of contraceptive methods. Contraception. 2016;93:406–11.

50. Schmidt EO, James A, Curran KM, Peipert JF, Madden T. Adolescent experiences with intrauterine devices: a qualitative study. J Adolesc Health. 2015;57:381–6.

51. Gomez AM, Clark JB. The relationship between contraceptive features preferred by young women and interest in IUDs: an exploratory analysis. Perspect Sex Reprod Health. 2014;46:157–63.

52. Contraceptive use in the United States. In: Guttmacher Institute [Internet]. 4 Aug 2004 [cited 19 Jan 2019]. Available: https://www.guttmacher.org/fact-sheet/contraceptive-use-united-states.

53. Pratt M, Searles GE. Using visual aids to enhance physician-patient discussions and increase health literacy. J Cutan Med Surg. 2017;21:497–501.

54. UCSF School of Medicine Bixby Center and Bedsider.org. How well does birth control work? [Internet]. [cited 19 Jan 2019]. Available: https://beyondthepill.ucsf.edu/sites/beyondthepill.ucsf.edu/files/Tiers_Chart_ENGLISH.pdf.

55. Fleming KL, Sokoloff A, Raine TR. Attitudes and beliefs about the intrauterine device among teenagers and young women. Contraception. 2010;82:178–82.

56. Potter J, Rubin SE, Sherman P. Fear of intrauterine contraception among adolescents in New York City. Contraception. 2014;89:446–50.

57. Whitaker AK, Johnson LM, Harwood B, Chiappetta L, Creinin MD, Gold MA. Adolescent and young adult women's knowledge of and attitudes toward the intrauterine device. Contraception. 2008;78:211–7.

Chapter 6
Just Do It: The When and How of IUD Insertion

Nicole Chaisson

Abbreviations

ACOG	American College of Obstetricians and Gynecologists
AYA	Adolescent and young adult
BMI	Body mass index
CDC	Centers for Disease Control and Prevention
EC	Emergency contraception
IUDs	Intrauterine devices
LARC	Long-acting reversible contraception
LNG	Levonorgestrel
MEC	Medical Eligibility Criteria
SPR	Selected Practice Recommendations
UPIC	Unprotected intercourse

Learning Objectives

Following completion of this chapter, you should be able to:

1. Discuss the appropriate timing of intrauterine device (IUD) placement, including use of the IUD as emergency contraception (EC).
2. Describe same-day insertion and Quick Start protocols that facilitate timely IUD provision.
3. Explore optimal IUD placement for patients who are postpartum, post-abortion, or breastfeeding.

N. Chaisson (✉)
Department of Family Medicine and Community Health, University of Minnesota, Minneapolis, MN, USA
e-mail: chai0027@umn.edu

© Springer Nature Switzerland AG 2019
M. S. Coles, A. Mays (eds.), *Optimizing IUD Delivery for Adolescents and Young Adults*, https://doi.org/10.1007/978-3-030-17816-1_6

Introduction

Intrauterine contraception is the most popular form of reversible contraception in the world [1]. IUDs and other forms of long-acting reversible contraception (LARC) should be offered routinely to all, including nulliparous individuals and adolescents, as highly effective and safe methods of contraception [2–4]. It is important to reduce barriers to insertion of IUDs in order to increase access to this method [5–7]. These include insertion at any time during the menstrual cycle as long as pregnancy can be reasonably excluded [8], use as a highly effective form of emergency contraception (EC) (Cu copper IUD) or in combination with oral EC (levonorgestrel (LNG) IUDs), and insertion following vaginal delivery, cesarean section, and abortion. At the same time, it is equally important to provide non-coercive counseling about all contraceptive methods, create a clinical space for shared decision-making about IUDs, and ensure that if adolescents and young adults (AYAs) chooses to have an IUD inserted, you are willing to remove it at any time if they opt to change to a different method.

Case 1

Sara is a 17-year-old cisgender female who presents to her primary care clinic for discussion about contraception. She has used oral contraceptive pills in the past, but recently read about IUDs online and likes the idea of something she doesn't have to take every day. Sara wants to know if you could insert an IUD today. She is particularly interested in one "with hormones in it" because she likes the idea of less periods over time. She is not exactly sure of her last menstrual period, but thinks it was about 2 weeks ago. Sara last had intercourse 4 days ago without condoms. Her urine pregnancy test today in clinic is negative.

Same-Day Insertion and Quick Start Protocols

In the past, clinicians traditionally placed IUDs during menses, as they thought it would both ensure that the patient was not pregnant, and ease the insertion due to relaxation of the cervical os during menses. However, **we now know that there are no documented advantages to inserting during menses** [9], and that with appropriate counseling and pregnancy assessment, IUDs can be inserted on the same day as an initial clinic visit [8]. IUDs can be placed at any time during the menstrual cycle, as long as pregnancy can be reasonably excluded and follow-up ensured if needed [8]. While many clinic protocols include universal urine pregnancy testing prior to initiation of any contraceptive method, the Centers for Disease Control and Preventions (CDC's) USA Selected Practice Recommendations

A health care provider can be reasonably certain that a patient is not pregnant if there are no symptoms of pregnancy, and any of the following criteria are met:

- It has been ≤ 7 days since the start of the last menses
- The patient has not had sexual intercourse since the start of the last menstrual period
- The patient has been correctly and consistently using a reliable method of contraception
- It has been ≤ 7 days after a spontaneous or induced abortion
- It is within 4 weeks postpartum
- The patient is fully or nearly fully breastfeeding (exclusively or ≥ 85% of feeds), amenorrheic, and <6 months postpartum

Fig. 6.1 Criteria that reasonably ensure a woman is not pregnant [8]

for Contraceptive Use (SPR) identifies several additional criteria that can be used to reasonably exclude pregnancy, *even without a urine pregnancy test result* (Fig. 6.1) [8].

In Case 1 above, our patient *does not* meet the criteria to reasonably exclude pregnancy. In fact, she has recently had unprotected intercourse. Is it still possible to insert her chosen IUD?

The SPR and USA Medical Eligibility Criteria for Contraceptive Use (MEC) support a guided conversation weighing the possible risk of an early, undetectable pregnancy with the benefits of taking oral EC medication (LNG or ulipristal, depending on timing of last intercourse and body mass index (BMI) of the patient) and offering options for same-day insertion of a hormonal IUD—versus later insertion and bridging with a different method of birth control until pregnancy can be ruled out (Fig. 6.2) [8, 10]. For methods such as hormonal IUD insertion that require a second visit, it is important to weigh the small risk that EC may be less effective with the risk of patients not returning to start a LARC method on another day. **It is both safe and effective to offer both ulipristal and oral LNG for EC at the same time as placement of a LNG IUD, if this is the patient's preference.**

As long as this patient understands the small, but potential, risk of an early, undetected pregnancy (and the need to follow up for repeat pregnancy testing in 2–3 weeks), it is reasonable to offer same-day insertion of the hormonal IUD as requested. Same-day initiation of IUDs increases the likelihood that AYAs will use the method, and also saves patients from needing additional office visits, which can be a barrier to use of LARC methods [12].

Case 2

Aliah is a 16-year-old cisgender female who comes to her high school school-based clinic asking for EC. She had unprotected intercourse (UPIC) 4 days ago. Her urine pregnancy test is negative and her last menstrual period was 2 weeks ago. Aliah had been thinking about getting an IUD, but wasn't sure what kind.

2. Progestin IUD or Implant

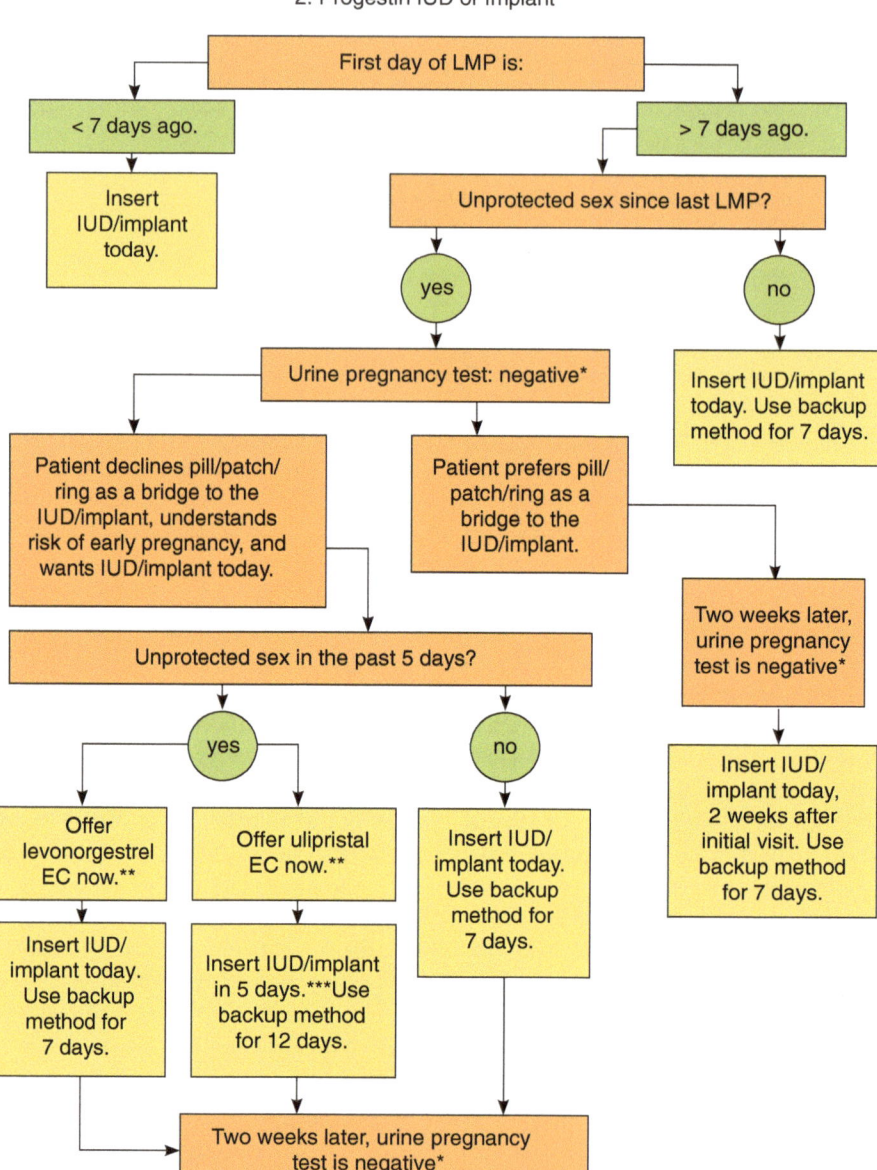

Fig. 6.2 Quick start algorithm for progestin IUD. (Protocols available online at https://www.reproductiveaccess.org/resource/quick-start-algorithm/ [11]). * If pregnancy test is positive, provide options counseling. ** For patients with BMI over 25, LNG EC works no better than placebo. For those who had unprotected sex 3–5 days ago, ulipristal EC has higher efficacy than LNG EC. *** Because ulipristal EC may interact with hormonal contraceptives, the new method should be started no sooner than 5 days after ulipristal EC. Consider starting injection/IUD/implant sooner if benefit outweighs risk

IUDs as EC

Time permitting and with proper counseling [13], the individual in Case 2 could receive both emergency and continuing contraception if she chose a same-day insertion of an IUD as previously discussed. Indeed, the copper IUD (Fig. 6.3) has been well studied as a method of EC, working in part to disrupt the normal development of a fertilized oocyte and to prevent implantation, with an efficacy of 99% up to 5–7 days after UPIC [14, 15]. Not only are copper IUDs the most effective method of EC available; they can also provide up to 12 years of highly effective and ongoing contraception [16]. Indeed, one study looking at pregnancy rates 1 year after use of EC of any type noted that 64% of patients who chose the copper IUD still had it in place and had significantly fewer pregnancies in that year than those who chose an oral EC pill [17].

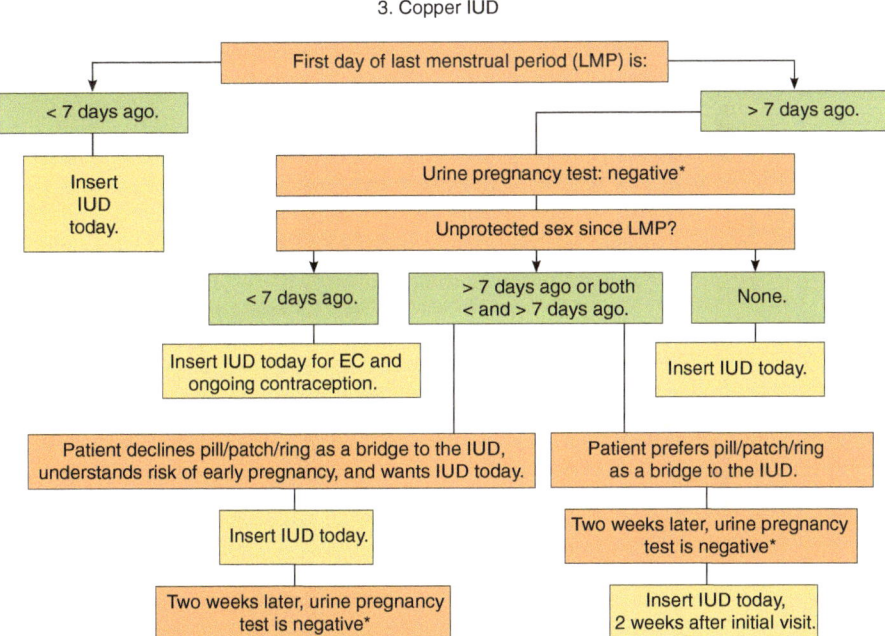

Fig. 6.3 Quick start algorithm for copper IUD. (Protocols available online at https://www.repro-ductiveaccess.org/resource/quick-start-algorithm/ [11]). ∗ If pregnancy test is positive, provide options counseling

As with adults, AYAs are often more likely to choose LNG IUDs rather than copper IUDs for a long-term contraceptive method [5, 18]. Current research is also evaluating the effectiveness of the LNG IUD for use as EC on its own [19, 20]. However, as previously noted, concomitant use of the hormonal IUD at the same time as ulipristal or oral LNG could also be an option if the individual is interested in that combination (Fig. 6.2). When specifically counseled, 64% of women chose the option of oral LNG for EC combined with same-day initiation of LNG IUD, versus same-day copper IUD placement [18].

Case 3

Jordan is a 19-year-old G1P0 cisgender female who comes to clinic at 36 weeks of gestation to discuss postpartum contraceptive options with her prenatal provider. She does not want to be pregnant again for at least a few years, and plans to breast-feed her baby. Jordan is thinking about an IUD and wants more information.

Postpartum IUD Insertion

The timing of IUD placement after either vaginal or cesarean delivery is largely determined by patient preference, experience of the provider, institutional support, and available provider reimbursement options depending on insurance require-ments [21]. The MEC for IUD use after pregnancy and while breastfeeding is noted in Fig. 6.4 [8]. Because of their ability to help prevent rapid repeat pregnancies (especially after cesarean section), the American College of Obstetricians and Gynecologists (ACOG) recommends immediate postpartum insertion as a best practice for those seeking LARC methods [21]. ACOG recommends prenatal coun-seling about this option. Resumption of ovulation varies widely after delivery, and many people report having unprotected intercourse before their 6-week postpartum visit [20]. While there is a slightly higher expulsion rate after immediate postpar-tum IUD placement compared to placement after 4–6 weeks postpartum, there are good data that suggest that as many as 40% of patients will miss their postpartum follow-up visit [22]. Attendance rates are even lower among populations with lim-ited resources [23], and AYA parents can be particularly at-risk.

Condition	Sub-Condition		Cu-IUD	LNG-IUD
Postpartum (in breastfeeding of non-breastfeeding women, including cesarean delivery)	<10 minutes after delivery of the placenta			
	a) Breastfeeding		1*	2*
	b) Not breastfeeding		1*	1*
	10 minutes after delivery of the placenta to <4 wks		2*	2*
	≥4 weeks		1*	1*
	Postpartum sepsis		4	4
Postabortion	First trimester		1*	1*
	Second trimester		2*	2*
	Immediate postseptic abortion		4	4

Key	
1. No restrictions to method	3. Theoretical of proven risks usually outweigh advantages
2. Advantages generally outweigh theoretical or proven risks	4. Unacceptable health risk (method not to be used)

Fig. 6.4 USA Medical Eligibility Criteria for postpartum and postabortion IUD use. (Source: [10, 24])

At present, the most significant barrier to providing immediate postpartum IUD placement is the ability for providers and hospitals to be reimbursed for the procedure, and even for the device itself. Most states pay for labor and delivery services as part of a "global package" under one Diagnosis Related Group (DRG) code that does not provide reimbursement for individual procedures or devices while the patient is in the hospital. Because of the higher cost of IUDs initially, providers and hospitals will not typically provide these devices without guarantee of reimbursement. In Colorado, a grant-funded pilot program offered immediate postpartum LARC methods to patients at no cost, and noted high demand for these options. Evaluation of teen mothers involved in this pilot study noted a reduction in unplanned pregnancies among those that chose immediate postpartum LARC placement. In this same cohort, early initiation of the etonogestrel implant in adolescents was more successful than early initiation of IUDs when offered after hospital discharge, regardless of contraceptive intent at the time of delivery. Reducing barriers to immediate postplacental placement of IUDs could increase the successful use of that method [25]. During this same period of time (2007–2010), while the overall repeat adolescent birth rate in the USA declined by 6.2%, the birth rate in Colorado dropped by 45% [26]. Because of these findings, several states have moved to unbundle family planning codes and reimbursement from the global labor and delivery package in an effort to decrease barriers to immediate postpartum LARC methods. It is important to note that immediate postplacental placement of IUDs requires a different technique than routine IUD insertion and is not discussed in this book. For further information and training regarding this procedure, please see training videos developed by the ACOG and Innovating Education in Reproductive Health [27].

IUDs and Breastfeeding

Breastfeeding is safe with both copper and hormonal IUDs. Since the copper IUD contains no hormones, the MEC places no restrictions on the method for breastfeeding (Category 1) [10]. The MEC rates LNG IUDs as Category 2 because of the theoretical risk of exogenous progesterone affecting initiation of milk production [10]. Data suggest no differences in milk production or breastfeeding rates between those choosing LNG IUDs over copper IUDs at 6–8 weeks postpartum [28]. While the effects of immediate postpartum LNG IUDs on breastfeeding are limited, data suggest that there is not an overall negative effect on breastfeeding outcomes [21]

Case 4

Gloria, a 15-year-old cisgender female, presents to clinic at 8 weeks of gestation for termination of pregnancy. She absolutely does not want to be pregnant again, and wants to talk about her about contraceptive options. You are aware that IUDs are highly effective at preventing pregnancy and are considered a safe choice for teens.

Postabortion IUD Insertion

Similar to the data on immediate postpartum IUD placement, facilitating access to immediate postabortal intrauterine contraception has been shown to reduce repeat abortions, and has the potential to reduce future unplanned pregnancies [29]. A systematic review of the literature noted that IUD insertion immediately after aspiration abortion is not associated with increased risk of side effects or adverse outcomes [30]. Rates of perforation (0.1%) and infection (0.4% for pelvic inflammatory disease) were comparable to those seen with IUD insertions at other times [31]. Expulsion rates (7%), however, have been seen to increase fourfold with increasing gestational age at time of abortion from the first to second trimester [30, 31]. In spite of higher rates of expulsion, patients with immediate postabortion IUD insertion still had higher rates of continued IUD use after 1-year follow-up, compared to those who intended to return for an IUD placement visit postabortion [32]. Low rates of postabortion follow-up have been well described in the literature, even among those who intended to return for IUD insertion at a follow-up visit [33, 34]. A study reviewing barriers to IUD placement after first-trimester abortion noted that only 32% of women who had intended to return for IUD placement after abortion had one in place at 6 months after the abortion [33]. The main reported barrier to postabortion IUD placement was the need for an additional visit. A 2014 Cochrane review reiterated that IUD insertion immediately following an elective or spontaneous abortion is both safe and convenient [35]. As seen in Fig. 6.4, the MEC recognizes that postabortion IUD placement is safe, except in the event of a septic abortion [10].

Optimizing Insertion Within a Reproductive Justice Framework

As noted in the previous chapters, multiple organizations have adopted guidelines and recommendations that list LARC methods, including IUDs, as a "first-line" contraceptive option for AYAs. While there are many advantages to IUDs in terms of effectiveness and ease of use after initiation, the lack of control over method discontinuation can be viewed as a major disadvantage—it often requires not only a provider visit but also trust that the provider will be willing to remove the device even if it's "too early." Qualitative research with young adult women noted that many believed that providers would be more likely to recommend LARC methods to socially marginalized communities over other groups and reported experiences of provider resistance to LARC removal [36]. Shared decision-making counseling at the time of IUD insertion is crucial, along with understanding the circumstances around which the decision about contraception is being made. Using a shared decision-making approach to contraceptive counseling as thoroughly discussed in Chap. 5—one that focuses on patient preferences—helps optimize the experience of counseling and satisfaction with method [37] and helps to avoid provider coercion.

In Case 4, a 15-year-old patient is presenting to clinic for an abortion. She may be highly motivated to not get pregnant again soon (or not); she may feel ashamed of the pregnancy in the first place (or not). Whatever the circumstances, it is important for the provider to create an open space for her or any individual to make the right decision about next steps in contraception for themselves, and not based on what the provider thinks is the best option. Both abortion care and adolescent pregnancy are stigmatized in USA society [38, 39]. Adolescents who present for abortion care and are considering options for ongoing contraception are particularly vulnerable to feeling pressured by the tier-based approach to contraceptive counseling. A recent qualitative study of women presenting for an abortion noted that almost half of the participants perceived some form of coercion around contraceptive counseling, particularly regarding specific methods, or the immediate initiation of those methods [40]. It was noted that abortion stigma itself may mediate those perceptions of coercion. In light of the potential for (intentional or unintentional) directive or coercive counseling, allowing time for careful consideration of all methods and encouraging questions—including self-reflection about one's own preferences—is integral in promoting and supporting reproductive autonomy and agency.

Summary

IUDs are safe and highly effective methods of LARC. While increased use of LARC methods has been associated with decreased rates of unintended pregnancy and abortion in AYAs, these methods require provider visits for method initiation (and often for discontinuation) that can be significant rate-limiting steps for method use. When AYAs choose an IUD for their contraceptive method, it is crucial that providers work to remove barriers to both initiation and discontinuation of these methods. For IUD insertions, proposing clinic and medical system policies that support same-day insertion of IUDs, immediate postpartum insertion, and immediate postabortion insertion can help reduce these barriers. Importantly, at time of insertion, and throughout use, it is essential to ensure that patients can choose to discontinue the method at any time—without question—in order to fully support their bodily and reproductive autonomy.

Clinical Pearls
- If chosen as the preferred method, it is considered best practice to insert IUDs on the same day as initial consultation for contraception.
- Quick Start algorithms in the SPR and from the Reproductive Health Access Project [8, 11] help determine strategies to support same-day insertion of IUDs with or without concomitant use of EC.
- Evidence supports the practice of placing IUDs immediately postpartum and postabortion, without increased risk of side effects.
- AYAs in general, and specifically youth of color and/or low-income youth, are impacted by reproductive coercion, making it crucial to provide non-directive counseling about **all contraceptive methods** to **all youth** using shared decision-making techniques.
- At the time of IUD insertion, it is imperative that providers reiterate that AYAs can have their *IUDs removed at any time, for any reason,* and *without question,* in order to provide complete autonomy in method choice.

References

1. United Nations, Department of Economic and Social Affairs, Population Division (2015). Trends in Contraceptive Use Worldwide 2015 (ST/ESA/SER.A/349). Available: https://www.un.org/en/development/desa/population/publications/pdf/family/trendsContraceptiveUse2015Report.pdf
2. World Health Organization. Medical eligibility criteria for contraceptive use. 2015. Available: http://www.who.int/reproductivehealth/publications/family_planning/MEC-5/en/.
3. World Health Organization. Medical eligibility criteria for contraceptive use. 2015.
4. Committee on Adolescence. Contraception for adolescents. Pediatrics. 2014;134:e1244–56.
5. McNicholas C, Madden T, Secura G, Peipert JF. The contraceptive CHOICE project round up: what we did and what we learned. Clin Obstet Gynecol. 2014;57:635–43.
6. Berenson AB, Tan A, Hirth JM, Wilkinson GS. Complications and continuation of intrauterine device use among commercially insured teenagers. Obstet Gynecol. 2013;121:951–8.
7. Society for Adolescent Health and Medicine. Improving knowledge about, access to, and utilization of long-acting reversible contraception among adolescents and young adults. J Adolesc Health. 2017;60:472–4.
8. Curtis KM, Jatlaoui TC, Tepper NK, Zapata LB, Horton LG, Jamieson DJ, et al. U.S. selected practice recommendations for contraceptive use, 2016. MMWR Recomm Rep. 2016;65:1–66.
9. Whiteman MK, Tyler CP, Folger SG, Gaffield ME, Curtis KM. When can a woman have an intrauterine device inserted? A systematic review. Contraception. 2013;87:666–73.
10. Curtis KM, Tepper NK, Jatlaoui TC, Berry-Bibee E, Horton LG, Zapata LB, et al. U.S. medical eligibility criteria for contraceptive use, 2016. MMWR Recomm Rep. 2016;65:1–103.
11. Reproductive Health Access Project. Quick start algorithm – reproductive health access project. In: Reproductive health access project [Internet]. [cited 1 Dec 2018]. Available: https://www.reproductiveaccess.org/resource/quick-start-algorithm/.
12. Bergin A, Tristan S, Terplan M, Gilliam ML, Whitaker AK. A missed opportunity for care: two-visit IUD insertion protocols inhibit placement. Contraception. 2012;86:694–7.
13. Schwarz EB, Papic M, Parisi SM, Baldauf E, Rapkin R, Updike G. Routine counseling about intrauterine contraception for women seeking emergency contraception. Contraception. 2014;90:66–71.
14. Turok DK, Godfrey EM, Wojdyla D, Dermish A, Torres L, Wu SC. Copper T380 intrauterine device for emergency contraception: highly effective at any time in the menstrual cycle. Hum Reprod. 2013;28:2672–6.
15. Cleland K, Zhu H, Goldstuck N, Cheng L, Trussell J. The efficacy of intrauterine devices for emergency contraception: a systematic review of 35 years of experience. Hum Reprod. 2012;27:1994–2000.
16. Wu JP, Pickle S. Extended use of the intrauterine device: a literature review and recommendations for clinical practice. Contraception. 2014;89:495–503.
17. Turok DK, Jacobson JC, Dermish AI, Simonsen SE, Gurtcheff S, McFadden M, et al. Emergency contraception with a copper IUD or oral levonorgestrel: an observational study of 1-year pregnancy rates. Contraception. 2014;89:222–8.
18. Turok DK, Sanders JN, Thompson IS, Royer PA, Eggebroten J, Gawron LM. Preference for and efficacy of oral levonorgestrel for emergency contraception with concomitant placement of a levonorgestrel IUD: a prospective cohort study. Contraception. 2016;93:526–32.
19. RAPID EC – Rct Assessing Pregnancy With Intrauterine Devices for EC – full text view – ClinicalTrials.gov [Internet]. [cited 1 Dec 2018]. Available: https://clinicaltrials.gov/ct2/show/NCT02175030.
20. Levonorgestrel intrauterine system for emergency contraception – full text view – ClinicalTrials.gov [Internet]. [cited 1 Dec 2018]. Available: https://clinicaltrials.gov/ct2/show/NCT01539720.

21. American College of Obstetricians and Gynecologists' Committee on Obstetric Practice. Committee opinion no. 670: immediate postpartum long-acting reversible contraception. Obstet Gynecol. 2016;128:e32–7.
22. Tully KP, Stuebe AM, Verbiest SB. The fourth trimester: a critical transition period with unmet maternal health needs. Am J Obstet Gynecol. 2017;217:37–41.
23. Bryant AS, Haas JS, McElrath TF, McCormick MC. Predictors of compliance with the postpartum visit among women living in healthy start project areas. Matern Child Health J. 2006;10:511–6.
24. CDC – summary – USMEC – reproductive health [Internet]. 2 Nov 2018 [cited 6 Jan 2019]. Available: https://www.cdc.gov/reproductivehealth/contraception/mmwr/mec/summary.html.
25. Tocce K, Sheeder J, Python J, Teal SB. Long acting reversible contraception in postpartum adolescents: early initiation of etonogestrel implant is superior to IUDs in the outpatient setting. J Pediatr Adolesc Gynecol. 2012;25:59–63.
26. Centers for Disease Control and Prevention (CDC). Vital signs: repeat births among teens – United States, 2007–2010. MMWR Morb Mortal Wkly Rep. 2013;62:249–55.
27. LARC insertion: immediate postpartum period – innovating education in reproductive health. In: Innovating education in reproductive health [Internet]. 25 Apr 2018 [cited 1 Dec 2018]. Available: http://innovating-education.org/2018/04/larc-insertion-immediate-postpartum-period/.
28. Shaamash AH, Sayed GH, Hussien MM, Shaaban MM. A comparative study of the levonorgestrel-releasing intrauterine system Mirena versus the Copper T380A intrauterine device during lactation: breast-feeding performance, infant growth and infant development. Contraception. 2005;72:346–51.
29. Goodman S, Hendlish SK, Reeves MF, Foster-Rosales A. Impact of immediate postabortal insertion of intrauterine contraception on repeat abortion. Contraception. 2008;78:143–8.
30. Steenland MW, Tepper NK, Curtis KM, Kapp N. Intrauterine contraceptive insertion postabortion: a systematic review. Contraception. 2011;84:447–64.
31. Stanwood NL, Grimes DA, Schulz KF. Insertion of an intrauterine contraceptive device after induced or spontaneous abortion: a review of the evidence. BJOG. 2001;108:1168–73.
32. McNicholas C, Hotchkiss T, Madden T, Zhao Q, Allsworth J, Peipert JF. Immediate postabortion intrauterine device insertion: continuation and satisfaction. Womens Health Issues. 2012;22:e365–9.
33. Madden T, Westhoff C. Rates of follow-up and repeat pregnancy in the 12 months after first-trimester induced abortion. Obstet Gynecol. 2009;113:663–8.
34. Stanek AM, Bednarek PH, Nichols MD, Jensen JT, Edelman AB. Barriers associated with the failure to return for intrauterine device insertion following first-trimester abortion. Contraception. 2009;79:216–20.
35. Okusanya BO, Oduwole O, Effa EE. Immediate postabortal insertion of intrauterine devices. Cochrane Database Syst Rev. 2014:CD001777.
36. Higgins JA, Kramer RD, Ryder KM. Provider bias in Long-Acting Reversible Contraception (LARC) promotion and removal: perceptions of young adult women. Am J Public Health. 2016;106:1932–7.
37. Dehlendorf C, Krajewski C, Borrero S. Contraceptive counseling: best practices to ensure quality communication and enable effective contraceptive use. Clin Obstet Gynecol. 2014;57:659–73.
38. Kumar A, Hessini L, Mitchell EMH. Conceptualising abortion stigma. Cult Health Sex. 2009;11:625–39.
39. Bonell C. Why is teenage pregnancy conceptualized as a social problem? A review of quantitative research from the USA and UK. Cult Health Sex. 2004;6:255–72.
40. Brandi K, Woodhams E, White KO, Mehta PK. An exploration of perceived contraceptive coercion at the time of abortion. Contraception. 2018;97:329–34.

Chapter 7
Consenting and Pre-procedural Counseling for IUD Insertion: What to Expect and What to Talk About

Katherine Blumoff Greenberg

Abbreviations

AYA   Adolescents and Young Adult
FDA   Federal Drug Administration
IUD   Intrauterine Device
LNG   Levonorgestrel
NSAID   Non-Steroidal Anti-Inflammatory Drugs
STI   Sexually Transmitted Infection

Learning Objectives
Following completion of this chapter, you should be able to:

1. Review how informed consent applies to Adolescents and Young Adults (AYAs), including those seeking IUD services.
2. Describe the risk and benefit profile of IUDs that should be included in the informed consent process.
3. Offer sample language of how to provide pre-procedural, pelvic exam, and IUD insertion counseling for patients seeking IUD placement.

Background

When consenting a patient prior to an intrauterine device (IUD) insertion, you will revisit many elements of comprehensive contraceptive counseling, including discussion of the overall risks and benefits of various contraceptive methods. As a visit for an IUD insertion may be the first time a young person is having a pelvic and/or

K. B. Greenberg (✉)
Departments of Pediatrics (Primary) and Obstetrics and Gynecology (Secondary),
University of Rochester Medical Center, Rochester, NY, USA
e-mail: Katherine_greenberg@urmc.rochester.edu

© Springer Nature Switzerland AG 2019
M. S. Coles, A. Mays (eds.), *Optimizing IUD Delivery for Adolescents and Young Adults*, https://doi.org/10.1007/978-3-030-17816-1_7

speculum exam, pre-procedural consent for adolescents and young adults (AYAs) includes not only specific procedural risks, but also details about the examination itself. With an eye toward using empowering language, the goal of this additional counseling is (1) to inform patients about the potential risks of the IUD insertion procedure and (2) to help them feel comfortable and affirmed during their pelvic exam experience. Some IUD providers may be inserting IUDs for patients who they themselves saw for contraceptive counseling, while other clinical sites may have health educators or non-clinician family planning staff provide contraceptive counseling. On the day of the IUD insertion, it is the responsibility of the clinician performing the procedure to cover the medical risks, benefits, and procedural steps in more detail.

Case

T is an 18-year-old (assigned female at birth) non-binary individual who has been on the patch off and on since age 13. They initially started the patch for heavy menstrual bleeding and cramping, but more recently have been using it for contraception. T's dysmenorrhea is better when they are on the patch, but they still feel like their monthly cycles are heavier and crampier than they would like them to be. T also reports that they are having some trouble remembering to change the patch at the same time every week, and are worried about how well it works for pregnancy prevention. They came in to see you for contraceptive counseling a few weeks ago to discuss their options. After doing this (using a shared decision making model), they decided on a levonorgestrel (LNG) IUD, but wanted to come back in for the placement in a few weeks with a friend for support. T is on your schedule today for their IUD insertion.

Informed Consent Process

Who Can Provide Informed Consent? Informed consent policies for sexual and reproductive healthcare services for patients under the age of 18 years vary highly from state to state [1]. Many states explicitly allow minors to make their own decisions about sexual and reproductive health care, without parental or guardian consent. These policies recognize that many minors will not use important healthcare services if they are not allowed to do so confidentially [1, 2]. That being said, parental or other adult involvement in decisions is common, and clinicians should welcome it whenever it is safe and supportive [3]. As of 2018, 26 states and the District of Columbia allowed all minors (12 years and older) to consent to contraceptive services. Twenty states allowed only certain categories of minors (often including those who are pregnant or parenting) to consent to contraceptive services. Four states had no relevant policy or case law [4]. It is important to be familiar with the laws in the state where you practice. If it is the parent or guardian who is giving consent, the patient must also provide informed assent if they are able to do so. Many informed consent forms include spaces for both patient and parent/guardian signatures. For more detailed information on the minor informed consent laws in your state, go to the Guttmacher Institute [5].

Counseling for informed consent All pre-procedural counseling should follow a similar outline, and cover the relevant information that the patient and/or guardian requires to make an informed decision. Much of this information may have been covered in initial comprehensive contraceptive counseling, but will need to be revisited in more detail on the day of the procedure.

Benefits of IUDs

IUDs have many benefits, which should be covered in comprehensive contraceptive counseling, and re-addressed during the pre-procedural consent. Several common benefits to address during the consent process include the **duration of action** and **potential changes in bleeding and cramping patterns**.

1. **Long duration of action**: IUDs are highly effective for contraception, and are effective for use over a long time frame. Evidence-based use may differ from the manufacturer's Federal Drug Administration (FDA) labeling, and it is important to share this information with patients. It is also important to remind patients that while IUDs have a very long duration of action, they can be removed at any time. Evidence-based durations for common IUDs are [6]:
   - CuT380A IUD is FDA approved for up to 10 years, but evidence-based protocols support its use for up to 12 years [7].
   - LNG 52 mg IUDs are FDA approved for up to five years. Evidence currently supports use for up to seven years [8].
   - LNG 19.5 mg IUD is FDA approved for up to five years. There is no evidence-based protocol currently extending its use.
   - LNG 13.5 mg IUD is FDA approved for up to three years. There is no evidence-based protocol currently extending its use.
2. **Changes to menstrual bleeding and cramping patterns** [6]: After the insertion of any type of IUD, there is an initial adjustment period of typically three to six months where individuals may have irregular bleeding and/or spotting. We tell patients that this happens, "while the uterus gets used to having something inside of it," and that this bleeding pattern tends to improve (lessen) over time. Bleeding patterns after this adjustment period vary based on the amount (or lack) of hormones in the IUD. Overall, IUDs will result in changes in bleeding for most individuals, and those with LNG IUDs often have less bleeding or cramping. We counsel patients as such:
   - As the CuT380A IUD has no hormones, patients continue to have periods on a regular basis. Many patients have periods that are slightly heavier, or slightly crampier than before the IUD was placed. This is typically easily treated with

ibuprofen or other non-steroidal anti-inflammatory drugs (NSAID)-type medications just before and during early menses. This IUD is a good choice for patients who want to maintain regular periods and/or avoid hormones.

- Many patients have little or no bleeding with the LNG 52 mg IUD in place, and heavy bleeding and dysmenorrhea symptoms are often much improved [9].
- About 38% of patients using LNG 19.5 mg IUD will have amenorrhea or very light spotting by the end of its first year of use [10]. Periods may become lighter and/or shorter, and may be regular or irregular.
- About a quarter of patients (26%) using LNG 13.5 mg IUD will have amenorrhea or very light spotting by the end of the first year of use [11]. Based on the available data and the mechanism of action, we counsel that periods may become lighter and/or shorter, and may remain regular.

Risks of IUDs

Review of procedural risks is also an important part of providing informed consent. However, it is incredibly important to present these risks in context, in order to allow patients to make decisions that are not unduly guided by fear or concern. We recommend discussing risks in the order below [6].

1. **Infection:** People tend to worry about getting infections from modern IUDs due to historical issues with prior generations of IUDs, most notably the Dalkon Shield [12] as discussed in Chap. 1. We find it helpful to explain risk of infection as follows: "The risk of infection is that placing an IUD could introduce an already existing, and often sexually transmitted, infection into your uterus. If you are not having symptoms, and your exam is normal, it's perfectly okay for us to do a test for infections, and also place the IUD today." Testing for asymptomatic STIs on the day of IUD placement is standard of care in many clinics, without any increase in rates of ascending pelvic infections with prompt treatment of positive test results [13]. There does seem to be a transiently increased risk of pelvic infection right after IUD placement, presumably due to seeding of bacteria from uterine instrumentation during the IUD placement. However, this increased risk is small and disappears after the first few weeks [14]. Patients should be counseled to return to care with any increase in vaginal discharge, pain, or unexpected bleeding in the first month after IUD placement.

2. **Expulsion:** One way to discuss expulsion is, "The uterus is such a strong muscle that it may push the IUD out." Rates of expulsion range from 2 to 5%, and young people are more likely to experience an expulsion than adults. If patients are having symptoms such as sudden cramping or pain, a change in bleeding pattern, and/or are unable to feel the strings, we recommend that they use a backup birth control method like condoms, take a home pregnancy test, and return to clinic for

additional evaluation in a timely fashion. Routine IUD string checks are no lon-ger recommended, as discussed in Chap. 11, though these can be helpful to have patients check if they call with concerns of expulsion.

3. **Pregnancy including ectopic pregnancy:** Patients have often heard that they can get pregnant with an IUD in place. We discuss that, "This [IUD] is really good at preventing pregnancy, but nothing is 100%." The risk of pregnancy with an IUD in place is less than one in one hundred [15], with lower rates of both intrauterine and ectopic pregnancies. However, because IUDs are so effective at preventing intrauterine pregnancies, if a patient does get pregnant with an IUD in place, the relative risk of an ectopic pregnancy is higher [16, 17].

4. **Perforation:** We describe this as, "The IUD moving someplace in the body that it shouldn't be, instead of staying in the body of the uterus." Perforation occurs in one in one thousand IUD placements [15]. Most perforations are simple, do not involve vascular structures, and require no intervention besides removing the IUD. It is important to let patients know that if there is a complete IUD perfora-tion, in which the IUD goes into the abdominal cavity, additional procedures may be needed to remove the IUD.

Standard Informed Consent Templates

Many institutions have standardized procedural informed consent templates, which are modified and standardized to different procedures. Some providers use consents that are free to download, and focus on patient-centered and easy-to-understand language, such as those available at the Reproductive Health Access Project [18].

Pre-procedural Counseling

Informed consent often dovetails into pre-procedural counseling. Pre-procedural counseling, particularly if it is also a young person's first pelvic exam, is conversa-tional in style, and includes highly important information about the procedure itself.

Pelvic exam counseling Approaching an AYA's first pelvic exam starts with acknowledgement of the awkwardness and uncertainty that the exam often entails. We typically ask patients what they have heard from family or friends; often the phrase "cold duckbill thing" is their first received impression of a speculum. Acknowledging that this exam can be "weird and uncomfortable" is an important step in forming an alliance and a sense of trust. We typically tell patients, "You may have heard or anticipate many things about this exam, but it's usually neither hor-rible, nor awesome. The exam is not painful, it can just be a bit uncomfortable." Counseling about the pelvic exam, as about the IUD, should happen when the patient is dressed (not gowned) and seated on a chair (not on an exam table). It is also essential to assess for experiences of sexual abuse, coercion, or violence, as personal experiences can greatly impact both patients' anxiety around and pain during exams. Keep in mind that patients may not disclose these experiences, so one must always be sure to use a trauma-informed approach to counseling and exams. Respecting our patient's physical boundaries is an important way of promoting autonomy and establishing rapport.

We then explain the pelvic exam in a step-by-step fashion:

1. "These are the footrests." Explain the exam table and the position you will ask the patient to be in during the procedure. Using phrases like, "let your knees fall out to the side" can be helpful for patients. Phrases like, "spread your legs wide open" can be uncomfortable for patients and should be avoided.
2. "I will perform an exam with two fingers in your vagina, and a hand on your lower abdomen or belly." Explaining the bimanual exam and its purpose is important. We tell patients that, "it helps me to determine the size, shape, and position of your uterus and ovaries."
3. "This is a speculum." Pull out a small or medium speculum and allow the patient to take a look at it or touch it if possible. If you are using a sterile metal speculum for the procedure, having a demo in the room can be helpful.
4. If also doing a pap smear and/or sexually transmitted infection (STI) testing, this is when we show the cytobrush, broom, or swabs to the patient.

IUD Insertion Counseling

Stemming from the introduction to the physical exam as above, I tell patients that "after I have done the bimanual exam and placed the speculum, I will then place your IUD."

How to talk about uterine anatomy "Your uterus is shaped like a pear or a yellow squash. The narrow end of the pear is the cervix, which is located at the top of the vagina. The wide end of the pear, which is the body of the uterus, points towards your belly button. The stem of the pear, which leads into the body of the uterus, is your cervical canal and is the natural opening into your uterus. This is where your IUD will be placed. I will place it through the cervix, and the cervical canal, and into the body of the uterus."

Explain the IUD insertion in three steps:

• **Step 1**. "I have to hold onto your cervix in order to place the IUD." You can use your hand clenched into a fist, with thumb and first finger forming a tight opening, and explain that the cervix looks like a little donut as represented by your hand. "I will clean your cervix using some big cotton swabs, and then use my cervix holder to hold on to your cervix so that I can keep it still." **A note on tenaculums: we do not typically show a tenaculum, or other parts of the IUD tray, to patients**.

- **Step 2.** "Next I measure how long the uterus is, so I know where to place the IUD." Some clinical practices use an endometrial sampling pipelle as a uterine sound, which has the benefit of being sterilely packaged outside of the IUD tray. We typically show these pipelles, or other types of plastic sounds to patients in order to demonstrate that they are narrow, plastic, and flexible.
- **Step 3.** "I will place the IUD, once I have held onto your cervix and measured how long your uterus is." We show a model IUD inserter to demonstrate how the IUD is placed into the flexible plastic tube of the inserter itself, and how it is released into the uterus. We are clear with patients that only the T of the IUD goes into the uterus, and that the rest of the inserter stays on the outside of the uterus and is thrown away.

What Patients Should Expect

Many patients wonder what the IUD placement will feel like. After explaining the three steps above, we address this by saying, "Everyone experiences different sensations when they get their IUD. Some of these steps may be crampy or uncomfortable, some may feel light pressure or stretching — depending on the person this pressure may feel pretty easy, or more intense. We gave you pain medication to help with the cramps after the insertion. During the procedure, we'll give you a heating pack to help you. If you are more uncomfortable than you expect, please let us know so we can talk about how to make this more comfortable for you." (Please see Chaps. 9 and 10 on IUD insertion pain management.)

Conclusion

It is important that providers are knowledgeable of the minor consent laws in their state regarding reproductive health care for AYAs, especially in regards to IUDs. Providers should have proficient knowledge of the risks and benefits of IUD placement to provide optimal pre- and post-procedural counseling for patients. As some AYAs have never had a pelvic exam, or may have experienced trauma in the past, it is imperative that providers approach these conversations in a sensitive, stepwise manner that optimizes patient education and comfort.

Clinical Pearls
- Informed consent begins with contraceptive counseling, and continues through the pre-procedural counseling.
- Informed consent needs to contain relevant information on the risks and benefits of the IUD insertion procedure, and is an important part of patient education.

References

1. English A. Sexual and reproductive health care for adolescents: legal rights and policy challenges. Adolesc Med State Art Rev. 2007;18:571–81, viii–ix.
2. Jones RK, Purcell A, Singh S, Finer LB. Adolescents' reports of parental knowledge of adolescents' use of sexual health services and their reactions to mandated parental notification for prescription contraception. JAMA. 2005;293:340–8.
3. Padon AA, Baren JM. Achieving a decision-making triad in adolescent sexual health care. Adolesc Med State Art Rev. 2011;22:183–94, vii.
4. An overview of minors' consent law. In: Guttmacher Institute [Internet]. 14 Mar 2016 [cited 1 Dec 2018]. Available: https://www.guttmacher.org/state-policy/explore/overview-minors-consent-law.
5. Minors' access to contraceptive services. In: Guttmacher Institute [Internet]. 14 Mar 2016 [cited 1 Dec 2018]. Available: https://www.guttmacher.org/state-policy/explore/minors-access-contraceptive-services.
6. Cason P, Goodman S. Protocol for provision of intrauterine contraception. San Francisco: UCSF Bixby Center Beyond the Pill. 2016 [Internet]. [cited 1 Dec 2018]. Available: https://beyondthepill.ucsf.edu/sites/beyondthepill.ucsf.edu/files/Beyond%20the%20Pill%20IUC%20Protocol.pdf.
7. Long-term reversible contraception. Twelve years of experience with the TCu380A and TCu220C. Contraception. 1997;56:341–352.
8. McNicholas C, Swor E, Wan L, Peipert JF. Prolonged use of the etonogestrel implant and levonorgestrel intrauterine device: 2 years beyond Food and Drug Administration-approved duration. Am J Obstet Gynecol. 2017;216:586.e1–6.
9. Mirena (levonorgestrel-releasing intrauterine system). Highlights of prescribing information [Internet]. [cited 1 Dec 2018]. Available: https://www.accessdata.fda.gov/drugsatfda_docs/label/2009/021225s027lbl.pdf.
10. Kyleena (levonorgestrel-releasing intrauterine system). Highlights of prescribing information [Internet]. [cited 1 Dec 2018]. Available: https://labeling.bayerhealthcare.com/html/products/pi/Kyleena_PI.pdf.
11. Skyla (levonorgestrel-releasing intrauterine system). Highlights of prescribing information [Internet]. [cited 1 Dec 2018]. Available: http://labeling.bayerhealthcare.com/html/products/pi/Skyla_PI.pdf.
12. Daniele MAS, Cleland J, Benova L, Ali M. Provider and lay perspectives on intra-uterine contraception: a global review. Reprod Health. 2017;14:119.
13. Sufrin CB, Postlethwaite D, Armstrong MA, Merchant M, Wendt JM, Steinauer JE. Neisseria gonorrhea and Chlamydia trachomatis screening at intrauterine device insertion and pelvic inflammatory disease. Obstet Gynecol. 2012;120:1314–21.
14. Farley TM, Rosenberg MJ, Rowe PJ, Chen JH, Meirik O. Intrauterine devices and pelvic inflammatory disease: an international perspective. Lancet. 1992;339:785–8.
15. Jatlaoui TC, Riley HEM, Curtis KM. The safety of intrauterine devices among young women: a systematic review. Contraception. 2017;95:17–39.
16. Li C, Zhao W-H, Zhu Q, Cao S-J, Ping H, Xi X, et al. Risk factors for ectopic pregnancy: a multi-center case-control study. BMC Pregnancy Childbirth. 2015;15:187.
17. Rossing MA, Daling JR, Voigt LF, Stergachis AS, Weiss NS. Current use of an intrauterine device and risk of tubal pregnancy. Epidemiology. 1993;4:252–8.
18. IUD insertion consent form. In: Reproductive health access project [Internet]. [cited 1 Dec 2018]. Available: https://www.reproductiveaccess.org/wp-content/uploads/2013/02/iud_consent.pdf.

Chapter 8
Integrating IUD Provision into Your Practice: Site Preparedness, Staff Training, and Procedural Steps

Lela R. Bachrach and Suzan Goodman

Abbreviations

AYA	Adolescent and young adult
BMI	Body mass index
CuT380A IUD	Copper IUD
EC	Emergency contraception
EHR	Electronic health record
IUD	Intrauterine device
LMP	Last menstrual period
STI	Sexually transmitted infection
UPIC	Unprotected intercourse

Learning Objectives

Following completion of this chapter, you should be able to:

- Identify initial steps to establish readiness for introducing Intrauterine device (IUD) services into a practice.
- Access proctoring supervision in order to successfully insert and remove IUDs.
- Compile supplies and materials necessary for IUD procedures.
- Utilize the detailed steps for IUD set-up, placement, and removal.

L. R. Bachrach (✉)
Department of Adolescent Medicine, UCSF Benioff Children's Hospital Oakland, Oakland, CA, USA

S. Goodman
Bixby Center for Global Reproductive Health, Department of Family and Community Medicine, UCSF, San Francisco, CA, USA

© Springer Nature Switzerland AG 2019
M. S. Coles, A. Mays (eds.), *Optimizing IUD Delivery for Adolescents and Young Adults*, https://doi.org/10.1007/978-3-030-17816-1_8

Background

The World Health Organization and most major national medical organizations advise that adolescent and young adults (AYAs) should have access to a wide range of contraceptive options, including IUDs [1–4]. Despite this guidance, many pediatric and adolescent primary care providers have received relatively little training regarding LARC methods [5–7]. One study found that only one-quarter of adolescent medicine clinicians were trained to insert IUDs or implants [8]. Education on updated recommendations and guidelines is critical.

Case

Blanca is a 19-year-old cisgender female who is parenting an 18-month-old and working full time. She has taken a day off from work and arranged childcare to come to clinic to discuss her birth control options. She had unprotected intercourse (UPIC) 3 days ago and likes the idea of a copper IUD for emergency and ongoing contraception. Unfortunately, the clinic's only IUD-trained provider is at another site today. There are other clinicians on site who have had IUD training on pelvic models and are interested in being proctored, but their clinic schedules have not allowed for this type of supervision. Blanca is offered a referral to another clinic that can provide her with same-day IUD placement, but she prefers her regular clinic. She takes an oral emergency contraception (EC) pill and makes a follow-up appointment in 2 weeks for an IUD.

On Blanca's second visit, she is told she must wait for insurance preauthorization and clinic stocking for her IUD, as well as have sexually transmitted infection (STI) screening labs done before the IUD placement. Blanca takes a prescription for birth control pills and reschedules her IUD placement.

On Blanca's third visit, a new medical assistant is working in clinic who does not have much experience with IUD appointments. She does not feel comfortable counseling Blanca about the various types of IUDs and does not know how to help with the procedure set-up. Blanca's provider does the counseling and shows the medical assistant how to set up for the procedure. When the provider goes to review Blanca's pregnancy test result, she realizes that the staff did not know that the patient needed this done, and Blanca just went to the bathroom. Blanca drinks three cups of water while her provider sees another patient. Eventually, Blanca provides a urine sample, and her pregnancy test is negative. She finally gets her IUD—4 weeks after her initial visit!

Points to consider:

- Is there adequate administrative buy-in, supervision, and staff training to integrate IUDs?
- Can patient education, insurance authorization, stocking, and STI testing occur in advance, or on the same day as visit?
  Which processes guide staff (especially new staff) to support providers and patients during IUD placement?

Assessing for Readiness and Developing a Plan for Sustainable Integration of IUDs

Equal access to all methods, including LARC, is the standard of care for AYAs. Respect for the AYA's right to choose or decline any method is critical. Patient preference should be the principal factor driving method choice. Each practice setting has its own process for incorporating a new service or procedure. It is important to have clinic champions, administrative buy-in, and both staff and stakeholders—including patients—on board [9]. The importance of timely access to IUDs is highlighted by studies that show that delays in scheduling IUD insertion increase risk of unplanned pregnancy [10, 11].

As you begin to consider integration of IUDs into your practice, it is important to determine elements of greatest need by reviewing current services and evaluating clinic quality improvement processes that may support practice change. Addressing staff and training needs—including time available for staff training and the clinic's ability to invest in an IUD program—can help move things forward. Additional areas for consideration include optimizing physical space, identifying and ordering affordable supplies and equipment, and optimizing reimbursement and revenue streams.

Keep in mind that service-delivery change:

- Requires **support** for those introducing and implementing it
- Requires **comprehensive** training for the entire clinical team (front desk staff, nursing, medical assistants, medical providers, health educators, etc.)
- Must be **sustainable** in order to have lasting impact
- May be a **complex** process, requiring persistence
- Must be tailored to the **site/system needs**

Identifying Champions and Involving Key Stakeholders

Maximize your efforts in developing new IUD services by identifying staff allies who may be part of a planning committee. Begin meeting regularly to discuss tasks, timelines, potential obstacles, and solutions. Tasks can include training staff in new skills/counseling techniques, updating protocols, refining clinic schedule templates, assigning administrative roles to research reimbursement, ordering supplies, developing forms, and setting up feedback systems.

Engage the support of key players at your institution in order to elicit buy-in and expertise in certain areas. These people may include:

- Chief executive officer—impact on bottom line, efficiency, overall game plan
- Medical director—expected volumes, clinical flow, screening
- Billing manager or chief financial officer—billing strategies, anticipated expenses and income
- Practice providers—proctoring, coverage for any complications
- Operations or nursing director—counseling, nursing, and support staff responsibilities

Financial Considerations for IUD Services

Addressing the financial implications of offering IUDs is critical to gaining support of your leadership. Although cost-effective over time, the acquisition costs of the devices are significantly higher than other contraceptives. While insurance coverage has improved for all contraceptive methods in the past decade, uncertainty regarding future healthcare restructuring poses coverage and reimbursement challenges, especially for safety-net providers.

Utilize the following resources:

- Reimbursement guides on coverage, stocking, and coding
- Quick coding guides
- A LARC Modeling Tool, which helps examine LARC cost assumptions to calculate if LARC costs will create profit, loss, or break-even based on an agency's current payer mix and reimbursement rates
- Cost-effective ways to make IUDs accessible to your clinic and patients:

    - Add IUDs to your formulary—for practices that are part of an academic medical center or hospital system, update the formulary via the pharmacy and therapeutics committee.
    - Explore discounts via 340B programs if you are a federally qualified and/or Title X health center.
    - Access group purchasing programs via your institutional umbrella or others (see Afaxys.com).
    - Utilize manufacturers' patient assistance programs.

- Develop IUD order sets (if your practice uses an Electronic health record (EHR)) that have all the relevant orders and billing codes easily accessible to providers.

Building Staff Knowledge and Skills

It is important to train **all staff** (providers, medical assistants, nursing, administrative staff, etc.) on *all contraceptive methods* including IUDs, as everyone plays an important role in supporting and streamlining contraceptive access. Staff answering phones must be trained on how to discuss contraception with patients, triage calls, and schedule appropriately. Empowering non-clinician staff to counsel, consent, and set up for procedures will facilitate same-day services and is recommended as the standard of care [12]. The following actions may help build the knowledge base of clinic staff members:

- Survey staff members to gauge knowledge and common misconceptions.
- Provide comprehensive contraceptive training for all staff members. Consider working with an outside training facilitator.
- Utilize online trainings, such as this one-hour training [13] designed for all staff members.

Procedural Competency

Growing literature supports the use of models and simulations in procedural training [14–17] (see Fig. 8.1). Limited patient encounters and a heightened focus on patient safety underscore the importance of using models and simulators and practicing complicated scenarios in advance of or in tandem with clinical care [18–21]. This can be applied to practicing IUD placements on patients. For various gynecologic procedures, working with models and simulators has led to improvements in medical knowledge, comfort in procedures, and improvements in performance during complications [22–25]. We recommend practicing on IUD models before proctored cases whenever possible, as this may help increase the speed of the provider gaining comfort and the safety of patients during IUD placements [26]. Procedural practice can be low-tech, such as papaya workshops that allow learners to practice placing IUDs [27]. High-tech virtual reality simulators can also be used to simulate various uterine positions and give feedback [28, 29]. **Regardless of the model of training, it is critically important for learners to be observed by experienced trainers, and to receive feedback** [35]. We recommend using an IUD competency checklist, such as the one included in the Resources section of this book [30].

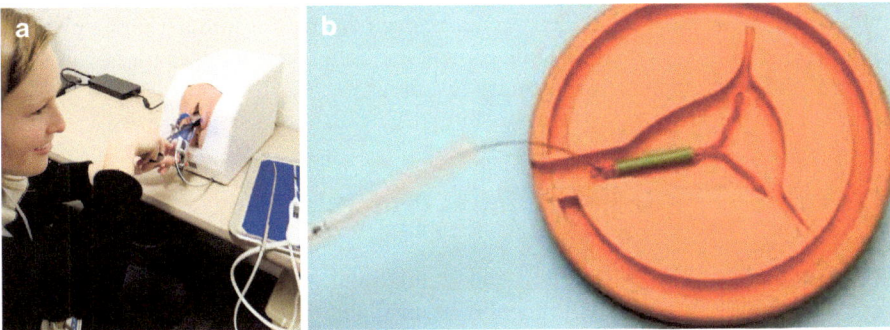

Fig. 8.1 Examples of a simulator (left) and a model (right) used in IUD procedure training. (Image sources: VirtaMed (left) and Bayer (right))

Proctoring Clinicians

It is ideal for clinicians to become competent with procedures during professional training. However, primary care fields have not routinely included LARC training [31, 32]. IUD skill acquisition, confidence, and competency are generally obtained after 3–10 proctored IUD placements, although this may vary by provider and specialty training [33].

On-site proctoring, supervised by experienced providers One option for skills training is proctoring—hands-on IUD placement training, supervised by experienced providers, during patient visits. This can be done in a number of different ways depending on the options in the area. Proctoring within your clinical setting, by existing clinical staff (when available), will minimize the need for outside credentialing, malpractice coverage, and memorandums of understanding [34].

Training in an off-site, high-volume setting If on-site proctoring is not available, training in a high-volume setting can be an option. The hands-on Reproductive Health Training Center through the Reproductive Health Access Project in New York City has developed a model for a regional, hands-on LARC training center in a primary care clinic. This allows for the development of competency in IUD insertions by completing a large volume of procedures in a short amount of time (once or twice a week over 6 weeks) and may be a blueprint for others to develop similar LARC training programs for practicing clinicians [35].

Clinic-wide training A California study that provided tailored clinic-wide IUD training and clinician proctoring on-site found that clinic staff and providers felt better prepared to place IUDs and provide same-day LARC services after participating in on-site proctoring [36]. Various organizations can help with logistical assistance and proctoring support, such as Get LARC, The Reproductive Health Access Project, Beyond the Pill team, or Upstream. Providers will often need to request new privileges for IUD procedures, even during this initial training phase. A sample form for requesting IUD placement and removal privileges for hospital settings is included in the supplementary resources.

Developing or Adapting Clinical Protocols

IUD protocols work by defining and standardizing clinical workflows for IUD provision. Sample clinical protocols are available via the Reproductive Health Access Project and Beyond the Pill. Some examples are noted below, including:

- Office visit lengths
- Required patient labs and testing
- On-site supplies
- Support staff available to assist during the procedure
- Complication management plans

Medical Documentation

Medical documentation is fundamental to patient care and risk management. Customizing your EHR or forms to allow quick and thorough documentation will help with successful IUD integration. Important IUD forms include:

- Patient education handouts
- Aftercare instructions post procedure
- Informed consents
- Procedure notes for placements and removals

Sources for excellent patient education materials are listed in the Supplementary Resources section at the end of this book.

Case 2

In the Groove with IUD Service.

Over the last few months, several clinic team members have become champions for improving contraceptive access. They organized an all-staff training on adding IUDs to the methods available in clinic, redistributed roles, and learned to optimize flow. Schedulers now use their judgment to adjust the schedule to accommodate walk-ins, beyond the reserved "same-day" appointment slots. The practice administrator learned to optimize billing and reimbursement—stocking and purchasing IUDs using the more affordable 340B status—so that now IUDs enhance the clinic revenue stream.

Shantell, a 20-year-old cisgender female, calls in to schedule a routine health maintenance visit. The staff member speaks with her by phone and finds out that Shantell is interested in learning more about her birth control options. Staff members guide Shantell to reliable online contraceptive information, along with testimonials from other patients regarding their experiences with various methods at www.bedsider.org, and schedule a clinic visit. During her brief wait in the clinic, Shantell looks at contraception educational pamphlets and posters. The health educator uses shared decision-making techniques to counsel her on method choice, provides her with a consent form, and informs the medical assistant and provider that Shantell would like to have an IUD placed today. The medical assistant sets up the room with supplies for an IUD insertion. As there is an IUD-trained clinician each day, Shantell gets her IUD placed without delay.

IUD Placement and Removal: Supplies and Procedures.
Adapted with permission [37]

Instruments and supplies Create or modify a list (see Supplementary Resources section at the end of the book) with photos of necessary instruments (see Fig. 8.2), supplies, and set-up for all staff, including new or cross-covering. Depending on access to autoclave and sterilization services, reusable versus disposable IUD insertion kits can be chosen. Clinics without sterilization services will find disposable kits convenient (see Fig. 8.3 below). It helps if the tenaculum in a disposable kit has metal tips. For sites that have autoclave or sterilization services, consider ordering enough supply sets to avoid the need to autoclave mid-day.

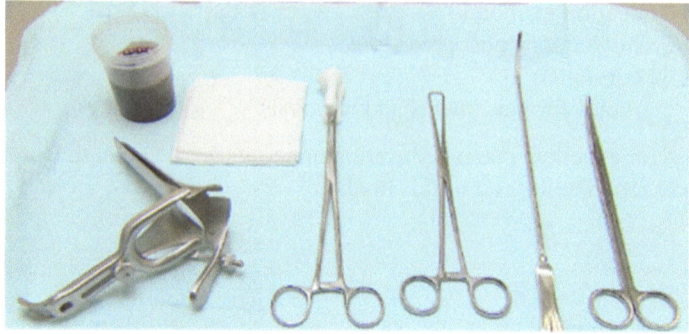

Fig. 8.2 A selection of IUD placement and removal equipment (from left to right): speculum, ring forceps with gauze, tenaculum, metal uterine sound, scissors

Fig. 8.3 A disposable IUD kit generally contains the items above. (Image source: MPM Medical Supply)

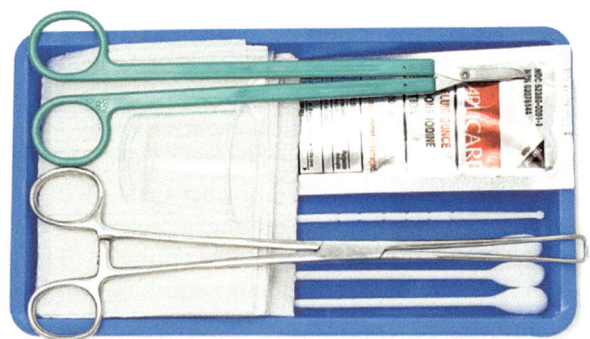

IUD Placement and Removal Equipment

IUD IUD shelf life ranges from 3 years (most LNG IUDs) to 7 years (copper IUD) from manufacturing date; printed expiration date indicates when sterile packaging expires, which does not indicate the end of contraceptive efficacy.

Exam gloves Most IUD placements can be performed with non-sterile gloves using *no-touch technique* (assuring portions of instruments entering the uterine cavity remain sterile) [38]. Some providers use sterile gloves to bend the end of a metal sound or load the CuT380A IUD.

Speculum Choosing shorter and wider specula allows for better visualization, while providing greater mobility and ability to straighten uterine flexion with a tenaculum under tension. The speculum does not have to be sterile for IUD insertion and can be plastic or metal. Cordless vaginal illuminator systems or specula with internal lights can also be helpful, especially when working with trainees or proctors.

Mayo stand (or flat surface) with sterile drape To place supplies including the IUD.

Water-based lubricant For a pelvic exam and to apply to speculum. Avoid application before vaginal testing.

Antiseptic solution (povidone-iodine or chlorhexidine).

Scopettes, swabs, 4 × 4 gauze pads or cotton balls These can be used for antiseptic prep or to remove blood or antiseptic solution after IUD placement. Swabs can help demarcate sound depth (as described in detail under sounding below) if needed.

Tenaculum The tenaculum stabilizes the cervix and straightens the uterine canal. These can be made of plastic or metal, and include single tooth or blunted types. Single-tooth tenaculum is usually the more commonly used, though blunted types can be helpful for multiparous cervices. If using a disposable tenaculum, we generally recommend using one that is metal or at least has metal tips for grasping the cervix.

Uterine sound Any of the following types of sterile uterine sounds can work well; a provider may prefer one type over another in different clinical situations:

- Plastic sound (often with markings for measuring depth)
- Metal sound
- Endometrial biopsy pipelle; generally a slightly smaller diameter (3 mm)

Ring forceps Ring forceps can be used to hold a cotton ball to cleanse the cervix, or retrieve IUD strings from the vagina during IUD removal. Curved (Kelly) forceps may substitute (10 inches).

Long curved scissors Used to cut IUD strings after placement. The sharpness of the scissors helps avoid incomplete cutting of the IUD strings, with possible displacement. The curvature of the scissor head is important to avoid cutting vaginal tissue.

Anesthetic supplies For use if you are going to provide pharmacologic anesthesia (see Chap. 9).

Sanitary napkins To give to patient after IUD placement if there is spotting, which is common after IUD placement.

Have available (not needed for most placements):

- **Endocervical cytobrush, os finder, and/or small metal or plastic dilators** (i.e., French 13/15): to aid in locating the external os, which sometimes can be visually distorted or difficult to distinguish.
- **Monsel's solution or silver nitrate sticks:** to provide chemical cauterization in the event of prolonged bleeding at tenaculum removal site.
- **Alligator forceps**: these can be very helpful for retrievals with missing strings.

Figure 8.3: Disposable IUD Kit Contents

- (1) Stainless steel tenaculum
- (1) Long handled plastic scissor, 8.5″
- (3) Swab, rayon 8″
- (1) Plastic uterine sound
- (1) Prep, PVP 1 oz solution
- (1) Drape/Towel 4-ply poly 17″ × 19″
- (1) Cup, 2 oz medicine (for solution)
- (1) Tray

Procedure for IUD placement. *Adapted with permission* [39].

Note: If providing pharmacologic pain management such as an NSAID, provide to the patient before beginning the procedure for IUD placement. See Chap. 9 for more details on pharmacologic pain management.

Step 1: Perform a bimanual exam to:

1. Determine uterine position and version (see Fig. 8.4)

   - Use non-sterile gloves and lubricating gel.
   - Place 2 fingers in vagina.
   - Place other hand on belly.
   - Determine location of cervix (anterior or posterior).
   - Palpate uterine fundus by applying gentle pressure to cervix.
   - Determine uterine position with the assistance of sweeping vaginal fingers to feel for uterine fullness anterior or posterior to cervix.

2. **Assess for signs that contraindicate placement** such as cervical motion tenderness, uterine tenderness, or adnexal tenderness on exam, or question of anatomic abnormalities that may require ultrasound assessment prior to placement.

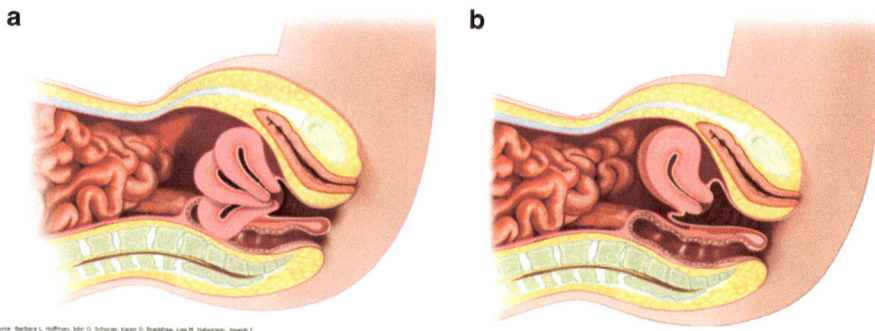

Fig. 8.4 A bimanual exam will determine uterine position, as seen below. (**a**) Uterine position may be anteverted, midplane, or retroverted. (**b**) As shown here, the uterine fundus can be flexed forward, and this is termed anteflexion. Similarly, the uterine fundus may be flexed backward to create a retroverted uterus. (Image source: McGraw Hill Education)

Step 2: Set up lighting.

1. Turn on light
2. Adjust light for maximal visualization

Step 3: Remove drape covering tray (if present) or open disposable IUD kit and set out.

Step 4 (optional): If using, put on sterile gloves.

1. Adjust instruments as needed
2. If using bendable sound, adjust curve as needed (can be done through sterile package)

Step 5: Place speculum.

1. Ask patient's permission to place the back of your hand on the interior of thigh, and let them know you are about to place speculum:

   • If vaginal muscles are tight, you can gently place 2 fingers on inferior portion of vagina and ask patient to squeeze and then relax the muscles you are touching.

2. Insert lubricated speculum fully prior to opening it, in order to place beyond vaginal folds.
3. If unable to see cervix in patients with an elevated body mass index (BMI):

   • Use a longer/wide speculum.
   • Place a condom with tip removed around the speculum.

4. **Assess for abnormal discharge and obtain samples for STI screening** per guidelines or clinic protocol if not already completed. Note: *If mucopurulent discharge is present, do not continue with IUD placement.* Treat for presumptive cervicitis, and have patient return for IUD placement in 1–2 weeks [40].

Step 6: Clean the cervix with povidone-iodine or chlorhexidine gluconate.

Step 7: If providing cervical anesthesia, see Chap. 9 for more details.

Step 8: Place the tenaculum.

Reasons to use a tenaculum:

1. *Straightens* the cervical canal to enable the uterine sound and the IUD inserter to pass more safely through the os.
2. *Aligns* the uterine body with the cervix, so that curves from anteflexion or retroflexion are straightened out to avoid perforation at the point of flexion.
3. *Stabilizes* the cervix and holds it in place, so that pressure from the sound or the IUD applicator does not push the cervix and uterus away from the instruments.

Where to position the tenaculum on the cervix:

1. Position the tenaculum horizontally or vertically, 1–2 centimeters above or below the external os.
2. Grasping the **anterior lip of an anteflexed uterus or the posterior lip of a retroflexed uterus** may be most helpful in aligning cervico-uterine angle.
3. If only a portion of the cervix is visible, grasp the visible lip of the cervix and bring the os into view with traction, re-grasping as necessary.

How to hold a tenaculum when placing it on the cervix:

1. Grasp with dominant hand.
2. Open and place the tenacular teeth on the surface of the cervix.
3. Once in contact with the cervix, with the tips 1–2 centimeters apart, squeeze together *slowly* to imbed teeth in the cervical tissue.

    • You can ask patient to cough, or take a deep breath as you close tenaculum.

4. Grasp a 1–2 centimeter width of cervical tissue with a bite that is 1–2 centimeters deep.

    • Do not take too shallow a bite. Adequate bite will prevent the tenaculum from pulling through the cervical epithelium when applying traction during sounding and IUD placement.

5. Close the tenaculum to the first or second ratchet.

    • Closing the tenaculum fully is unnecessary and can cause more bleeding with tenaculum removal.

6. Lay the tenaculum down gently to rest on the posterior blade of the speculum, in order to pick up the sound or IUD.
7. Use the non-dominant hand to apply good traction with the tenaculum during sounding and when placing the IUD, in order to assure the sound or IUD inserter is at the fundus (rather than the back wall of a flexed uterus).

Step 9: Sounding the uterus.

Sounding the uterus (see Fig. 8.5 for an image of sound use) prior to IUD insertion is important for a number of reasons. First of all, sounding documents the ability to pass something through the cervical os and measures uterine depth—both observations are needed in order to place the IUD. **Note**: We recommend that you do not open the IUD package until you have successfully passed the sound. This timing avoids making the IUD unsterile. Sounding also assists in assuring that the uterine size is consistent with the size noted on bimanual exam. Lastly, some IUD manufacturers suggest the uterus should measure specific depth for adequate IUD placement, as listed below. **Note** that you should also use your clinical judgment with these guidelines, as many providers place devices if the uterus sounds ≥5.5 centimeters with no upper limit. If the uterus sounds >10–11 centimeters, it is

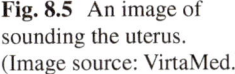

Fig. 8.5 An image of
sounding the uterus.
(Image source: VirtaMed.)

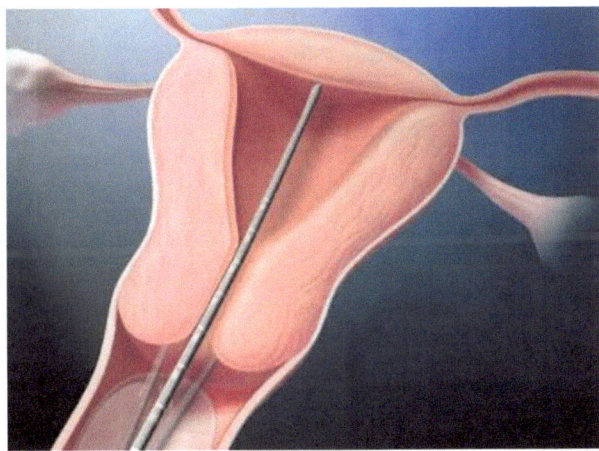

important to correlate with bimanual exam and clinical circumstance (postaspiration, postpartum, fibroids, etc.) and to also consider perforation.

- 6–9 centimeters for Copper IUD (CuT380A IUD)
- 6–10 centimeters for Mirena
- No less than 5.5 centimeters for Liletta (with no upper limit specified)
- Depth not specified for LNG 13.5 mg or 19.5 mg IUDs

Sounding technique:

1. Gentle traction should be applied to the tenaculum throughout sounding to straighten the uterus.

    (a) If using a metal sound, consider bending the distal few centimeters to mimic the uterine flexion.
    (b) To maintain sterility, only adjust sound through sterile packaging or with sterile gloves.

2. Hold the sound like a pencil, or like throwing a dart, using wrist and finger (not elbow) action to move sound.
3. If it is difficult to pass through the internal os, try repositioning the sound at various angles in the os to find the direction of the pathway.
4. For patient comfort, minimize repeated tapping of the fundus with the sound.
5. Note the depth sounded in centimeters.

    (a) Most sounds have centimeter markings on them, or may be held up to a measuring tape at the "line of glistening" where blood, mucous, or betadine is visible.
    (b) Remember to note the sound depth in your procedure note.

Step 10: Inserting the IUD.

IUD placement for Bayer-branded LNG-IUDs (such as Mirena, Skyla, etc.):

1. Sterile loading of device into inserter.

   - Load the IUD arms into the inserter **no more than** 2–5 minutes before placement.
   - Push the slider completely forward in the direction of the arrow to load the IUD into the inserter.
   - The tips of the arms will meet to form a rounded end extending slightly beyond the insertion tube.
   - Keep pressure with your thumb or forefinger on the slider at all times, and in the fully forward-most position.
   - DO NOT move the slider back at this time, as this may prematurely release the IUD.
   - Once the slider is moved below the mark, the IUD cannot be reloaded.

2. Adjust the flange

   - Use the notches in the sterile packaging to set the upper edge of the flange to the corresponding uterine depth (in centimeters) measured during sounding.

3. Apply traction to the tenaculum with the non-dominant hand.
4. Pass the inserter through the internal os.
5. Advance the loaded inserter until the flange is 1.5–2 centimeters below the external os.
6. Retract the slider down to the "first mark."
7. Wait 10–15 seconds in this position (for the device to resume its "T" shape).

   - This step ensures that the arms have fully opened before advancing, and helps prevent perforation.

8. Advance the inserter to the fundus. When the inserter is at the fundus, the flange will be touching or close to the cervix.

   - Once you encounter fundal resistance, stop, as the IUD is now in the fundal position.

9. Holding the inserter firmly in place, release the IUD by moving the slider all the way down.
10. Continue to hold the slider all the way down while gently withdrawing the inserter from the uterus.

IUD placement for Allergan-branded hormonal IUD (Liletta) [41]

1. Adjust the flange.

   - Use one of the notches in the sterile packaging to set the upper edge of the flange to the corresponding uterine depth (in centimeters) measured during sounding.

2. Load the inserter.

- Remove the inserter, and hold it with the buttons facing up.
- Ensure both sliders are pushed fully forward, and aligned with their respective markings.
- To load the IUD into the inserter, maintain forward pressure on the BLUE slider, and pull the threads until you feel a hard stop.
- Pull—and lock—the threads into the cleft at the bottom of the handle.

3. Insert IUD into the uterus.

- Apply traction to the tenaculum with the non-dominant hand.
- Pass the inserter through the internal os.
- Maintain forward pressure on the BLUE slider throughout the insertion process.
- Advance the loaded inserter until the upper edge of the flange is 1.5–2 centimeters below the external os.

4. Release IUD into the uterus.

- Gently slide only the BLUE slider back until the BLUE and GREEN sliders are together and wait 10 seconds—this will allow the IUD arms to fully open.
- While maintaining the slider position, advance the inserter to the fundal position—the flange should now be at the top of the cervix.

5. Complete the insertion.

- Move both sliders down the handle until it clicks.
- The GREEN indicator at the bottom of the handle should now be visible.
- Remove the inserter from the uterus.
- Look at the cleft to ensure the threads were properly released; if not released, grab the threads and gently pull the threads out of the cleft.
- Cut the threads perpendicularly, leaving about 3 centimeters outside the cervix.

IUD placement for ParaGard (CuT380A IUD, or copper IUD)

1. Sterile loading of copper IUD into insertion tube.

- Load the IUD into the inserter no more than 2–5 minutes before placement.
- Use either sterile gloves or the no-touch technique (by loading the IUD while still in the package) to ensure sterility of the IUD.
- Fold the two horizontal arms down, and tuck the tips of the arms into the insertion tube. The copper collars will be outside the tube.
- Slide the solid-white stabilizing rod into the insertion tube until it is touching the bottom of the IUD within the tube, while maintaining gentle pressure at the tip of the IUD to ensure it is not pushed out.

2. Set flange.

   - Set the flange to the sound depth measured either through the sterile packaging, or with sterile gloves.
   - The wide aspect of the flange is designed to be in the same plane as the arms of the IUD, which is also the same plane as the arms of the patient.

3. Insert IUD into the uterus.

   - Apply traction to the tenaculum with the non-dominant hand.
   - Hold the insertion tube with the dominant hand, and advance the tube gently to the fundus until resistance is met.

4. Let go of the tenaculum and let it rest on the speculum.
5. Hold onto the white solid rod with your non-dominant hand, and keep it immobile. It functions as a stabilizer to hold the IUD in place (the white rod is never used as a plunger).
6. Pull the insertion tube back until it touches the ring of the rod to release the arms of the copper IUD at the fundal position.
7. Re-advance the insertion tube to the fundus to "re-seat" the IUD, and ensure high fundal placement.
8. Remove the white solid rod before removing the insertion tube—this prevents inadvertently pulling the IUD down into the lower uterine segment or even expelling the IUD.
9. Remove the insertion tube.

Step 11: Cutting the IUD strings.

1. Use the insertion tube as a guide to hold and cut the strings using long, curved, blunt scissors, before removing tube from vagina.
2. Use blunt (not pointed), but sharp scissors to avoid IUD displacement with multiple cutting attempts.
3. Cut straight across strings to minimize sharply pointed tips that may poke the partner.

   - Most providers will cut IUD strings at 3–4 centimeters to allow the strings to wrap around the posterior lip of the cervix.
   - Trimming strings shorter can be considered for those experiencing reproductive or sexual coercion, or for those who wish to conceal IUD use from a partner.
   - Document length of strings in chart.
   - Consider letting the patient hold a piece of the extra string that will be discarded so they know what it feels like.

Step 12: Remove tenaculum.

1. Open tenaculum so that teeth are fully removed from cervix.
2. Very gently rock the tenaculum to get teeth out of the cervix if stuck.

Step 13: Check for bleeding at os and tenaculum site.

1. Visualize cervix for 5–10 seconds.
2. Minimal bleeding from the tenaculum site will often stop with pressure from the vaginal walls.
3. If bleeding occurs:

   - Hold pressure with a scopette or gauze in ring forceps for 30 to 60 seconds and re-evaluate.
   - Apply the tip of a silver nitrate stick, or cotton ball of Monsel's solution to the bleeding area for a few seconds and re-evaluate (do not touch any other tissue).

Step 14: Remove speculum.

1. Loosen washer to close speculum (if metal) or unlock (if plastic).
2. Remove speculum.

Step 15: Postprocedure care.

1. Have patients rest and relax for 5–10 minutes, until they are feeling back to baseline. Rarely, if patients get up too quickly, they may faint due to vagal stimulation.
2. Provide wipes to remove any lubricant or blood from the procedure, and a sanitary pad for underwear.
3. Provide a confidential after-visit summary to include: the date of IUD placement, information regarding care after IUD placement, and how to get in touch if questions come up later. **Note:** if the patient does not want a paper copy, one can verbally give patient instructions that patients can type into their phone
4. Encourage a follow-up visit in approximately 1–2 weeks to check in, remind patient of menstrual side effects, or answer any questions they may have.

IUD Removal Procedure

The majority of IUD removals are quick and uncomplicated. For a review of how to manage complicated IUD removals, please see Chap. 12. Note that if the patient has had intercourse without condoms in the 5 days prior to IUD removal, there is a theoretical risk of pregnancy. Make sure to discuss this with patients, and offer another birth control method or EC at time of IUD removal.

Uncomplicated removals:

1. Perform speculum exam to fully visualize cervical os with strings in view.
2. Clasp IUD strings with ring forceps close to os (make sure you clasp *both* strings).
3. Pull straight toward clinician with a steady direct movement.

Summary

Many resources exist on how to optimize IUD service delivery and guide clinics in developing IUD programs and training providers. Implementing IUD services will go more smoothly if all stakeholders are involved, and all clinic staff members are operating at their highest skill level. Clinics can streamline access to patients' preferred method by optimizing clinic-wide training in IUD skills, counseling, and operationalization. Having a standardized approach to IUD insertion and removal procedures, which takes into account both behavioral components and cognitive reasoning, helps providers improve standard IUD provision and to work through complications if they arise.

Clinical Pearls
1. Assessing your clinical site readiness to implement IUD procedures is important; engage all clinical staff members, administrative leadership, and other key stakeholders.
2. Creating a structured process for training your entire clinical team will help to streamline and standardize IUD delivery at your site.
3. Understanding not just the steps in IUD insertions and removals, but also the rationale for each step, will help you problem solve in the case of challenging procedures.

References

1. World Health Organization Department of Reproductive Health and Research (WHO/RHR) and Johns Hopkins Bloomberg School of Public Health/Center for Communication Programs (CCP). Knowledge for health project. Family planning: a global handbook for providers (2018 update). Baltimore/Geneva: CCP and WHO; 2018. [Internet]. [cited 1 Dec 2018]. Available: http://apps.who.int/iris/bitstream/handle/10665/260156/9780999203705-eng.pdf.
2. ACOG Committee Opinion No. 735. Adolescents and long-acting reversible contraception: implants and intrauterine devices. Obstet Gynecol. 2018;131:e130–9.
3. Society for Adolescent Health and Medicine. Improving knowledge about, access to, and utilization of long-acting reversible contraception among adolescents and young adults. J Adolesc Health. 2017;60:472–4.
4. Ott MA, Sucato GS, Committee on Adolescence. Contraception for adolescents. Pediatrics. 2014;134:e1257–81.
5. Harper CC, Rocca CH, Thompson KM, Morfesis J, Goodman S, Darney PD, et al. Reductions in pregnancy rates in the USA with long-acting reversible contraception: a cluster randomised trial. Lancet. 2015;386:562–8.
6. Harper CC, Stratton L, Raine TR, Thompson K, Henderson JT, Blum M, et al. Counseling and provision of long-acting reversible contraception in the US: national survey of nurse practitioners. Prev Med. 2013;57:883–8.
7. Thompson KMJ, Rocca CH, Kohn JE, Goodman S, Stern L, Blum M, et al. Public funding for contraception, provider training, and use of highly effective contraceptives: a cluster randomized trial. Am J Public Health. 2016;106:541–6.

8. Greenberg KB, Makino KK, Coles MS. Factors associated with provision of long-acting reversible contraception among adolescent health care providers. J Adolesc Health. 2013;52:372–4.
9. LB Presler, RS Fehrman, R Gordon, K Turner. Mentoring for service-delivery change: a trainer's handbook. Chapel Hill, NC: Ipas; 2006. [Internet]. [cited 1 Dec 2018]. Available: https://www.go2itech.org/HTML/CM08/toolkit/links/print/Mentoring/Mentoring_Handbook_Ipas.pdf.
10. Bergin A, Tristan S, Terplan M, Gilliam ML, Whitaker AK. A missed opportunity for care: two-visit IUD insertion protocols inhibit placement. Contraception. 2012;86:694–7.
11. Pritt NM, Norris AH, Berlan ED. Barriers and facilitators to adolescents' use of long-acting reversible contraceptives. J Pediatr Adolesc Gynecol. 2017;30:18–22.
12. Gavin L, Pazol K. Update: providing quality family planning services - recommendations from CDC and the U.S. office of population affairs, 2015. MMWR Morb Mortal Wkly Rep. 2016;65:231–4.
13. Online training | Beyond the pill [Internet]. [cited 1 Dec 2018]. Available: http://beyondthepill.ucsf.edu/online-training.
14. Bartz D, Paris A, Maurer R, Gardner R, Johnson N. Medical student simulation training in intrauterine contraception insertion and removal: an intervention to improve comfort, skill, and attitudes. Contracept Reprod Med. 2016;1:3.
15. Dodge LE, Hacker MR, Averbach SH, Voit SF, Paul ME. Assessment of a high-fidelity mobile simulator for intrauterine contraception training in ambulatory reproductive health centres. J Eur CME. 2016;5:30416.
16. Nitschmann C, Bartz D, Johnson NR. Gynecologic simulation training increases medical student confidence and interest in women's health. Teach Learn Med. 2014;26:160–3.
17. Khadivzadeh T, Erfanian F. The effects of simulated patients and simulated gynecologic models on student anxiety in providing IUD services. Simul Healthc. 2012;7:282–7.
18. Motola I, Devine LA, Chung HS, Sullivan JE, Issenberg SB. Simulation in healthcare education: a best evidence practical guide. AMEE guide no. 82. Med Teach. 2013;35:e1511–30.
19. Lofaso DP, DeBlieux PM, DiCarlo RP, Hilton C, Yang T, Chauvin SW. Design and effectiveness of a required pre-clinical simulation-based curriculum for fundamental clinical skills and procedures. Med Educ Online. 2011;16. https://doi.org/10.3402/meo.v16i0.7132.
20. Ziv A, Wolpe PR, Small SD, Glick S. Simulation-based medical education: an ethical imperative. Acad Med. 2003;78:783–8.
21. Okuda Y, Bryson EO, DeMaria S Jr, Jacobson L, Quinones J, Shen B, et al. The utility of simulation in medical education: what is the evidence? Mt Sinai J Med. 2009;76:330–43.
22. Stitely ML, Cerbone L, Nixon A, Bringman JJ. Assessment of a simulation training exercise to teach intrauterine tamponade for the treatment of postpartum hemorrhage. J Midwifery Womens Health. 2011;56:503–6.
23. Daniels K, Lipman S, Harney K, Arafeh J, Druzin M. Use of simulation based team training for obstetric crises in resident education. Simul Healthc. 2008;3:154–60.
24. Ennen CS, Satin AJ. Training and assessment in obstetrics: the role of simulation. Best Pract Res Clin Obstet Gynaecol. 2010;24:747–58.
25. Goodman S, McNeil S, Shih G. Simulation for managing hemorrhage as a complication of uterine aspiration. MedEdPORTAL. 2015; https://doi.org/10.15766/mep_2374-8265.10296.
26. Goodman S. UCSF Bixby beyond the pill: protocol for the provision of IUD; LARC proctoring toolkit [Internet]. 2018 [cited 6 Jan 2019]. Available: https://beyondthepill.ucsf.edu/clinic-tools.
27. Steinauer J, Preskill F, Robertson P. Training medical students in intrauterine procedures using papayas. Med Educ. 2007;41:1099–100.
28. Levine AI, DeMaria S Jr, Schwartz AD, Sim AJ. The comprehensive textbook of healthcare simulation. New York: Springer Science & Business Media; 2013.
29. Sanders A, Wilson RD. Simulation training in obstetrics and gynaecology residency programs in Canada. J Obstet Gynaecol Can. 2015;37:1025–32.

30. IUD competency checklist. In: Beyond the pill [Internet]. [cited 2 Dec 2018]. Available: http://beyondthepill.ucsf.edu/sites/beyondthepill.ucsf.edu/files/Beyond%20the%20Pill%20 IUD%20Competency%20Checklists.pdf.
31. Gubrium AC, Mann ES, Borrero S, Dehlendorf C, Fields J, Geronimus AT, et al. Realizing reproductive health equity needs more than Long-Acting Reversible Contraception (LARC). Am J Public Health. 2016;106:18–9.
32. Higgins JA. Celebration meets caution: LARC's boons, potential busts, and the benefits of a reproductive justice approach. Contraception. 2014;89:237–41.
33. Potter J, Koyama A, Coles MS. Addressing the challenges of clinician training for long-acting reversible contraception. JAMA Pediatr. 2015;169:103–4.
34. MOU LARC clinical placement agreement template. In: Reproductive health access project [Internet]. [cited 1 Dec 2018]. Available: http://www.reproductiveaccess.org/wp-content/ uploads/2015/02/LARC-Clinical-Placement-Agreement-Template.doc.
35. Rubin SE, Maldonado L, Fox K, Rosenberg R, Wall J, Prine L. Establishing and conducting a regional, hands-on long-acting reversible contraception training center in primary care. Womens Health Issues. 2018;28:375–8.
36. Mays A, Harper C, Freeman L, Biggs MA. The role of proctoring to increase LARC access in community health centers. 2016 American public health conference; 2016 Nov.
37. Cason P, Goodman S. Protocol for provision of intrauterine contraception. San Francisco: UCSF Bixby Center Beyond the Pill; 2016. [Internet]. [cited 2 Dec 2018]. Available: https:// beyondthepill.ucsf.edu/sites/beyondthepill.ucsf.edu/files/Beyond%20the%20Pill%20 IUC%20Protocol.pdf.
38. This is how I teach: no touch technique for copper IUD - innovating education in reproductive health. In: Innovating education in reproductive health [Internet]. 17 Oct 2018 [cited 10 Jan 2019]. Available: https://innovating-education.org/2018/10/ this-is-how-i-teach-no-touch-technique-for-cooper-iud/.
39. Coles MS. IUD insertion task analysis. Developed through funding by the Society of Family Planning; Report no.: SFP5–11.
40. Curtis KM, Tepper NK, Jatlaoui TC, Berry-Bibee E, Horton LG, Zapata LB, et al. U.S. medical eligibility criteria for contraceptive use, 2016. MMWR Recomm Rep. 2016;65:1–103.
41. LILETTA insertion refresher sheet [Internet]. [cited 14 Dec 2018]. Available: https://www. lilettahcp.com/Content/pdfs/SHI_Refresher_Sheet.pdf.

Chapter 9
Pharmacologic Approaches to Pain Management with IUD Insertion

Aletha Y. Akers

Abbreviations

AYA	Adolescent and young adult
EMLA	Eutectic mixture of local anesthetics
IUD	Intrauterine device
NSAID	Non-steroidal anti-inflammatory agents

Learning Objectives

Following completion of this chapter, you should be able to:

- Discuss the complex nature of pain in gynecological procedures, including IUD placement.
- Review clinical guidelines to assist AYAs with pain control during procedures.
- Describe evidence-based pharmacological pain control modalities that can be used during IUD procedures.

Introduction

Patient fears that they may experience discomfort during gynecologic procedures are common and are one of the many identified barriers for younger patients considering intrauterine devices (IUDs) [1, 2]. While pain control options during gynecologic procedures are well studied, there is relatively limited information about these for adolescent and young adult (AYA) patients, particularly for those choosing IUDs.

A. Y. Akers (✉)
The Craig Dalsimer Division of Adolescent Medicine, The Children's Hospital of Philadelphia, Philadelphia, PA, USA
e-mail: akersa@email.chop.edu

© Springer Nature Switzerland AG 2019
M. S. Coles, A. Mays (eds.), *Optimizing IUD Delivery for Adolescents and Young Adults*, https://doi.org/10.1007/978-3-030-17816-1_9

Case

Miranda is a 15-year-old, sexually active, cisgender female who has never been pregnant, coming into clinic today for contraceptive counseling. At the end of her visit, she expresses interest in having a hormonal IUD placed. However, Miranda has never had a pelvic exam and confides in you that she is very nervous about the procedure. She states that her friend had an IUD placed; her friend said it hurt, and she was very uncomfortable for several days after the insertion.

Fear of Pain: The Role of Anxiety and Other Pain-Associated Manifestations

Young patients' concerns regarding pain during IUD insertion have been well described, and were noted as the primary reason younger patients were not interested in using an IUD in two national studies [1, 3]. Levels of pain that patients experience during IUD insertions vary widely in published reports. Clinical predictors of pain include the following [4, 5]:

- Nulliparity (patients who have never had a baby)
- Young age (<30 years)
- A longer interval since last pregnancy, or since last menses
- A history of dysmenorrhea

Psychosocial factors also influence reports of pain. Most notably, patients who report *higher levels of expected pain* prior to the IUD insertion procedure *are more likely to report experiencing higher pain during the procedure* [6]. In addition, AYAs have less experience with pelvic exams and other gynecologic procedures compared to adult patients, which may heighten anxiety and lower pain tolerance during procedures [1–3].

Although the literature on pain control during IUD insertion is substantial, the data have largely been inconclusive. Previous studies, including systematic reviews and meta-analyses, have evaluated various medications for controlling pain, including non-steroidal anti-inflammatory agents (NSAIDs), narcotics, anxiolytics, anesthetic spray or gel, nitroprusside, and misoprostol (a cervical softening agent); none of these were conclusively shown to be beneficial [4, 7–13]. Similarly, a 2015 Cochrane systematic review examining the efficacy of various medications for controlling pain during IUD insertion did not identify any method that conclusively reduced pain [14]. More recent studies showed mainly mixed results [15–17]. However recent studies suggest that local anesthetics may be beneficial.

Although research has not been conclusive in identifying specific pain control measures for AYAs having IUD insertions, pain perception is complex and multifactorial. Thus, we do recommend taking preventative measures to reduce patient pain during IUD placement. In this chapter, we examine **pharmacologic** pain control options to highlight to care for a patient like Miranda (from the case above). We begin by presenting guidelines for performing procedures with AYA patients, and continue by reviewing the neuroanatomy of pain responses during IUD insertion procedures. Non-pharmacologic pain management strategies will be addressed in the following chapter (Chap. 10).

Guidelines for AYA Procedures

A procedural experience can be stressful for any patient, regardless of age [18]. Guidelines for creating adolescent-centered procedural environments exist and have identified several key features that may be beneficial for AYA patients [19]. These are shown in Table 9.1 below. We recommend that providers assess and address patient fears and/or communication issues, educate about the procedure and the procedural environment, maintain privacy and confidentiality, identify and include key sources of social support (as appropriate), and serve as patient advocates.

There are some important differences when supporting AYA patients, as compared to adult patients, before and during procedures. For example, it is specifically recommended that young patients be allowed to examine the equipment to be used, to control the pace of the procedure, to have the opportunity to ask as many questions as needed prior to (and during) the procedure, and to have a support person(s) present [19]. Though these differences in the philosophical approach to structuring care experiences for AYA patients may affect procedure length, they ensure the highest level of both patient satisfaction and quality of care. Table 9.1 lists strategies clinicians can employ to help patients feel more comfortable during the IUD procedure.

Table 9.1 Some existing guidelines for creating adolescent-centered procedural environments

Key features of procedural case management that may benefit AYA patients	
Goals	Strategies
Procedural phases	
Reduce stress response Assess, address, and alleviate anxiety Identify barriers to communication Assess coping mechanisms Identify sources of social support	Provide education about the procedure Provide education about the procedural environment Advocate for the patient Encourage a sense of control Maintain privacy and confidentiality Answer questions Validate fears and concerns
Post-procedural phase	
Minimize pain Provide anticipatory guidance	Assess and address pain Provide education about the procedure and post-procedure guidance Ensure patient safety Encourage key social supports

Source: [19]

Anatomy of Pain (Brain, Nerves, and Uterus)

Pain during IUD insertion is relayed through multiple nerve fibers. Cervical pain is mediated by the S2 to S4 parasympathetic nerves, while the T10 to L1 sympathetic fibers innervate the uterine fundus. Therefore, pain during IUD insertion procedure is under different types of pain control (sympathetic and parasympathetic systems) and may be most responsive to **multimodal therapies.**

Multiple components of the IUD insertion procedure may result in patient pain or discomfort. These include:

- Insertion of the speculum
- Application of the tenaculum to the cervix
- Passage of the uterine sound
- Advancement of the inserter tube through the cervix
- Deployment of the IUD within the endometrial cavity

Uterine size may also play a role in the pain response. The size of a patient's uterus changes throughout the first two decades of life, with full adult morphology not achieved until most patients are in their early to mid-twenties [20]. Although the mean uterine size among AYAs is sufficient to accommodate an IUD, younger patients may be more likely to experience pain during IUD insertion, due to smaller average uterine size compared to older adult patients.

Understanding the **neurological basis** of pain during IUD insertion helps us to understand the potential utility of various pain mitigation approaches. Many types of pain reduction interventions have been trialed, including, but not limited to, oral narcotics NSAIDs, amide-anesthetics, and complementary and alternative approaches. The rationale for each of these methods is rooted in the neurologic and cognitive origins of the pain response. For example, paracervical infiltration of local anesthetic drugs interrupts the visceral sensory fibers of the lower uterus, cervix, and upper vagina (T10-L1) as they pass through the uterovaginal plexus on each side of the cervix. Acupuncture disrupts neurologic transmission of pain sensations via alternative mechanisms, which will be discussed in Chap. 10. The hopeful and planned end result of each of these methods is the same—less acute pain responses and a more positive overall procedural experience for the patient.

What pain reduction method(s) is/are selected will likely depend on patient factors (age, medical comorbidities) as well as logistical factors, such as what resources are readily available in a clinic setting. The next section reviews the evidence for various pharmacologic options.

Pharmacologic Pain Control

Table 9.2 summarizes the interventions, with evidence supporting their effectiveness at reducing pain during the IUD insertion procedure, along with the dose and route, or administration steps.

Table 9.2 Pharmacologic pain interventions

Effective pharmacologic options for managing pain
Pre-procedure administration of 550 mg oral naproxen, 50 mg oral tramadol, or 20–30 mg of oral ketorolac.
Notably, naproxen will likely be much easier for most clinical sites to obtain than ketorolac or tramadol. Also, tramadol is a controlled substance and may not be easily available in non-hospital-based clinical care sites.
Paracervical administration of 10–12 ml of 1% lidocaine, administered as:
1-2 mL at the tenaculum site.
Remainder given in divided doses at the 4 o'clock and 8 o'clock positions at the cervico-vaginal junction.
Topical 10% lidocaine spray administered as 3–4 sprays to the cervical surface, with one spray directed toward the cervical os.
EMLA cream (2.5% lidocaine and 2.5% prilocaine) administered as 5 g on the cervix and cervical opening 7 minutes before device insertion.

Source: [8, 14, 16, 21, 28, 32, 33, 40, 41]

NSAIDs Several studies have evaluated NSAIDs for pain control around IUD insertions. Eleven randomized, controlled trials have been published [4, 8, 13, 16, 17, 21–25] and do not provide convincing or consistent evidence that NSAIDs reduce pain *during* IUD insertion. There is good evidence that NSAIDs, **particularly naproxen**, *do reduce post-insertional pain* [8, 16]. If providers choose to use an NSAID, we recommend that clinicians administer the following doses:

- **Naproxen 550 mg, given at least 60 minutes prior to IUD insertion.**
- **Ketorolac 20–30 mg PO, given 40–60 minutes prior to IUD insertion.**

Tramadol Tramadol is a narcotic receptor agonist, with evidence from one trial supporting its value in reducing pain control during IUD insertion [21]. If providers choose to use tramadol, we recommend that clinicians administer the following dose:

- **Tramadol 50 mg, 60 minutes prior to IUD insertion.**

Lidocaine paracervical nerve blocks Paracervical blocks provide clinically significant pain control during many gynecologic procedures, including IUD placement [12, 26–29]. If providers choose to use a lidocaine paracervical block, we recommend that the following be administered:

- **2 mL of 1% lidocaine given at the tenaculum site, followed by 4–5 mL of 1% lidocaine at 4 o'clock and 8 o'clock at the cervico-vaginal junction, at least 3–5 minutes prior to the IUD insertion procedure (total of 10–12 mL of 1% lidocaine).**

Intracervical lidocaine One study of nulliparous adult women examined the effect of 1.8 mL of a 2% intracervical block, given 5 minutes prior to IUD insertion, as compared to 400 mg of oral ibuprofen given 1 hour prior to IUD insertion [30].

The study arms did not differ in mean pain scores assessed immediately after insertion, nor at 2 and 6 hours after IUD insertion.

- **Based on available data, *we do not recommend* using 2% intracervical lidocaine prior to IUD insertion as a pain reduction intervention.**

Intrauterine lidocaine infusion Nelson et al. [31] examined the effect of a 2% lidocaine intrauterine infusion (1.2 mL), compared to a 0.9% saline intrauterine infusion administered 3 minutes prior to IUD insertion. No effect was noted.

- **Based on available data, *we do not recommend* intrauterine infusion of 2% lidocaine as a pain reduction intervention prior to IUD insertion.**

Topical lidocaine spray Two studies have examined the effect of a 10% lidocaine spray on pain during IUD insertion [32, 33]. One study examined the effect of a 10% lidocaine spray (each spray delivers 0.1 mL, 10 mg of lidocaine), administered 3 minutes prior to the procedure on pain during IUD insertion among parous patients [32]. The 10% lidocaine spray was administered as three puffs to the cervical surface, and one puff toward the cervical os, for a total of 40 mg. Those receiving the lidocaine spray noted lower pain scores than the placebo group. If providers choose to use a 10% lidocaine spray, we recommend that the following be administered:

- **10% lidocaine spray administered as three (30 mg lidocaine) to four (40 mg lidocaine) sprays to the cervical surface, with at least one spray directed toward the cervical os.**

G. Lidocaine gel Five trials examined 2% topical lidocaine gel, compared to placebo [34–38]. None showed a reduction in pain at IUD insertion, although lidocaine gel may reduce pain with tenaculum placement. A more recent pilot study looking at a novel formulation of lidocaine gel demonstrated pain reduction with IUD placement procedures [39].

- **Based on available data, *we do not recommend* routine application of 2% lidocaine gel as a pain reduction intervention prior to IUD insertion.**

EMLA cream Three trials compared Eutectic mixture of local anesthetics EMLA cream (2.5% lidocaine and 2.5% prilocaine) to placebo, and noted significant reductions in pain [40, 41]. Investigators applied 5 g on the cervix and cervical opening, 7 minutes before intrauterine device insertion. If providers choose to use a EMLA cream, we recommend:

- **Administering 5 g of EMLA on the cervix and cervical opening *7 minutes* before IUD insertion.**

Nitrous oxide donors (nitroprusside and nitroglycerin ointment) Three studies have assessed medical treatments that serve as nitrous oxide donors [7, 42, 43]. One study evaluated intracervical administration of 10% nitroprusside aqueous gel [7], a second study administered nitroglycerin ointment [42], and a third study compared inhaled oxygen (O_2) to a mixture of 50% nitrous oxide and 50% oxygen through a nasal mask. None of these studies showed a benefit of nitrous oxide donors on pain during IUD insertion.

- **Based on available data,** *we do not recommend* **use of nitrous oxide donors as a pain reduction intervention prior to IUD insertion.**

Misoprostol Eleven trials have evaluated the effect of 400 mg of misoprostol on pain during IUD insertion, when administered orally, buccally, vaginally, or sublingually from 60 minutes to 8 hours prior to IUD insertion [9–11, 25, 44–49]. Findings from a meta-analysis showed no benefit, and potentially greater cramps and pain, while findings from four trials not included in the meta-analysis were mixed [9, 47, 48].

- **Based on available data,** *we do not recommend* **routine use of misoprostol as a pain reduction intervention prior to IUD insertion.**

Other methods Several trials have used randomized, controlled study designs to manipulate other aspects of the IUD insertion procedure to examine the effect on patient-reported pain. *One trial compared different types of cervical stabilizers (vulsellum, or a single-tooth tenaculum)* and found no difference in pain [50].

Special Considerations

Most patients can have their IUD placed in an outpatient setting with the aforementioned proactive pharmacologic pain control measures, in addition to the non-pharmacological pain control measures to be discussed in Chap. 10. However, providers should consider that there are some individuals who may benefit from additional tailoring of the procedural experience, such as those with cognitive delay, physical disabilities, very young age (ages 11–13 years), severe anxiety, trauma, gender dysphoria, or pain disorders. In particular, with patients who may be experiencing gender dysphoria, it is important to not make assumptions about prior vaginal penetration and comfort with speculum placement or intrauterine procedures. Individual patient needs should be considered prior to procedural scheduling, as the logistics for IUD placement in an operative room, and/or under light-to-moderate sedation may be more complicated and many require advanced planning for the patient or their family.

Additional considerations for pain management may be needed for young people with select medical conditions. For example, some young people with contraindications to NSAIDs may be able to be allowed by their subspecialty provider to take one dose of NSAID prior to the procedure. This should be confirmed before the procedure. Others should have tramadol ordered prior to the procedure. Providers for patients with bleeding disorders should discuss IUD placement with the hematologist prior to the procedure regarding strategies for minimizing bleeding during placement.

Conclusion

Concerns about pain during IUD insertion are a major barrier to uptake of IUDs among AYA patients who may otherwise be interested in this method. Although few studies of pain control options have been conducted in this population, available data suggest that several pharmacologic interventions discussed in this chapter may be beneficial (see Table 9.2). Pre-procedure naproxen, ketorolac, or tramadol can help to reduce post-procedure discomfort. Paracervical nerve blockage with lidocaine-based anesthetics, topical lidocaine spray, or EMLA cream also appear to reduce pain with IUD insertion. Intravaginal 2% lidocaine gel may reduce pain with tenaculum placement. Multimodal therapies that include both pharmacologic and non-pharmacologic options, as addressed in the following chapter, may be the most beneficial.

Clinical Pearls
- Perception of pain varies across individuals and is multifaceted, including anatomic, physiologic, and psychologic inputs.
- Though pharmacologic options for pain management with IUDs have been well studied, ongoing research continues to identify promising medical interventions to reduce pain.
- NSAIDs, tramadol, and lidocaine (administered as a paracervical injection, or topically to the cervix) are evidence-based options for reducing pain during (or after) IUD insertions.
- Multimodal therapies, including pharmacologic and non-pharmacologic approaches, will best support patients through their IUD placements.

References

1. Fleming KL, Sokoloff A, Raine TR. Attitudes and beliefs about the intrauterine device among teenagers and young women. Contraception. 2010;82:178–82.
2. Kavanaugh ML, Frohwirth L, Jerman J, Popkin R, Ethier K. Long-acting reversible contraception for adolescents and young adults: patient and provider perspectives. J Pediatr Adolesc Gynecol. 2013;26:86–95.
3. Kavanaugh M, Frohwirth L, Jerman J, Popkin R, Ethier K. Long-acting reversible contraception for adolescents and young adults: service availability, provider attitudes and patient perspectives. J Adolesc Health. 2013;52:S88–9.
4. Hubacher D, Reyes V, Lillo S, Zepeda A, Chen P-L, Croxatto H. Pain from copper intrauterine device insertion: randomized trial of prophylactic ibuprofen. Am J Obstet Gynecol. 2006;195:1272–7.
5. Kaislasuo J, Heikinheimo O, Lähteenmäki P, Suhonen S. Predicting painful or difficult intrauterine device insertion in nulligravid women. Obstet Gynecol. 2014;124:345–53.
6. Murty J. Use and effectiveness of oral analgesia when fitting an intrauterine device. J Fam Plann Reprod Health Care. 2003;29:150–1.

7. Bednarek PH, Micks EA, Edelman AB, Li H, Jensen JT. The effect of nitroprusside on IUD insertion experience in nulliparous women: a pilot study. Contraception. 2013;87:421–5.
8. Massey SE, Varady JC, Henzl MR. Pain relief with naproxen following insertion of an intrauterine device. J Reprod Med. 1974;13:226–31.
9. Heikinheimo O, Inki P, Kunz M, Parmhed S, Anttila A-M, Olsson S-E, et al. Double-blind, randomized, placebo-controlled study on the effect of misoprostol on ease of consecutive insertion of the levonorgestrel-releasing intrauterine system. Contraception. 2010;81:481–6.
10. Dijkhuizen K, Dekkers OM, Holleboom CAG, de Groot CJM, Hellebrekers BWJ, van Roosmalen GJJ, et al. Vaginal misoprostol prior to insertion of an intrauterine device: an RCT. Hum Reprod. 2011;26:323–9.
11. Edelman AB, Schaefer E, Olson A, Van Houten L, Bednarek P, Leclair C, et al. Effects of prophylactic misoprostol administration prior to intrauterine device insertion in nulliparous women. Contraception. 2011;84:234–9.
12. Tangsiriwatthana T, Sangkomkamhang US, Lumbiganon P, Laopaiboon M. Paracervical local anaesthesia for cervical dilatation and uterine intervention. Cochrane Database Syst Rev. 2013;2013:CD005056.
13. Bednarek PH, Creinin MD, Reeves MF, Cwiak C, Espey E, Jensen JT, et al. Prophylactic ibuprofen does not improve pain with IUD insertion: a randomized trial. Contraception. 2015;91:193–7.
14. Lopez LM, Bernholc A, Zeng Y, Allen RH, Bartz D, O'Brien PA, et al. Interventions for pain with intrauterine device insertion. Cochrane Database Syst Rev. 2015;2015:CD007373.
15. Fouda UM, Salah Eldin NM, Elsetohy KA, Tolba HA, Shaban MM, Sobh SM. Diclofenac plus lidocaine gel for pain relief during intrauterine device insertion. A randomized, double-blinded, placebo-controlled study. Contraception. 2016;93:513–8.
16. Ngo LL, Ward KK, Mody SK. Ketorolac for pain control with intrauterine device placement: a randomized controlled trial. Obstet Gynecol. 2015;126:29–36.
17. Ngo LL, Braaten KP, Eichen E, Fortin J, Maurer R, Goldberg AB. Naproxen sodium for pain control with intrauterine device insertion: a randomized controlled trial. Obstet Gynecol. 2016;128:1306–13.
18. Bailey L. Strategies for decreasing patient anxiety in the perioperative setting. AORN J. 2010;92:445–57; quiz 458–60.
19. Monahan JC. Using an age-specific nursing model to tailor care to the adolescent surgical patient. AORN J. 2014;99:733–49.
20. Sultan C. Pediatric and adolescent gynecology: evidence-based clinical practice. Basel: Karger Medical and Scientific Publishers; 2012.
21. Karabayirli S, Ayrim AA, Muslu B. Comparison of the analgesic effects of oral tramadol and naproxen sodium on pain relief during IUD insertion. J Minim Invasive Gynecol. 2012;19:581–4.
22. Jensen HH, Blaabjerg J, Lyndrup J. Prophylactic use of prostaglandin synthesis inhibitors in connection with IUD insertion. Ugeskr Laeger. 1998;160:6958–61.
23. Chor J, Bregand-White J, Golobof A, Harwood B, Cowett A. Ibuprofen prophylaxis for levonorgestrel-releasing intrauterine system insertion: a randomized controlled trial. Contraception. 2012;85:558–62.
24. Crawford M, Davy S, Book N, Elliott JO, Arora A. Oral ketorolac for pain relief during intrauterine device insertion: a double-blinded randomized controlled trial. J Obstet Gynaecol Can. 2017;39:1143–9.
25. Elkhouly NI, Maher MA. Different analgesics prior to intrauterine device insertion: is there any evidence of efficacy? Eur J Contracept Reprod Health Care. 2017;22:222–6.
26. Hindocha A, Beere L, O'Flynn H, Watson A, Ahmad G. Pain relief in hysterosalpingography. Cochrane Database Syst Rev. 2015;2015:CD006106.
27. Renner RM, Jensen JT, Nichols MD, Edelman AB. Pain control in first-trimester surgical abortion: a systematic review of randomized controlled trials. Contraception. 2010;81:372–88.

28. Akers AY, Steinway C, Sonalkar S, Perriera LK, Schreiber C, Harding J, et al. Reducing pain during intrauterine device insertion: a randomized controlled trial in adolescents and young women. Obstet Gynecol. 2017;130:795–802.
29. Perez-Lopez FR, Martinez-Dominguez SJ, Perez-Roncero GR, Hernandez AV. Uterine or paracervical lidocaine application for pain control during intrauterine contraceptive device insertion: a meta-analysis of randomised controlled trials. Eur J Contracep Reprod Health Care. 2018;23:207–17.
30. Castro TVB, Franceschini SA, Poli-Neto O, Ferriani RA, Silva de Sá MF, Vieira CS. Effect of intracervical anesthesia on pain associated with the insertion of the levonorgestrel-releasing intrauterine system in women without previous vaginal delivery: a RCT. Hum Reprod. 2014;29:2439–45.
31. Nelson AL, Fong JK. Intrauterine infusion of lidocaine does not reduce pain scores during IUD insertion. Contraception. 2013;88:37–40.
32. Aksoy H, Aksoy Ü, Ozyurt S, Açmaz G, Babayigit M. Lidocaine 10% spray to the cervix reduces pain during intrauterine device insertion: a double-blind randomised controlled trial. J Fam Plann Reprod Health Care. 2016;42:83–7.
33. Karasu Y, Cömert DK, Karadağ B, Ergün Y. Lidocaine for pain control during intrauterine device insertion. J Obstet Gynaecol Res. 2017;43:1061–6.
34. Allen RH, Raker C, Goyal V. Higher dose cervical 2% lidocaine gel for IUD insertion: a randomized controlled trial. Contraception. 2013;88:730–6.
35. Maguire K, Davis A, Rosario Tejeda L, Westhoff C. Intracervical lidocaine gel for intrauterine device insertion: a randomized controlled trial. Contraception. 2012;86:214–9.
36. Mohammad-Alizadeh-Charandabi S, Seidi S, Kazemi F. Effect of lidocaine gel on pain from copper IUD insertion: a randomized double-blind controlled trial. Indian J Med Sci. 2010;64:349–55.
37. McNicholas CP, Madden T, Zhao Q, Secura G, Allsworth JE, Peipert JF. Cervical lidocaine for IUD insertional pain: a randomized controlled trial. Am J Obstet Gynecol. 2012;207:384.e1–6.
38. Rapkin RB, Achilles SL, Schwarz EB, Meyn L, Cremer M, Boraas CM, et al. Self-administered lidocaine gel for intrauterine device insertion in nulliparous women: a randomized controlled trial. Obstet Gynecol. 2016;128:621–8.
39. Abd Ellah NH, Abouelmagd SA, Abbas AM, Shaaban OM, Hassanein KMA. Dual-responsive lidocaine in situ gel reduces pain of intrauterine device insertion. Int J Pharm. 2018;538:279–86.
40. Tavakolian S, Doulabi MA, Baghban AA, Mortazavi A, Ghorbani M. Lidocaine-prilocaine cream as analgesia for IUD insertion: a prospective, randomized, controlled, triple blinded study. Glob J Health Sci. 2015;7:399–404.
41. Abbas AM, Abdellah MS, Khalaf M, Bahloul M, Abdellah NH, Ali MK, et al. Effect of cervical lidocaine-prilocaine cream on pain perception during copper T380A intrauterine device insertion among parous women: a randomized double-blind controlled trial. Contraception. 2017;95:251–6.
42. Micks EA, Jensen JT, Bednarek PH. The effect of nitroglycerin on the IUD insertion experience in nulliparous women: a pilot study. Contraception. 2014;90:60–5.
43. Singh RH, Thaxton L, Carr S, Leeman L, Schneider E, Espey E. A randomized controlled trial of nitrous oxide for intrauterine device insertion in nulliparous women. Int J Gynaecol Obstet. 2016;135:145–8.
44. Ibrahim ZM, Sayed Ahmed WA. Sublingual misoprostol prior to insertion of a T380A intrauterine device in women with no previous vaginal delivery. Eur J Contracep Reprod Health Care. 2013;18:300–8.
45. Sääv I, Aronsson A, Marions L, Stephansson O, Gemzell-Danielsson K. Cervical priming with sublingual misoprostol prior to insertion of an intrauterine device in nulliparous women: a randomized controlled trial. Hum Reprod. 2007;22:2647–52.
46. Scavuzzi A, Souza ASR, Costa AAR, Amorim MMR. Misoprostol prior to inserting an intrauterine device in nulligravidas: a randomized clinical trial. Hum Reprod. 2013;28:2118–25.

47. Lathrop E, Haddad L, McWhorter CP, Goedken P. Self-administration of misoprostol prior to intrauterine device insertion among nulliparous women: a randomized controlled trial. Contraception. 2013;88:725–9.
48. Espey E, Singh RH, Leeman L, Ogburn T, Fowler K, Greene H. Misoprostol for intrauterine device insertion in nulliparous women: a randomized controlled trial. Am J Obstet Gynecol. 2014;210:208.e1–5.
49. Swenson C, Turok DK, Ward K, Jacobson JC, Dermish A. Self-administered misoprostol or placebo before intrauterine device insertion in nulliparous women: a randomized controlled trial. Obstet Gynecol. 2012;120:341–7.
50. Doty N, MacIsaac L. Effect of an atraumatic vulsellum versus a single-tooth tenaculum on pain perception during intrauterine device insertion: a randomized controlled trial. Contraception. 2015;92:567–71.

Chapter 10
Nonpharmacologic Approaches to Pain Management with IUD Insertion

Rachel C. Passmore and Melanie A. Gold

Abbreviations

AYA   Adolescent and Young Adult
IUD   Intrauterine Device
SBHC   School-Based Health Center

Learning Objectives
Following completion of this chapter, you should be able to:

1. Describe the range of nonpharmacologic treatment options available for IUD-related pain.
2. Identify which nonpharmacologic treatment options best fit within your practice setting when providing IUD services.
3. Create a plan for how you can integrate nonpharmacologic treatment options into pain management in your clinical practice.

Introduction

There are a number of nonpharmacologic approaches one can offer to help adolescent and young adults (AYAs) manage anxiety, discomfort, and pain related to bimanual and speculum exams and intrauterine device (IUD) insertions. These may include diaphragmatic breathing, hypnotic language, music, heat packs, social support ("IUD doula"), aromatherapy, acupressure, and acupuncture. Given the clear

R. C. Passmore (✉)
Department of Population and Family Health, Columbia University Mailman School of Public Health, New York, NY, USA

M. A. Gold
Department of Pediatrics, Division of Child and Adolescent Health, Columbia University Irving Medical Center/New York–Presbyterian Hospital, New York, NY, USA

© Springer Nature Switzerland AG 2019
M. S. Coles, A. Mays (eds.), *Optimizing IUD Delivery for Adolescents and Young Adults*, https://doi.org/10.1007/978-3-030-17816-1_10

and direct relationship between anxiety and pain perception [1], any nonpharmaco-logic approaches that reduce anxiety have the potential to reduce pain associated with IUD insertions.

Case

KC is a 16-year-old, cisgender female who comes to your office requesting an IUD for contraception. She has been sexually active with a single male partner for the past 3 months and reports using condoms every time she has sex. But last time she had sex (2 weeks ago), the condom broke. KC took an oral emergency contraceptive pill the next day; she now worries more about getting pregnant and wants a better form of contraception. She read online about all the methods, and decided she wants a hormonal IUD. KC has never had a pelvic exam before.

After confirming her knowledge and understanding of the method, you explain the IUD insertion procedure and obtain patient consent. KC seems nervous, but in control. You begin to do the bimanual exam, and KC clenches her legs together, raises her hips off the table, and starts to cry and hyperventilate. You stop the procedure and talk with her, and KC is able to slow her breathing down and stop crying. You complete the bimanual exam, but it takes over 10 minutes to do this. When you attempt to insert the speculum, she cries and hyperventilates. You stop. What do you do next?

Breathing and Isometric Muscle Exercises

Diaphragmatic Breathing Diaphragmatic breathing is performed by contracting the diaphragm. Air enters the lungs, and the chest rises and the belly expands during this type of breathing. Diaphragmatic breathing encourages full oxygen exchange—the beneficial trade of incoming oxygen for outgoing carbon dioxide [2]—and is recommended to help patients feel more comfortable during IUD insertions, as well as with other gynecologic procedures [3].

Here is a diaphragmatic breathing technique that you can use with your patients:

- **Begin by asking the patient's permission** to walk them through a breathing exercise, and explain that the patient can then utilize this technique throughout the procedure.
- Ask the patient to focus on their breathing cycles, and to imagine each 'rise and fall of the chest' breathing cycle to be like a wave.
- Explain to the patient that they can breathe in through their nose for 3 seconds, watching their diaphragm and chest rise, and then breathe out through their mouth for 6 seconds, watching their chest and diaphragm fall.
- Support the patient by counting aloud for the first few breathing cycles, until the patient no longer needs support to maintain the breathing focus.

Yoga-Based Exercises Yoga uses breathing techniques in combination with physical movements. The "breathing exercises used in yoga can also reduce pain [as] exhalation can help produce relaxation and reduce tension. Awareness of breathing helps to achieve calmer, slower respiration and aid in relaxation and pain management" [4]. This can help to reduce dysmenorrhea intensity and pain duration [4].

Isometric Exercises Isometric exercises use deep breathing in the supine position, along with muscle contraction, and can help relieve the pain and duration of primary dysmenorrhea symptoms [5].

Here is a method for talking a patient through an isometric exercise [6]:

- Instruct the patient to intensely grip arm, hand, leg, and foot muscles, while at the same time keeping the abdominal muscles soft and relaxed. There is no need to bring the legs together, no need to change position on the examination table—just ask the patient to strongly tense the muscles.
- Demonstrate which muscles the patient should tense by touching the lower leg, foot, knee, lower thigh, hand, and arm.
- You can say: "Tense up your muscles here, all of the muscles in your hands and arms and feet and legs—you don't need to move them at all—just grip your muscles really strongly. Now hold it … hold it."
- Advise the patient to hold the contraction until you think they may be getting tired and, then, have them take a break for a moment. "And now grip your muscles again, really tightly!" You can continue to do this for as many cycles as is necessary, but often once or twice is sufficient.

It is reasonable to offer patients support and instruction on the above breathing techniques during and after IUD procedures to help ameliorate pain. It may also be helpful to time the placement of the tenaculum with the patient's slow, rhythmic breathing (not when coughing) and to gently rock the tenaculum in place during slow exhalation rather than quickly pinching the tenaculum onto the cervix.

Pelvic and Gluteal Muscle Contraction and Release

A quick muscle contraction-release exercise similar to that discussed above can be useful for patients with pre-placement anxiety, or for those with a heightened sense of pain or discomfort with bimanual exam or speculum placement. The goal of the exercise is to identify the pelvic floor and gluteal muscles that can reflexively contract in an anxious patient, and to help the patient relax and release those muscles in order to decrease discomfort during the procedure.

An example of how to guide patients through pelvic and gluteal muscle contraction and release:

- **Begin by asking the patient's permission** to walk through a simple muscle relaxation exercise that will help them to relieve tension and make placement of their IUD more comfortable.

- While the patient is lying on the examining bed, ask the patient to take a deep breath in and contract or squeeze the gluteal or "butt" muscles and hold for 3 seconds.
- Place your hands on the patient's contracted gluteal muscles. When the patient releases the contracted gluteal muscles, use gentle pressure downward, allowing the muscles of the pelvic floor and gluteus to relax, with the goal of the gluteal muscles releasing down into the table.
- Next, introduce the bimanual exam fingers, one finger at a time, just inside the vaginal introitus, placing gentle posterior vaginal wall pressure.
- Instruct the patient to take a breath in, contract the gluteal muscles, and hold that contraction for 2–3 seconds.
- As the patient releases the breath, give gentle downward pressure on the posterior vaginal introitus and vaginal walls, allowing those muscles to relax and release.

Hypnotic Language

Hypnotherapy is also called clinical hypnosis and entails a trance-like state in which one has heightened focus and concentration [7]. **Guided imagery** is a language-based imagery intervention similar to hypnosis. **Pleasant imagery** is a specific type of guided imagery, in which patients listen to scripts that instruct them to focus all of their senses on a specific, relaxing scene (such as beach or mountain landscape).

Here are the some details for using these techniques with patients:

- Prior to the procedure, inquire about past experiences with gynecologic exams and/or procedures, as well as any issues of sexual abuse or assault and issues around control.
- As you start the examination and conduct the procedure, tell the patient what you will do before you do it, not as you are doing it or after you have done it. It can be helpful to suggest: "You can listen to what I am saying… and at the same time tune out and go to a place where you feels relaxed, comfortable, and in control."
- Encourage patient participation during the exam, and convey that the patient has a clear role during exam—this is not done *to* the patient, but *with* the patient. One way to incorporate hypnotic imagery into the IUD procedure is to ask the AYA to identify a favorite place and an activity that the AYA enjoys doing there.
- Give suggestions for feeling comfort and control, such as "now you might notice the feeling of the bed supporting your back, the crinkling sound of the clean white paper," and "you may find it helpful to place your hand on your own abdomen and feel that deep breath into your belly—you breathe in comfort, and breathe out tension."

- As you examine the patient, tell them what you are looking for and what you find; reassure when findings are normal, and calmly notify when abnormalities are found. It has been suggested that using open-ended statements such as "you may feel something now" allows for patients' widely varying responses to stimuli and is less likely to invoke a nocebo reaction [8].
- Avoid language that sets up an expectation of pain, such as "if anything is painful or hurts, tell me," or "this will not hurt." Opt for statements like, "now you may notice a different feeling, it may be like pressure, or pulling, or stretching — or like you have to pee, but if it bothers you, let me know. What does it feel like to you?"

It is particularly helpful to have the AYA patient lay flat, not upright, on the table *during the IUD procedure* to avoid vasovagal response. It is also useful to suggest that the patient push their hips into the table whenever they feel the urge to "do something," rather than pull away or up toward the head of the bed. At the conclusion of the procedure, the medical provider can suggest, "it may surprise you to notice how much easier each future gynecologic exam may be…now that you know how to help yourself relax with your breathing and feel better," and to remind patients that "you can practice diaphragmatic breathing whenever you want to help yourself feel calmer and more relaxed."

Music

Music can be considered therapeutic; it can be calming as well as distracting; therefore, music may reduce patients' anxiety and/or pain related to procedures. One expert recommends that music interventions be non-lyrical, slow (under 80 beats per minute), and low in volume (under 60 decibels), last for at least 30 minutes, and be chosen by the patient with informed support from the provider [9]. *We recommend offering to play soothing music during IUD insertion procedures.* This is best done when music is played *in the room*, rather than by headphones, as music has the capacity to reduce the anxiety of everyone in the room [10], including the patient, provider, and medical assistant.

Heat Therapy

It is common practice to offer heat packs to patients, to place on their lower abdomen, both during and after IUD insertion. Use of heat therapy to temporarily relieve dysmenorrhea is a common practice around the world [11–13]. Although high-quality research trials do not exist, *we recommend offering heat therapy*, in the form of hot packs or similar modalities, as a treatment for gynecologic procedures such as IUD insertions.

Social Support: "IUD Doula"

Social support, such as hand-holding or verbal assurance by a doula or medical assistant, has not been researched in relation to IUD or other gynecological procedures, with the exception of abortion. Qualitatively, trials [14–16] found that abortion support or the presence of doulas positively impacted patients' experience. In our experience, it is beneficial for *standard of care* to include a staff member, such as a medical assistant or a supportive peer, to serve as a *patient support or "IUD doula" during the IUD procedure*. It can be useful to suggest that the support person offer the patient two fingers to hold and ask them to "squeeze and put all the scary or nervous feelings into those fingers."

Acupressure and Acupuncture

Acupoints—points on the body through which qi energy flows—can be stimulated in a variety of ways, including by pressure from fingers or seeds/pellets (acupressure) and by needles with or without electricity (acupuncture), heat, or lasers. Recently, a randomized trial on pain management in first-trimester abortion patients showed that auricular acupuncture, which includes stimulating acupoints to subside uterine cramping, was successful in alleviating pain as compared to placebo and standard care groups [17]. When acupressure has been used to treat uterine cramping from dysmenorrhea, meta-analyses show improvements in pain relief compared with placebo, nonsteroidal anti-inflammatory medications and Chinese herbs [18, 19], without significant adverse effects. Given this, *acupressure can be a reasonable first line nonpharmacologic treatment* option to offer AYAs during, and post-IUD insertion.

Acupressure has been incorporated into the standard of care for AYA patients receiving IUD insertions at the New York-Presbyterian Hospital School-Based Health Centers (SBHCs) since February 2018. Pressing bilaterally for 2 minutes on the acupoint called Spleen 6 (Sanyinjiao), located four fingers above the top of the inner ankle bone (medial malleolus), has been shown to alleviate uterine pain and related stress in a safe manner [20–22]. Figure 10.1 shows an educational handout about Spleen 6 acupressure for post-IUD insertion-related pain.

Aromatherapy

Anxiety before and during IUD procedures is common, and aromatherapy can help patients to manage these feelings. While the exact mechanism of action for aromatherapy is still under investigation, it has been suggested that "when a scent is inhaled, its molecules cause the release of different neurotransmitters, such as enkephalin, endorphins, noradrenaline, and serotonin, which ultimately results in decrease in anxiety [24]."

The essential oil blends we recommend are "Clear" containing peppermint, lemon, orange, and eucalyptus or "Balance" containing lavender, ylang-ylang, mar-

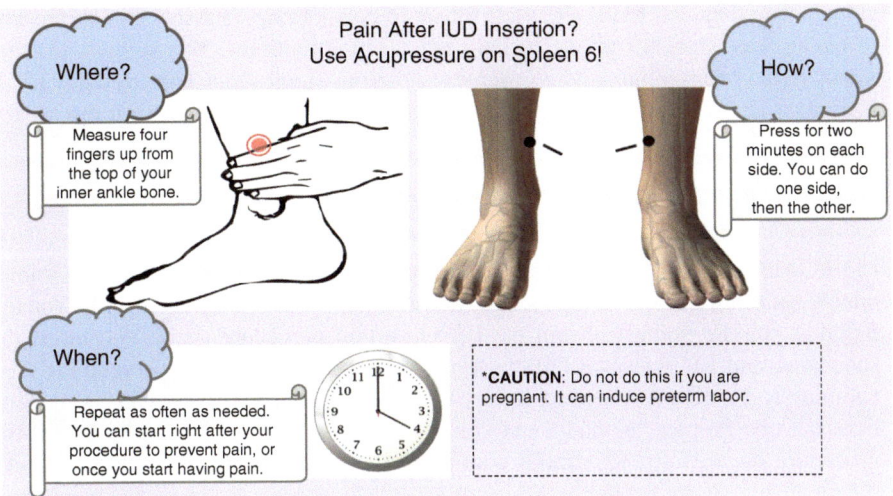

Fig. 10.1 An educational handout describing acupressure on Spleen 6 [23]

joram, and cedarwood. From personal clinical experience, aromatherapy is useful in three ways:

1. Diffusing (using water or dry diffuser) in the room where the IUD procedure will take place
2. Placing an essential oil on a gauze pad for the patient to inhale
3. Placing a drop of a specific essential oil on acupoints on the ears, hands, wrists, ankles, and feet to decrease anxiety and pain

Aroma Acupoint Therapy™ The Aroma Acupoint Therapy™ Protocol for Tense Conditions [25], entails placing a drop of the essential oils listed below bilaterally by fingertip application on each point for 90 seconds in the sequence given below. We have been using this protocol with great clinical success for dysmenorrhea in SBHCs, and have begun to offer it for IUD-related anxiety and pain management with plans to conduct research on its efficacy.

- Bergamot oil on the ear acupoint called Shen Men in the triangular fossa.
- Lavender oil on the dorsum of the hand at Large Intestine 4 (LI4 or Hegu).
- Roman Chamomile oil on the dorsum of the foot at Liver 3 (LIV3 or Taichong).
- Lavender oil on Pericardium 6 (PC6 or Neiguan).
- Atlas Cedarwood oil on Kidney 3 (KI3 or Taixi).

Case

You consider nonpharmacologic options. First, you ask KC if she would like to use aromatherapy to help her body relax. She agrees and you offer her a gauze pad with three drops of lavender oil on it to inhale. She takes a few inhalations and looks a bit calmer. You then ask KC if she finds music to be soothing, and she says she listens to ocean waves on her phone to help her sleep sometimes. You suggest playing music in the background, and KC agrees with your suggestion. Then you ask KC if it is okay if the medical assistant holds her hand and helps her breath during the procedure. She says she would like that.

You play soothing music on your computer while the medical assistant moves up to the head of the exam table and tells KC that she will guide her in some deep breathing exercises to help her feel more relaxed and comfortable during the procedure. KC begins to take slow, deep breaths as the medical assistant holds KC's hand. You immediately see more tension leave KC's body and her hips relax on the exam table. You tell KC that you are going to begin the IUD insertion procedure again. You insert the speculum, and KC winces a little between breaths but does not hyperventilate. You continue and notice KC holding tightly onto the medical assistant's fingers, but she does not cry. Progress is made, and you are able to swiftly complete the rest of the procedure successfully. KC smiles with relief once the procedure is over and thanks the medical assistant for her help. You offer KC a heat pack and show her how to use acupressure by pressing on Spleen 6 bilaterally if she has any post-procedural pain. After KC is dressed, you give her an extra heat pack to use at home and ask if she has any questions. She says she has only one: "Can you give this same support and these same treatments to my friend when she comes in for her IUD appointment next week?"

Conclusion

Nonpharmacologic modalities for pain and anxiety prevention and management related to IUD insertion are numerous, and many are easy to use. These modalities, ranging from diaphragmatic breathing to acupuncture, have the potential to support AYA patients in combination with pharmacologic modalities or on their own when pharmacologic modalities are contraindicated, ineffective, or unavailable.

Clinical Pearls
- Strategies including diaphragmatic breathing, isometric muscle contraction, hypnotic language, music, heat, and aromatherapy are effective adjunct, and stand-alone methods to reduce pain and anxiety during IUD insertions.
- Most nonpharmacologic pain reduction strategies are achievable in nearly all clinical settings without significant additional training.
- Acupressure, acupuncture, and acupoint aromatherapy can be highly effective at reducing IUD insertion-related pain by following emerging clinical guidelines (as noted in this chapter), with minimal additional training needs.

References

1. Rhudy JL, Meagher MW. Fear and anxiety: divergent effects on human pain thresholds. Pain. 2000;84:65–75.
2. Harvard Health Publishing. Learning diaphragmatic breathing – Harvard Health. In: Harvard Health [Internet]. [cited 2 Dec 2018]. Available: https://www.health.harvard.edu/lung-health-and-disease/learning-diaphragmatic-breathing.
3. Wu J, Chaplin W, Amico J, Butler M, Ojie MJ, Hennedy D, et al. Music for surgical abortion care study: a randomized controlled pilot study. Contraception. 2012;85:496–502.
4. Rakhshaee Z. Effect of three yoga poses (cobra, cat and fish poses) in women with primary dysmenorrhea: a randomized clinical trial. J Pediatr Adolesc Gynecol. 2011;24:192–6.
5. Azima S, Bakhshayesh HR, Kaviani M, Abbasnia K, Sayadi M. Comparison of the effect of massage therapy and isometric exercises on primary dysmenorrhea: a randomized controlled clinical trial. J Pediatr Adolesc Gynecol. 2015;28:486–91.
6. No more fainting in your practice [Internet]. [cited 2 Dec 2018]. Available: https://providers.bedsider.org/articles/no-more-fainting-in-your-practice.
7. Hypnosis – Mayo Clinic [Internet]. 1 Nov 2018 [cited 2 Dec 2018]. Available: https://www.mayoclinic.org/tests-procedures/hypnosis/about/pac-20394405.
8. Krauss BS. "This may hurt": predictions in procedural disclosure may do harm. BMJ. 2015;350:h649.
9. Nilsson U. The anxiety- and pain-reducing effects of music interventions: a systematic review. AORN J. 2008;87:780–807.
10. Bradt J, Dileo C, Shim M. Music interventions for preoperative anxiety. Cochrane Database Syst Rev. 2013:CD006908.
11. O'Connell K, Davis AR, Westhoff C. Self-treatment patterns among adolescent girls with dysmenorrhea. J Pediatr Adolesc Gynecol. 2006;19:285–9.
12. Wong CL, Ip WY, Lam LW. Self-care strategies among Chinese adolescent girls with dysmenorrhea: a qualitative study. Pain Manag Nurs. 2016;17:262–71.
13. Eryilmaz G, Ozdemir F. Evaluation of menstrual pain management approaches by northeastern Anatolian adolescents. Pain Manag Nurs. 2009;10:40–7.
14. Dennis A, Manski R, Blanchard K. A qualitative exploration of low-income women's experiences accessing abortion in Massachusetts. Womens Health Issues. 2015;25:463–9.
15. Kimport K, Cockrill K, Weitz TA. Analyzing the impacts of abortion clinic structures and processes: a qualitative analysis of women's negative experience of abortion clinics. Contraception. 2012;85:204–10.
16. Altshuler AL, Ojanen-Goldsmith A, Blumenthal PD, Freedman LR. A good abortion experience: a qualitative exploration of women's needs and preferences in clinical care. Soc Sci Med. 2017;191:109–16.
17. Ndubisi C, Danvers A, Gold MA, Morrow L, Westhoff CL. Auricular acupuncture as an adjunct for pain management during first trimester abortion: a randomized, double-blinded, three arm trial. Contraception. 2018. https://doi.org/10.1016/j.contraception.2018.11.016.
18. Smith CA, Armour M, Zhu X, Li X, Lu ZY, Song J. Acupuncture for dysmenorrhoea. Cochrane Database Syst Rev. 2016;4:CD007854.
19. Woo HL, Ji HR, Pak YK, Lee H, Heo SJ, Lee JM, et al. The efficacy and safety of acupuncture in women with primary dysmenorrhea: a systematic review and meta-analysis. Medicine. 2018;97:e11007.
20. Chung Y-C, Chen H-H, Yeh M-L. Acupoint stimulation intervention for people with primary dysmenorrhea: systematic review and meta-analysis of randomized trials. Complement Ther Med. 2012;20:353–63.
21. Kashefi F, Khajehei M, Ashraf AR, Jafari P. The efficacy of acupressure at the Sanyinjiao point in the improvement of women's general health. J Altern Complement Med. 2011;17:1141–7.
22. Pouresmail Z, Ibrahimzadeh R. Effects of acupressure and ibuprofen on the severity of primary dysmenorrhea. J Tradit Chin Med. 2002;22:205–10.

23. Warren L, Passmore RC. Educational handout on spleen 6 for SBHC patients. 2018.
24. Nikjou R, Kazemzadeh R, Rostamnegad M, Moshfegi S, Karimollahi M, Salehi H. The effect of lavender aromatherapy on the pain severity of primary dysmenorrhea: a triple-blind randomized clinical trial. Ann Med Health Sci Res. 2016;6:211–5.
25. Holmes P. About aroma acupoint therapy TM [Internet]. 2011 [cited 2 Dec 2018]. Available: http://www.snowlotus.org/about-aroma-acupoint-therapy-tm/.

Chapter 11
Follow-Up After IUD Insertions: Managing IUD Expectations, Addressing Side Effects, and Providing Post-Insertion Counseling

Mandy S. Coles

Abbreviations

AYA   Adolescent and Young Adult
BV   Bacterial Vaginosis
CDC   Centers for Disease Control
IUD   Intrauterine Device
LNG   Levonorgestrel
NSAIDs   Nonsteroidal Anti-inflammatory drugs
STI   Sexually Transmitted Infection

Learning Objectives
Following completion of this chapter, you should be able to:

1. Explain the rationale for scheduled versus problem-based visits after intrauterine device (IUD) insertion.
2. Describe the common and less common patient concerns after IUD insertion.
3. Utilize information presented to help manage IUD concerns.
4. Integrate a reproductive justice framework into discussions around IUD removal.

M. S. Coles (✉)
Department of Pediatrics, Boston University Medical Center, Boston, MA, USA
e-mail: mcoles@bu.edu

© Springer Nature Switzerland AG 2019   133
M. S. Coles, A. Mays (eds.), *Optimizing IUD Delivery for Adolescents and Young Adults*, https://doi.org/10.1007/978-3-030-17816-1_11

Introduction

Providers who place IUDs often ask patients to come back for a follow-up visit after their IUD insertions. Reasons for routine follow-up visits can include evaluating satisfaction with method choice, addressing method-associated side effects and patient concerns, reviewing prior education on what to expect with an IUD, and offering screening for pregnancy or sexually transmitted infections (STIs) as needed. While routine follow-up visits are not recommended [1]—due to a lack of consistent evidence that routine follow-up visits improve contraceptive method continuation rates or impact patient satisfaction [2–6]—they may be beneficial in the initial post-insertion periods and under some circumstances [7, 8]. Additionally, we know that it is clinical practice at many sites to offer routine follow-up visits. For these reasons, this chapter will provide guidelines for scheduled follow-up visits, as well as address how to manage patient-initiated visits for concerns after IUD placement.

Case

Alicia, a 17-year-old, gender queer youth, comes in to clinic for an urgent visit. They got their hormonal IUD 2 months ago. Alicia is worried about their health after hearing lots of negative things about IUDs from peers (especially around hormones). Alicia was scheduled to come back 4 weeks after insertion for a follow-up visit, but missed it because "things came up." Today, Alicia raises concerns around bleeding, weight gain, and mood changes.

Timing of IUD Follow-Up Visits

Initial post-insertion visits If you choose to routinely offer follow-up visits after IUD placement, the time frame for this visit may depend on patient population, perceived pregnancy risk, patient level of concern, encouragement of method continuation, or other factors. Many providers who care for adolescent and young adults (AYAs) find this initial follow-up visit especially important, though there is variation in the time frame that they have patients return. Some experts advocate for return visits in 1–2 weeks after insertion to address whatever it is that patients are feeling (cramping, bleeding) or hearing from others. Other experts recommend follow-up visits in the 4–6-week time frame. Individual patient factors, such as ability to come to clinic due to transportation or concerns around visit confidentiality, may make sooner (or in-person) follow-up visits more challenging. Alternatives for clinic-based follow-up visits include telephone calls by nursing staff, family planners, or providers or communication through electronic health record systems or text messages [9–11].

Additional scheduled follow-up visits Some clinicians will have patients return every 6–12 months for more routine follow-up visits. These may be helpful as opportunities to talk about general reproductive and sexual health, especially if patients are happy with their IUDs.

"Something isn't right" In addition to scheduled follow-up visits, patients should always be advised to contact their providers with any questions or concerns if, and when, they arise [1]. Patients may come back to clinic with concerns around pain with sex, or because their mother told them their IUD was causing weight gain; these young people are often unhappy with their IUDs and come in requesting IUD removal [12, 13]. If patients can get their concerns addressed in a more timely fashion, providers have found that they are much more open to continuing their IUDs, or at least having a conversation about contraceptive options. Providers often observe that the longer patients have been unhappy with their IUDs, the more difficult it becomes to address patient concerns with information or medication treatment options—and the more likely patients will choose IUD removal. For these reasons, we recommend repeating the message, "please contact us if you have any questions or concerns" as much as possible during IUD insertions and at any scheduled follow-up visits. Data show that AYA satisfaction around the initial adjustment and reassessment period after IUD insertion can be influenced by the amount of external support they receive, including from medical providers and clinic staff [13].

Material to Address During IUD Follow-Up Visits with AYAs

As clinicians, we all ensure that patients receive counseling before they have an IUD placed. This counseling may vary in terms of the information presented and the format (in person, paper, video, or online), as well as *who* is providing the counseling. Counseling is covered in detail in Chaps. 5 and 7. However, it is worth repeating that providing thorough pre-insertion contraceptive counseling [14, 15] is integral in helping patients to set expectations and to navigate the adjustment phase once they have their IUDs [13].

Should I be spotting? Is it normal to have cramps? Does this really work for birth control? These are just some of the questions that patients may ask you during follow-up appointments. And while patients may not remember discussing any of this information previously, these are all questions that you likely answered during your pre-insertion counseling. One way to think about framing follow-up visits is to review the information that was already discussed with patients. These conversations might start with, "Do you remember that we talked about…?" And while the answer may be "no," patients often repeat back the salient pre-insertion counseling messages that we focused on. *If the pre-insertion counseling is seen as an opportunity to set expectations, post-insertion follow-up visits can be seen as an opportunity to (re)set expectations.*

Some providers find it helpful to have a general script to use when they see patients for either a planned or an unplanned follow-up. A script allows a provider to elicit common concerns and also to assess patient satisfaction and potential points of discomfort that may not be brought up otherwise. In addition to gathering information from patients, this type of script can also be useful as a framework to provide anticipatory guidance around what to expect with an IUD moving forward. It can be helpful to start any routine or problem-based IUD follow-up visit by reviewing with patients their initial reasons for choosing an IUD. One recent study looking at counseling needs of nulliparous adolescents found that, in spite of any experienced side effects, the majority of individuals reported motivation to continue their IUD [13]. Some of the reported reasons included a strong desire to prevent pregnancy and prior experiences or dissatisfaction with other contraceptive methods. Table 11.1 presents one template for IUD follow-up visits.

Table 11.1 One general script template for an IUD follow-up visit	Template for follow-up after IUD insertion
	1. Reasons for choosing IUD
	2. Bleeding pattern
	3. Cramping
	4. Other side effects or concerns
	5. Unprotected sex since insertion and timing (to address pregnancy risk since placement)
	6. Method satisfaction
	7. String checks (not mandatory)
	8. Overall reproductive health (i.e. relationship safety, condom use, STI screening, etc.)
	Source: M. Coles

Case (continued)

You ask Alicia about their bleeding pattern. Alicia reports that they have spotting on most days, but it is starting to slow down. You use this as an opportunity to reassure them that this is a very normal bleeding pattern ("your uterus getting used to having something inside of it") and also remind them that they should expect to continue to have less bleeding over the next few weeks. You tell them that about half of people do not have any bleeding by about a year after insertion. Then, you inquire if their current bleeding pattern bothers Alicia, who answers, "As long as it stops soon, I can manage. Bleeding makes me feel really down, so if it doesn't stop sooner, I'm not going to be happy. I might want this IUD out."

Asking if [*fill in the* patient reported symptom *here*] bothers the patient can help to guide the amount of discussion around a specific topic, the plan (reassurance, close follow-up, treatment, or IUD removal), and timing of next visit.

Common Concerns and How to Address Them

Irregular or annoying bleeding Bleeding changes are one of the common concerns that young people report after having an IUD placed, with bleeding patterns ranging from no bleeding, to irregular bleeding, to menstrual-like bleeding. Specific bleeding patterns based upon IUD type are reviewed in Chaps. 3, 5, and 7, and can be viewed in detail. When seeing patients for follow-up, practitioners generally think about bleeding by (1) how recently the IUD was placed and (2) type of device.

Bleeding by time since placement

- *Up to 1 week after IUD insertion:* Bleeding or spotting immediately after IUD placement is common for both hormonal and copper IUDs, can last a few days, and should not be much heavier than a normal period [16, 17]. Any bleeding that is heavy—commonly described as needing to change a pad or tampon in less than 2 hours [18]—is atypical after an IUD insertion and needs to be further evaluated.
- *Weeks to months after IUD insertion:* We tend to think about this time period as an "IUD adjustment period" where people may experience irregular or intermenstrual bleeding within the first few months after placement [19]. This can be described as the uterus "getting used to having an IUD inside of it" and can occur with both hormonal and copper IUDs. This bleeding tends to be on the lighter side—think one to two pads, pantiliners, or tampons a day.
- *More than 3 months after IUD insertion:* Bleeding after the first few months varies by IUD type. It is reasonable to further evaluate any change in usual bleeding pattern, as discussed below.

Bleeding by type of IUD

- *Copper IUD:* Menstrual bleeding with a copper IUD may be similar to normal menses, but may also be heavier or last longer due to an increase in endometrial prostaglandin release [20]. Clinical pearl: Some experts recommend use of non-steroidal anti-inflammatory drugs (NSAIDs) around the time of menses for the first 6 months after copper IUD placement to reduce bleeding amount. Studies have found that menstrual-related symptoms (including cramping and bleeding) decrease over time [21, 22], supporting this interval for prophylactic medication. However, further research is needed regarding whether prophylactic treatment impacts continuation rates [23].
- *Hormonal IUDs:* Users may experience bleeding that is the same or lighter than their regular menses, and some will stop having menstrual bleeding within a year of placement [24]. Bleeding with a hormonal IUD will vary based on the amount of progesterone in the IUD, with less bleeding associated with higher levonorgestrel (LNG) delivery [25–27]. Spotting can also occur and is normal.

Managing patient response to bleeding pattern Even if a patient's bleeding pattern is normal or expected based upon time frame after IUD insertion or IUD type, the patient may not be happy with their bleeding pattern. Data demonstrate that people with heavier bleeding, or increased bleeding frequency were less likely to be satisfied with their method [17, 22], despite overall high rates of satisfaction. For this reason, we find it helpful to work with patients with nuisance bleeding in a step-by-step approach, as follows:

1. Acknowledge and validate patient concerns.
2. Evaluate if there is an underlying cause of the bleeding, such as IUD malpositioning, sexually transmitted infection, pregnancy, or new pathologic uterine condition [1].
3. Provide reassurance, and determine if this improves the individual's satisfaction with their IUD.
4. Inquire if the patient is interested in medication treatment to reduce or stop nuisance bleeding (see Table 11.2).
5. Ask if the patient wants to continue their IUD.

Table 11.2 Some medications that might aid in reducing nuisance bleeding

Medications to treat nuisance bleeding				
Medication	Dosing	Mechanism of action	Clinical pearls	Notes
Doxycycline	100 mg BID × 5 days (consider 10–14-day course if worried about endometritis)	Matrix metalloproteinase inhibitors	Use if concerned for underlying subacute infection	[32]
Tranexamic acid	1300 mg TID × 5 days	Antifibrinolytic	Consider for patients who need bleeding to stop as soon as possible, do not want hormones, and are not at high risk for blood clots	[34] Aminocaproic acid is an alternative option
Tamoxifen	10 mg BID × 5–10 days	Selective estrogen receptor modulator	This works well as a first-line option for a short-term method	[33]
Naproxen	500 mg BID × 5–10 days	Prostaglandin synthetase inhibitor	May work better for copper than hormonal IUDs	[29] Other NSAIDs may be used
Combined hormonal contraception (pill, patch, ring)	1. Short term for 7–14 days 2. Continuous use for up to 3 months	Stabilize endometrial lining	Consider for patients who want bleeding to stop, are okay with hormones, and are okay using a medication for months (instead of days)	[35, 36]

Sources indicated in the table

Clinical evaluation and management for underlying causes of nuisance bleeding We recommend that every patient who presents after IUD insertion, regardless of bleeding pattern, has a pregnancy test. The risk of pregnancy with an IUD in place is incredibly small [28], but does still exist. Additional evaluation of nuisance bleeding is well documented in the Centers for Disease Control and Prevention (CDC) Selected Practice Recommendations, which recommends considering an underlying gynecological problem, such as intrauterine device (IUD) displacement, STI, pregnancy, or new pathologic uterine conditions (e.g., polyps or fibroids) [1]. If an underlying gynecological problem is found, we recommend that you treat the condition or refer for care.

Case (continued)

You review Alicia's pregnancy test results, which are negative, and offer Alicia repeat STI testing, which they agree to. Based on Alicia's response that their bleeding makes them feel dysphoric and may be a reason for them to remove their IUD, you ask Alicia if they would like to talk about medication options to stop or slow down the bleeding. Alicia looks up and answers, "yes."

For individuals who experience nuisance or annoying bleeding without underlying cause (as above), it is reasonable to offer medication treatment options to try to reduce or stop the bleeding. A variety of medications have been studied as treatments of contraceptive-related unscheduled bleeding, though there is limited research looking specifically at IUD users. A review article that evaluated medication for treatment of bleeding irregularities in copper IUD noted that NSAIDs may reduce the amount menstrual blood loss, or the length of bleeding episodes [29]. Evidence suggests that NSAIDs function as prostaglandin synthetase inhibitors and thus help to decrease endometrial prostaglandin release and bleeding [24]. The authors also identified anti-fibrinolytics as potentially effective medications [29], and more recent research lends additional support to this [30]. At present, the CDC only recommends short-term use of NSAIDs for bleeding management, solely for copper IUD users [1], with no medications recommended for hormonal IUD users. While clearly an area that could benefit from additional research, in our clinical experience, medications that have been used to reduce nuisance bleeding in users of other contraceptive methods [31–33] may also be helpful for IUD users as well. These medications (listed in Table 11.2) may be reasonable to try in patients who would like treatment for bleeding and who do not have any medication-specific contraindications.

Case (continued)

You and Alicia discuss medications that can be used short term for 5–10 days, which "might stop or slow down the bleeding," and 3-month options, which " should stop the bleeding." Alicia initially says that they want a medicine that will stop the bleeding, but then looks uncomfortable when you talk about combined hormonal contraception, which contains estrogen. Alicia changes their mind and asks about the short-term options. After reviewing them, Alicia opts to try tranexamic acid because it will work quickly and does not have any hormones in it. They make a 2-week follow-up appointment to see how things are going.

If patients would like medication, we often ask them to decide if they want to start with a 3-month option or a 5- to 10-day option—often patients are guided by how much the bleeding is bothering them and how long they want to use another medication—and then go through the specific options. It is also important to have a follow-up plan if the bleeding or spotting continues, and to consider individual insurance coverage when making decisions around medication.

Uterine cramping or pain Cramping is another common complaint for AYAs who have IUDs. As with bleeding, there can be an adjustment period when patients may have increased cramping while the uterus gets used to having an IUD inside of it. We also know that pain perception is complex and multifactorial and may be influenced by anxiety and psychosocial factors as described in Chaps. 9 and 10. Specific cramping patterns based upon IUD type are also reviewed in Chap. 7 on consenting and can be viewed in detail. Concerns of cramping can be thought about based on (1) how recently the IUD was placed and (2) by the type of IUD.

Cramping by time since placement

- *Up to 1 week after IUD insertion:* Cramping tends to be most intense at the time of insertion and for many people quickly improves thereafter [37–39]. However, some people do experience a longer period of more intense cramping, which can last up to 5 days [39]. Clinical pearl: We recommend that patients take ibuprofen 600 mg every 6 hours for the initial 24 hours after IUD insertion and as needed thereafter (unless there is a contraindication to NSAIDs). Any cramping that is severe, described as worse than with a bad period, and is not improved with NSAIDS, is atypical after an IUD insertion and needs to be further evaluated.
- *Weeks to months after IUD insertion:* Some patients report intermittent cramping during this adjustment period. This can be described as the uterus "getting used to having an IUD inside of it" and can occur with both hormonal and copper IUDs.
- *More than 3 months after IUD insertion:* Cramping after the first few months varies by IUD type and may or may not be happen at the same time as bleeding. Intermenstrual cramping can also occur and is normal for all IUD types. It is reasonable to further evaluate any change in usual cramping pattern, as discussed below.

Cramping by type of IUD

- *Copper IUD:* Cramping with a copper IUD may be similar to a normal menses, but may also be stronger or last longer [17], due to an increase in endometrial prostaglandin release [20]. As discussed above, some experts recommend routine use of NSAIDs around the time of menses for the first 6 months after copper IUD placement to reduce cramping.

- *Hormonal IUDs:* Users may experience cramping that is the same or less than their regular menses, and some will stop having cramping altogether [17, 40]. The amount of cramping with a hormonal IUD will vary based on the amount of progesterone in the IUD.

Although cramping after an IUD insertion may be normal and expected, it can be quite uncomfortable; uncommonly, *this may be a sign that the IUD is malpositioned* [41]. If AYAs are concerned that pain means their IUD is out of place, this anxiety may increase both their awareness and perception of pain [42], as well as their desire for IUD removal. It is also worth noting that evidence is mixed as to whether IUD malpositioning leads to uterine symptoms. Experts suggest that addressing patient concerns and providing reassurance—including that the IUD is likely to be correctly positioned in the uterus [43], that cramping will improve over time, and that IUD continues to provide high contraceptive efficacy—are adequate interventions for most patients. That being said, studies demonstrate that people with increased cramping were less likely to be very happy with their IUD [17] and may be more likely to seek early IUD removal [44, 45].

Case (continued)

Alicia comes back to clinic 2 weeks later. Their bleeding has stopped, which they are very thankful for. But they are now worried about whether their IUD has moved. Last night they had a couple of hours of bad cramping, and they are having some mild cramping now despite taking ibuprofen. On further conversation, Alicia shares that they also had a new partner a few days ago and had sex without a condom and are worried and want to make sure that "everything is okay."

In addition to providing reassurance as discussed above, it is also reasonable to further evaluate uterine pain or cramping that continues to be concerning to patient, as well as any pain or cramping that is different from a patient's regular pattern or is severe in nature. Using a stepwise approach (such as suggested below) may help to identify IUD malposition or infection and can also provide additional reassurance to the patient. I usually start by asking patients if they have checked their IUD strings (discussed further below). If they can feel their IUD strings, I tell them that their IUD is likely in the right place. If they have not done a string check, I offer them the opportunity to do one in clinic themselves, or to have one done by a provider. For some patients, knowing that their IUD strings are palpable and of the correct length is reassuring. Others share that they will still be concerned, which leads to a conversation around a provider-performed bimanual exam to assess for uterine, adnexal, or cervical motion tenderness. STI testing via patient or provider collected vaginal swab can be done at this time or done via urine testing if a patient opts not to have an examination or string check. For those who will still be concerned about their cramping despite a potentially normal exam, we discuss the pros and cons of having a (likely transvaginal) ultrasound to confirm IUD placement.

Using this stepwise and patient-directed approach to evaluating concerning uterine cramping can provide reassurance for many of your patients. Some patients, however, feel that they will be worried regardless of the outcome of any imaging or examination and really would just like their IUD removed. In these cases, it is especially important to provide evidence-based information about IUD side effects and safety to ensure patient understanding and also to remove the IUD if the patient wishes.

Case (continued)

After a conversation with you, including the normalcy of cramping in the first month after IUD insertion and that this will likely improve over time, Alicia is still worried about their IUD. They choose to do a vaginal self-swab and also to try and do a string check themself, "anything to avoid something in my vagina again," they say. You provide some education on how to do string checks, give them with a vaginal swab, and leave the room after pulling the privacy curtain closed. You return a few minutes later, and Alicia shares that they felt their strings, are feeling better, and would like to know the results of their STI testing as soon as possible.

We do not recommend routine IUD string checks. Data show that the majority of IUD users did not check their IUD strings even when advised [46], and the CDC notes that providers should "*consider* performing an examination to check for the presence of the IUD strings," [1] without a mandate to do so. While not given as much emphasis as in the past, we do still talk with patients about string checks during follow-up visits to make sure that they at least know *how* to do them. The rationale for this, as noted above, is that if a patient calls with concerns about cramping or bleeding, one of the first questions will be, "Have you done a string check?" For some patients, string checks can also be helpful to reassure them that their IUD is still there. For individuals who have never done string checks, practitioners can explain them in the following way and offer them opportunity to try doing a string check in the office.

- Reassure: "It is okay to touch your own vagina."
- Educate: Your cervix feels like your nose—soft and squishy. Strings should be near the soft and squishy cervix.
- Explain: Different positions may make string checks easier (i.e., squatting, on your back with knees up, etc.).
- Acknowledge: Sometimes it can be difficult to feel strings. If you do not feel your IUD strings, do not panic.

Empower: If your IUD strings are bothering you or your partner, it is okay to push them back up into your vagina and toward your cervix. We can also trim them shorter if you would like.

Less Common IUD Concerns

The following concerns are less commonly reported by patients with IUDs (<10%). Some of these issues may not be related to the IUD itself, but may be perceived to be by patients. Clinicians need to ensure that all patients' concerns are heard and addressed.

Hormone-related concerns While the hormones in LNG IUDs work predominantly locally in the endometrial cavity and are unlikely to be present systemically at significant levels, especially after the first year [47], some individuals do complain of potentially hormone-related concerns. The most commonly reported of these in pre-market clinical trials include abdominal pain, headache, acne, mood changes, and breast tenderness [48]. Even if a provider believes that a patient's symptoms are unlikely to be caused by their IUD, it is clearly important to acknowledge and validate their concerns [13]. I will often say, "In my experience, I haven't see an IUD cause [*symptom*], but I hear that this is bothering you," or "I don't think that your IUD is causing [*symptom*], but I can never be 100% sure." Patients may be reassured by this or may be willing to continue their hormonal IUD for now, with a plan to follow up in the near future and continue to monitor their symptoms; others may still be concerned and seek IUD removal. I also let patients know that they can remove their IUD themselves and at home if they so decide. Studies have shown that even knowledge of self-removal can increase patient satisfaction with IUDs [49].

Weight gain Weight gain is another concern often raised by AYAs both before and after choosing an IUD. Though studies have not identified an association between IUD use and weight gain [50, 51], sharing this information may or may not reassure patients. As above, acknowledging concerns can help to maintain the patient-provider relationship and allow for ongoing conversations around contraception.

Increased vaginal discharge or odor AYAs may also come in to clinic complaining of an increase in vaginal discharge or odor since IUD placement. As with any AYA presenting with these concerns, we recommend screening for STIs, vaginitis, and bacterial vaginosis (BV). It is also important to explain to patients that hormonal IUDs increase cervical mucus and that they may note this as an increase in vaginal discharge. Others have suggested that copper IUD use may increase the kinds of bacteria more common in BV [52]. In addition, some studies have identified an association between IUD use and BV, which is mediated by irregular vaginal bleeding [53], which can be common in the first few months after IUD insertion. Medications that can stop or slow down irregular bleeding (see Table 11.2) may thus be helpful in addressing vaginal odor consistent with BV.

Future fertility It can also be important to reassure individuals that their IUD will not have any impact on future fertility. In fact, the majority of people who are seeking pregnancy will become pregnant within months to a year after removal of their IUD [54, 55].

Requests for IUD Removals

Patients may seek IUD removal earlier than their IUD removal date, and this is even more likely with AYAs. As discussed, side effects including cramping and bleeding are common reasons AYAs seek early IUD removal [44]. While addressing patient concerns through evidence-based information and providing reassurance is key to providing patient-centered care, it is also imperative to listen to the concerns of patients who seek IUD removal. IUD users expressed feelings of loss of control and disengagement with their medical provider when they felt that providers did not hear their concerns and discouraged removal [13]. And while patients can remove their own IUDs, the vast majority of people view IUDs as provider-controlled devices, which require both an office visit and a willing clinician to take out. Just as the principles of reproductive justice guide us in counseling around IUDs, they can also guide conversations around IUD removal. As noted in "Celebration Meets Caution:"

> Our ultimate reproductive justice endgame is to enhance the health, social well-being and bodily integrity of all our contraceptive clients … Let us also respect [individuals'] decisions not to use LARC, their ability to have LARC removed when they wish … Let us remember that [individuals] themselves know better than funders or practitioners do about where contraception fits into their lives, relationships and long-term goals at any particular moment. [56]

Patients should not need to justify changing or stopping contraception, even (and especially) long-acting reversible contraceptive (LARC) methods.

For patients calling to request IUD removal, I encourage staff to schedule an appointment in a timely manner and to inform patients that the provider will discuss their concerns prior to IUD removal. Providers can use these visits to determine and address motivation/concerns, as well as revisit pregnancy intention and reasons for choosing an IUD, *and* also remove the IUD if patient continues to desire removal. If patients choose IUD removal, it is important to discuss recent sexual activity, as ovulation often continues [47, 57] and there is a very small chance of unintended pregnancy if an IUD is removed less than 7 days after unprotected (condomless) penis in vagina intercourse [58]; some patients may delay removal for an additional week to reduce this risk. In addition, if patients are still not seeking pregnancy, it is also helpful to have a patient-centered discussion around ongoing contraception after IUD removal.

Case (continued)

Alicia comes in to clinic 1 year after their last visit with a chief complaint of "IUD removal." They have been happy with their IUD, but feel like they just want to have some time without any hormones in their body. Alicia also has some concerns about acne and headaches and is not sure if these are related to their IUD or not. You share information about likely versus unlikely side effects and that you are not sure that the headaches and acne are related to their IUD. You also inquire about recent sex and plans for future fertility. Alicia denies sex in the past month, is not seeking pregnancy right now, and reports that their recent partners have been female, "so

I'm not worried about it." Alicia has their IUD removed without incident. Before they leave, you give them some condoms and discuss how to access EC if they need.

Conclusion

While routine visits after IUD insertion are not recommended by evidence-based guidelines, they can present valuable opportunities to answer patient questions, review method-specific information, and offer routine reproductive health care. It is important for providers to be aware of the range of bleeding and cramping that happens after IUD placement, by both timing and type of device. This knowledge helps clinicians provide reassurance, as well as the treatment options available for those whose symptoms are bothersome. Understanding additional IUD-related symptoms and how to counsel on these in a patient-centered manner can help to maintain the ongoing patient-clinician relationship and improve method satisfaction.

Clinical Pearls
- Remind patients to call with any concerns or questions about their IUDs at any time and as frequently as needed.
- The sooner concerns are addressed, the more likely a patient may be to keep their IUD.
- Acknowledging patient concerns—even if they are not clearly causally related to their IUD—can help maintain the patient-provider relationship and allow for ongoing conversations around contraception and fertility planning.
- It is essential to use the principles of reproductive justice to guide conversations around IUD removal in order to maintain patient autonomy in method choice.

References

1. Curtis KM, Jatlaoui TC, Tepper NK, Zapata LB, Horton LG, Jamieson DJ, et al. U.S. selected practice recommendations for contraceptive use, 2016. MMWR Recomm Rep. 2016;65:1–66.
2. Steenland MW, Zapata LB, Brahmi D, Marchbanks PA, Curtis KM. The effect of follow-up visits or contacts after contraceptive initiation on method continuation and correct use. Contraception. 2013;87:625–30.
3. Herceg-Baron R, Furstenberg FF Jr, Shea J, Harris KM. Supporting teenagers' use of contraceptives: a comparison of clinic services. Fam Plan Perspect. 1986;18:61–6.
4. Kirby D, Raine T, Thrush G, Yuen C, Sokoloff A, Potter SC. Impact of an intervention to improve contraceptive use through follow-up phone calls to female adolescent clinic patients. Perspect Sex Reprod Health. 2010;42:251–7.
5. Neuteboom K, de Kroon CD, Dersjant-Roorda M, Jansen FW. Follow-up visits after IUD-insertion: sense or nonsense? A technology assessment study to analyze the effectiveness of follow-up visits after IUD insertion. Contraception. 2003;68:101–4.

6. Bernard A, Satterwhite CL, Reddy M. Frequency of 6-week follow-up appointment scheduling after intrauterine device insertion. BMJ Sex Reprod Health. 2018;44:33–6.
7. Draper IB, Haque MS, McManus RJ. Routine intrauterine device checks: are they advisable? J Fam Plann Reprod Health Care. 2012;38:15–8.
8. Hameed W, Azmat SK, Ali M, Ishaque M, Abbas G, Munroe E, et al. Comparing effectiveness of active and passive client follow-up approaches in sustaining the continued use of Long Acting Reversible Contraceptives (LARC) in rural Punjab: a multicentre, non-inferiority trial. PLoS One. 2016;11:e0160683.
9. L'Engle KL, Mangone ER, Parcesepe AM, Agarwal S, Ippoliti NB. Mobile phone interventions for adolescent sexual and reproductive health: a systematic review. Pediatrics 2016;138. https://doi.org/10.1542/peds.2016-0884.
10. Chernick LS, Stockwell MS, Wu M, Castaño PM, Schnall R, Westhoff CL, et al. Texting to increase contraceptive initiation among adolescents in the emergency department. J Adolesc Health. 2017;61:786–90.
11. Haider S, Dodge LE, Brown BA, Hacker MR, Raine TR. Evaluation of e-mail contact to conduct follow-up among adolescent women participating in a longitudinal cohort study of contraceptive use. Contraception. 2013;88:18–23.
12. Alnakash AH. Influence of IUD perceptions on method discontinuation. Contraception. 2008;78:290–3.
13. Brown MK, Auerswald C, Eyre SL, Deardorff J, Dehlendorf C. Identifying counseling needs of nulliparous adolescent intrauterine contraceptive users: a qualitative approach. J Adolesc Health. 2013;52:293–300.
14. Dehlendorf C, Krajewski C, Borrero S. Contraceptive counseling: best practices to ensure quality communication and enable effective contraceptive use. Clin Obstet Gynecol. 2014;57:659–73.
15. Schivone GB, Glish LL. Contraceptive counseling for continuation and satisfaction. Curr Opin Obstet Gynecol. 2017;29:443–8.
16. Ylikorkala O, Kauppila A, Siljander M. Anti-prostglandin therapy in prevention of side-effects of intrauterine contraceptive devices. Lancet. 1978;2:393–5.
17. Diedrich JT, Desai S, Zhao Q, Secura G, Madden T, Peipert JF. Association of short-term bleeding and cramping patterns with long-acting reversible contraceptive method satisfaction. Am J Obstet Gynecol. 2015;212:50.e1–8.
18. Fraser IS, Critchley HOD, Broder M, Munro MG. The FIGO recommendations on terminologies and definitions for normal and abnormal uterine bleeding. Semin Reprod Med. 2011;29:383–90.
19. Suvisaari J, Lähteenmäki P. Detailed analysis of menstrual bleeding patterns after postmenstrual and postabortal insertion of a copper IUD or a levonorgestrel-releasing intrauterine system. Contraception. 1996;54:201–8.
20. Ylikorkala O. Prostaglandin synthesis inhibitors in menorrhagia, intrauterine contraceptive device-induced side effects and endometriosis. Pharmacol Toxicol. 1994;75(Suppl 2):86–8.
21. Hubacher D, Chen P-L, Park S. Side effects from the copper IUD: do they decrease over time? Contraception. 2009;79:356–62.
22. Sanders JN, Adkins DE, Kaur S, Storck K, Gawron LM, Turok DK. Bleeding, cramping, and satisfaction among new copper IUD users: a prospective study. PLoS One. 2018;13:e0199724.
23. Hubacher D, Reyes V, Lillo S, Pierre-Louis B, Zepeda A, Chen P-L, et al. Preventing copper intrauterine device removals due to side effects among first-time users: randomized trial to study the effect of prophylactic ibuprofen. Hum Reprod. 2006;21:1467–72.
24. Grimes DA, Hubacher D, Lopez LM, Schulz KF. Non-steroidal anti-inflammatory drugs for heavy bleeding or pain associated with intrauterine-device use. Cochrane Database Syst Rev. 2006:CD006034.
25. Nelson AL. LNG-IUS 12: a 19.5 levonorgestrel-releasing intrauterine system for prevention of pregnancy for up to five years. Expert Opin Drug Deliv. 2017;14:1131–40.
26. Mejia M, McNicholas C, Madden T, Peipert JF. Association of baseline bleeding pattern on amenorrhea with levonorgestrel intrauterine system use. Contraception. 2016;94:556–60.

27. Skyla (levonorgestrel-releasing intrauterine system). Highlights of prescribing information [Internet]. [cited 17 Dec 2018]. Available: http://labeling.bayerhealthcare.com/html/products/pi/Skyla_PI.pdf.
28. Mansour D, Inki P, Gemzell-Danielsson K. Efficacy of contraceptive methods: a review of the literature. Eur J Contracept Reprod Health Care. 2010;15(Suppl 2):S19–31.
29. Godfrey EM, Folger SG, Jeng G, Jamieson DJ, Curtis KM. Treatment of bleeding irregularities in women with copper-containing IUDs: a systematic review. Contraception. 2013;87:549–66.
30. Friedlander E, Kaneshiro B. Therapeutic options for unscheduled bleeding associated with long-acting reversible contraception. Obstet Gynecol Clin N Am. 2015;42:593–603.
31. Abdel-Aleem H, d'Arcangues C, Vogelsong KM, Gaffield ML, Gülmezoglu AM. Treatment of vaginal bleeding irregularities induced by progestin only contraceptives. Cochrane Database Syst Rev. 2013:CD003449.
32. Zigler RE, McNicholas C. Unscheduled vaginal bleeding with progestin-only contraceptive use. Am J Obstet Gynecol. 2017;216:443–50.
33. Simmons KB, Edelman AB, Fu R, Jensen JT. Tamoxifen for the treatment of breakthrough bleeding with the etonogestrel implant: a randomized controlled trial. Contraception. 2017;95:198–204.
34. Ylikorkala O, Viinikka L. Comparison between antifibrinolytic and antiprostaglandin treatment in the reduction of increased menstrual blood loss in women with intrauterine contraceptive devices. Br J Obstet Gynaecol. 1983;90:78–83.
35. Guiahi M, McBride M, Sheeder J, Teal S. Short-term treatment of bothersome bleeding for etonogestrel implant users using a 14-day oral contraceptive pill regimen: a randomized controlled trial. Obstet Gynecol. 2015;126:508–13.
36. Hou MY, McNicholas C, Creinin MD. Combined oral contraceptive treatment for bleeding complaints with the etonogestrel contraceptive implant: a randomised controlled trial. Eur J Contracept Reprod Health Care. 2016;21:361–6.
37. Akers AY, Steinway C, Sonalkar S, Perriera LK, Schreiber C, Harding J, et al. Reducing pain during intrauterine device insertion: a randomized controlled trial in adolescents and young women. Obstet Gynecol. 2017;130:795–802.
38. Ngo LL, Braaten KP, Eichen E, Fortin J, Maurer R, Goldberg AB. Naproxen sodium for pain control with intrauterine device insertion: a randomized controlled trial. Obstet Gynecol. 2016;128:1306–13.
39. Rapkin RB, Achilles SL, Schwarz EB, Meyn L, Cremer M, Boraas CM, et al. Self-administered lidocaine gel for intrauterine device insertion in nulliparous women: a randomized controlled trial. Obstet Gynecol. 2016;128:621–8.
40. Imai A, Matsunami K, Takagi H, Ichigo S. Levonorgestrel-releasing intrauterine device used for dysmenorrhea: five-year literature review. Clin Exp Obstet Gynecol. 2014;41:495–8.
41. Golightly E, Gebbie AE. Low-lying or malpositioned intrauterine devices and systems. J Fam Plann Reprod Health Care. 2014;40:108–12.
42. Rhudy JL, Meagher MW. Fear and anxiety: divergent effects on human pain thresholds. Pain. 2000;84:65–75.
43. Jatlaoui TC, Riley HEM, Curtis KM. The safety of intrauterine devices among young women: a systematic review. Contraception. 2017;95:17–39.
44. Dickerson LM, Diaz VA, Jordon J, Davis E, Chirina S, Goddard JA, et al. Satisfaction, early removal, and side effects associated with long-acting reversible contraception. Fam Med. 2013;45:701–7.
45. Maguire K, Joslin-Roher S, Westhoff CL, Davis AR. IUDs at 1 year: predictors of early discontinuation. Contraception. 2015;92:575–7.
46. Davies A, Fleming C. Do intrauterine device/intrauterine system users check their threads? J Fam Plann Reprod Health Care. 2014;40:122–5.
47. Apter D, Gemzell-Danielsson K, Hauck B, Rosen K, Zurth C. Pharmacokinetics of two low-dose levonorgestrel-releasing intrauterine systems and effects on ovulation rate and cervical function: pooled analyses of phase II and III studies. Fertil Steril. 2014;101:1656–62.e1–4.

48. Mirena (levonorgestrel-releasing intrauterine system). Highlights of prescribing information [Internet]. [cited 13 Jan 2019]. Available: https://www.accessdata.fda.gov/drugsatfda_docs/label/2009/021225s027lbl.pdf.
49. Raifman S, Barar R, Foster D. Effect of knowledge of self-removability of intrauterine contraceptives on uptake, continuation, and satisfaction. Womens Health Issues. 2018;28:68–74.
50. Lopez LM, Ramesh S, Chen M, Edelman A, Otterness C, Trussell J, et al. Progestin-only contraceptives: effects on weight. Cochrane Database Syst Rev. 2016:CD008815.
51. Silva Dos Santos PN, Madden T, Omvig K, Peipert JF. Changes in body composition in women using long-acting reversible contraception. Contraception. 2017;95:382–9.
52. Achilles SL, Austin MN, Meyn LA, Mhlanga F, Chirenje ZM, Hillier SL. Impact of contraceptive initiation on vaginal microbiota. Am J Obstet Gynecol. 2018;218:622.e1–622.e10.
53. Madden T, Grentzer JM, Secura GM, Allsworth JE, Peipert JF. Risk of bacterial vaginosis in users of the intrauterine device: a longitudinal study. Sex Transm Dis. 2012;39:217–22.
54. Stoddard AM, Xu H, Madden T, Allsworth JE, Peipert JF. Fertility after intrauterine device removal: a pilot study. Eur J Contracept Reprod Health Care. 2015;20:223–30.
55. Girum T, Wasie A. Return of fertility after discontinuation of contraception: a systematic review and meta-analysis. Contracept Reprod Med. 2018;3:9.
56. Higgins JA. Celebration meets caution: LARC's boons, potential busts, and the benefits of a reproductive justice approach. Contraception. 2014;89:237–41.
57. Faundes A, Segal SJ, Adejuwon CA, Brache V, Leon P, Alvarez-Sanchez F. The menstrual cycle in women using an intrauterine device. Fertil Steril. 1980;34:427–30.
58. Nielsen D, Christensen OM, Nielsen R, Larsen J. Unwanted pregnancy after removal of the IUD. Ugeskr Laeger. 1990;152:3172–3.

Chapter 12
Challenging IUD Procedures

Amy Yoxthimer and Rebecca H. Allen

Abbreviations

AYA	Adolescent and young adults
BMI	Body mass index
CuT380A IUD	Copper IUD
IUD	Intrauterine device
LNG	Levonorgestrel

Learning Objectives

Following completion of this chapter, you should be able to:

1. Provide clinical strategies to address the common factors that contribute to challenging Intrauterine device (IUD) placements for Adolescent and young adults (AYAs).
2. Describe techniques to facilitate IUD placement in challenging scenarios.
3. Discuss approaches to manage difficult IUD removals.

Background

Several studies have shown that when barriers such as cost and education are removed, IUD utilization and satisfaction among adolescents is high [1–3]. Despite these findings, IUD use among AYAs in the USA remains low, at around 3% [4, 5]. Gaps in provider knowledge and training can lead to low IUD service provision and result in

A. Yoxthimer (✉)
Department of Women's Health, Open Door Family Medical Centers, Brewster, NY, USA

R. H. Allen
Department of Obstetrics and Gynecology, Women and Infants Hospital, Brown University, Providence, RI, USA

© Springer Nature Switzerland AG 2019   149
M. S. Coles, A. Mays (eds.), *Optimizing IUD Delivery for Adolescents and Young Adults*, https://doi.org/10.1007/978-3-030-17816-1_12

**Common Provider Misconceptions Regarding Placing IUDs for
Adolescent and Nulliparous Patients**

1. *Providers fear difficult IUD placements due to stenotic cervix and endocervical resistance*
   - *FACT: Adolescents and nulliparous patients have similar ease of insertion and first attempt success rates compared to older and parous individuals [8,10].*
2. *Providers fear increased pain at the time of insertion*
   - *FACT: 79–85% of nulliparous individuals rated their insertion-related pain as no more than 'moderate' [9,11].*
3. *Providers fear increased risk of perforation*
   - *FACT: Adolescence and nulliparity do not increase risk for uterine perforation. Perforation during IUD placement is rare and rates are similar at 0.1%, for both adolescents and older individuals [12–13].*

Fig. 12.1 Common provider misconceptions regarding placing IUDs for AYA and nulliparous patients [12, 13]

low IUD utilization among adolescents [6]. Providers' misconceptions about IUD placement with teens also affect their willingness to follow best practice family planning guidelines [7]. Adolescence and nulliparity are not risk factors for challenging IUD placement and should not be barriers to accessing effective family planning methods when desired (Fig. 12.1). The majority of IUD procedures among AYAs are successful and uncomplicated and do not require any additional advanced skill training [8–10], though occasional challenges may arise regardless of patient age or parity. Additionally, while there are several types of devices currently available, there is no evidence to support recommendation of any particular IUD over another as more effective or easier to place with AYA patients. This chapter will discuss challenges that can develop with IUD procedures, as well as review basic and advanced techniques that can increase provider success with placement and removal.

Factors Contributing to Challenging IUD Placement

One of the most important factors leading to successful IUD placement is provider experience. One study noted that inexperienced clinicians had three times the failure rate, compared to experienced clinicians, where inexperienced clinicians were defined as less than 5 years of experience and less than 12 IUD placements per year [14]. Anatomical and physiologic factors may also contribute to challenging IUD placements. Anatomic and physiological factors include the following:

No prior vaginal delivery, including those with cesarean deliveries While nulliparous individuals have similar first attempt success rates and ease of insertion compared to parous individuals, sometimes challenges can arise due to cervical resistance in those who have never had a vaginal delivery. Vaginal delivery leads to stretching of the cervical orifice (os) and canal, which contributes to easier sounding and placement of the device [11, 14, 15].

Preplacement and placement anxiety and fear Patient fear of a painful procedure can lead to an exaggerated experience of pain during the procedure, as well as pre-syncopal and syncopal events [16, 17]. Anxiety and fear can also result in patients contracting and tensing pelvic floor muscles, decreasing the flexibility of the vaginal introitus and vaginal canal muscles—and leading to increased patient discomfort. Pelvic floor muscle contraction during the procedure can also make visualization of the cervix more difficult for the provider.

Cervix flush with the vagina or stenotic cervix Small cervices and narrow cervical canals can be normal physiologic variants [18]. Techniques can be applied to facilitate successful IUD placement in these cases.

Severe uterine version or flexion (Fig. 12.2) Anteverted and retroverted describe the angle of the body of the uterus and cervix to the vagina and are common uterine variations. Most individuals have an anteverted uterus—where the body of the uterus and cervix tilts forward onto the urinary bladder. The remainder have either a mid-position uterus (where the uterus and cervix may only tilt slightly forward) or a retroverted uterus (where the uterus and cervix tilt backward toward the rectum). The angle between the cervix and uterus itself can also be flexed, leading to anteflexed or retroflexed uteruses. The angle between the cervix and the uterus may be more acute and can therefore affect the ease of IUD placement.

Large body habitus While obese AYAs are excellent candidates for IUDs [20], large body habitus can contribute to challenging IUD placements in several ways [21]. First, the bimanual exam may be inconclusive in a patient with an obese abdomen such that determining uterine position and ruling out abnormalities of the uterus may be difficult. Second, a large, heavy pannus can create increased resistance to opening a speculum, as well as increased resistance entering the uterine

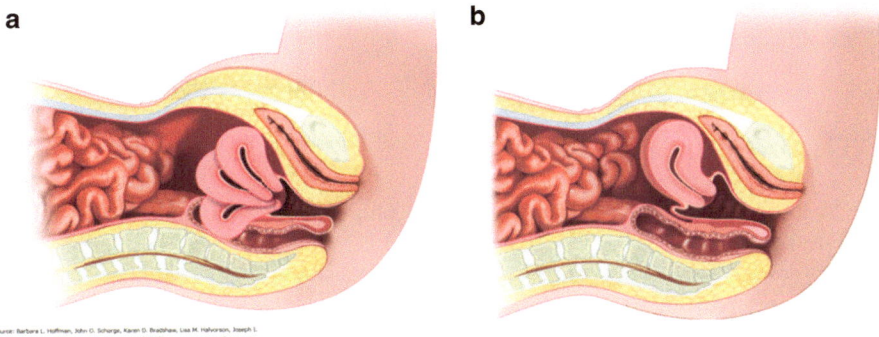

Fig. 12.2 Uterine positions. (a) Uterine position may be anteverted, midplane, or retroverted. (b) The uterine fundus can be flexed forward, and this is termed anteflexion. Similarly, the fundus may be flexed backward to create retroflexion [19]. (Image source: McGraw-Hill Education Material)

cavity during sounding and placement of the device. Third, vaginal wall prolapse can lead to challenges with visualization of the cervix.

Bradycardia, syncope, or presyncope Presyncope, syncope, and bradycardia can occasionally occur during IUD placement, due to cervical manipulation and pain. *Patients who have significant cervical stenosis or endocervical resistance may be at increased risk* for these challenges to occur [14]. Individuals may experience facial pallor, cold or sweaty extremities, feelings of dizziness or weakness, and numbness or tingling in extremities.

Uterine cavity distortion due to a congenital anomaly Uterine anomalies in the general population are estimated to be 0.5% and are often unknown prior to gynecologic procedures [22]. Depending on the type of anomaly, challenges can develop with IUD placement (e.g., septate uterus) or lead to decreases in IUD effectiveness (e.g., bicornuate uterus).

Uterine cavity distortion secondary to fibroid uterus Fibroids are uncommon in AYAs, but may result in an inability to sound, or to errors in sounding that lead to malposition of the IUD.

Strategies for Challenging IUD Placements: Maximizing the Basic Skill Set

As discussed above, there are some potential challenges to IUD placement. However, many of these can be overcome with a set of basic skills that do not require additional training or instrumentation. Optimizing provider comfort and proficiency with IUD placement can take some time. However, having some basic gynecologic procedural skills and knowledge of when to use them can help to make most IUD placements successful. The following section outlines potential challenges in IUD placement and steps to address them.

Case

Anna is a 17-year-old, cisgender female (G0P0, Body mass index (BMI) 34), referred for a copper IUD insertion after having a failed insertion attempt at her health center. The referral states: "unable to pass sound due to endocervical resistance. Patient also had a syncopal episode at end of procedure." She is nervous but very interested in obtaining a copper IUD. She presents to the health center today for repeat attempt at IUD placement.

Step 1: Managing preplacement anxiety For more information on anxiety and pain management during IUD placement, see Chaps. 10 and 11 on pain management. In addition, see Fig. 12.3.

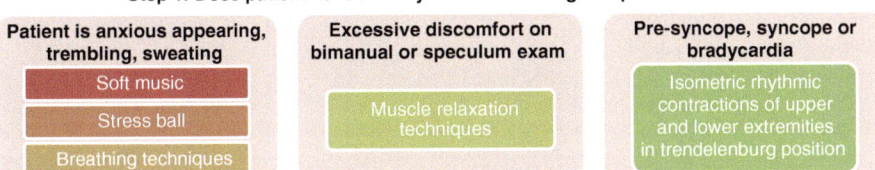

Fig. 12.3 Some suggestions for managing patient anxiety. (Image source: Yoxthimer, Allen, Coles)

Presyncope can occur at any point during an IUD placement procedure, either due to anxiety or secondary to pain and manipulation of the cervix, leading to a vagal response and bradycardic episode. One strategy that can be used to prevent a syncopal event is rhythmic, isometric contractions of upper extremities and lower extremities. If identified early, the isometric contractions can prevent a syncopal episode and distract the patient from pain as well. This can be done by having the medical assistant or provider instruct the patient to try and tense up and make muscle in both their arms and legs, to hold these contractions of hands and feet (and upper and lower extremities) for a 10 second count, and then to relax and repeat a few more times or until the patient is feeling better. See Chap. 11 for a further description of such methods.

Step 2: Challenges visualizing the cervix   Four common challenges to visualizing the cervix are presented in this section (see Fig. 12.4 for a quick guide to challenges and strategies). Common challenges to visualizing the cervix include:

1. **Vaginal Wall Prolapse:** Vaginal wall prolapse (when the vaginal walls collapse inward on the vaginal cavity during speculum exam) can often occur in patients with large body habitus or those that have had multiple vaginal deliveries. To

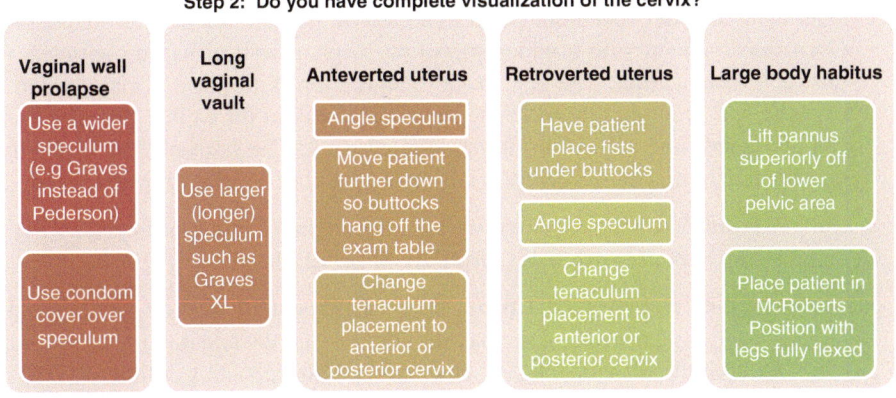

Fig. 12.4 A quick guide to strategies that may help gain visualization of the cervix. (Image source: Yoxthimer, Allen, Coles)

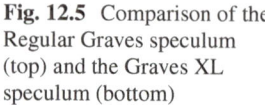

Fig. 12.5 Comparison of the Regular Graves speculum (top) and the Graves XL speculum (bottom)

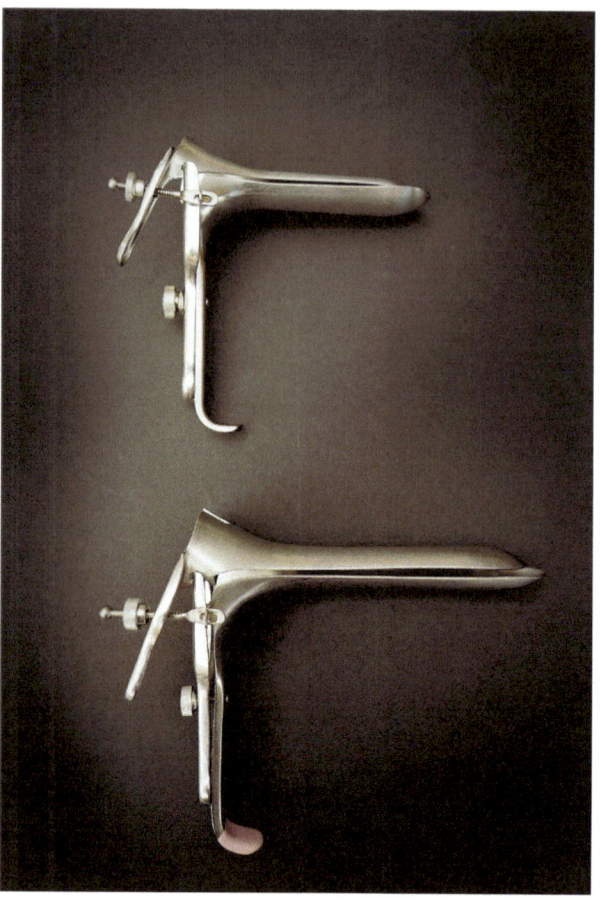

visualize the cervix in this instance, ensure appropriate speculum size and consider using a wider speculum (such as a Graves, instead of a smaller Pederson). Occasionally, even with a wider speculum, vaginal wall prolapse continues to obstruct visualization. The next basic intervention is to place a male condom over the speculum and then cut the tip of the condom off so that the speculum can be opened and placed inside the vaginal vault. The sidewalls of the vagina will be maintained by the lateral walls of the condom covering the speculum.

2. **Long Vaginal Vault:** In a patient with a long vaginal vault, consider utilizing a longer speculum size such as a Graves XL (Fig. 12.5).

3. **Anteverted or Retroverted Uterus with Displacement of the Cervix:** Begin the procedure by positioning the patient very low on the exam table, so the buttocks are partially off the table and continue to adjust patient position as needed. Low table position of the patient will allow increased vaginal vault flexibility with speculum and tenaculum for better visualizing of the cervix. If the individual has a retroverted uterus with a severely displaced cervix, you can ask the

patient to place their fists under their buttocks during the procedure. This will help to move both the uterus and cervix to a more midline position.

If traditional placement of the speculum does not allow the cervix to be fully visualized, we recommend trying to angle the speculum. With the speculum closed in the vault, turn the speculum 45° in either direction superiorly or inferiorly and then gradually open the speculum to isolate the cervix. If angling the speculum allows for full visualization, but the cervix remains severely displaced, then tenaculum use will allow for repositioning of the cervix and optimal visualization during the procedure. We recommend that providers place the tenaculum on whichever lip of the cervix is best visualized (or closest), and give gentle downward or upward traction on the tenaculum to allow for complete visualization of the cervix during sounding and IUD placement.

4. **Large Body Habitus:** Repositioning of a patient with large body habitus may require additional medical assistants. If opening the speculum is made difficult because of the heavy pannus, explain to the patient that an assistant can help to remove the pressure by gently moving the pannus toward the patient's head and away from the pelvis. If this improves the ability to open the speculum, but the cervix cannot be fully visualized, then attempt McRoberts positioning (Fig. 12.6). In McRoberts positioning (image below), medical assistants will gently bring the patients legs back (toward patient midline) in a fully flexed position.

Step 3: Challenges to introducing a sound into the cervical os A visually small cervical opening does not necessarily mean cervical stenosis. Figure 12.7 gives a summary of steps providers can take when faced with difficulty introducing a sound. A cervical opening may appear small but have good flexibility, which allows passing of the sound without difficulty. If the cervix does not allow introduction of a uterine sound, then the provider can gently introduce a cytobrush tip (Fig. 12.8) or a cervical os finder (Fig. 12.9) into the cervical os. We recommend trying to place the cytobrush tip, or the smooth lower tip, of the os finder into the cervical opening for about 10 seconds, as this may allow for gentle dilation to occur. **Do not advance the cytobrush or the os finder deep into the endocervical canal**, as this could result in creation of a false endocervical tract and significant pain to the patient. If you are using a metal sound (Fig. 12.10) and the os appears more dilated, but you are still

Fig. 12.6 McRoberts positioning. (Reprinted with permission [23])

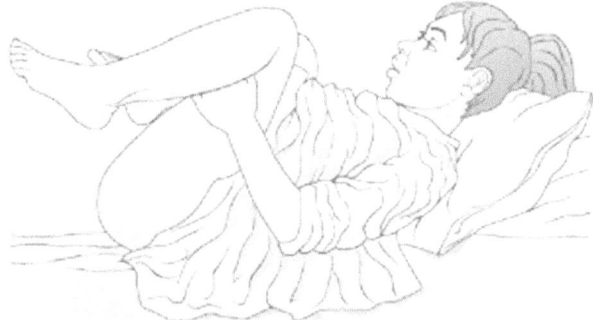

unable to pass the metal sound, we recommend trying a smaller endometrial biopsy pipelle (Fig. 12.11) or plastic uterine sound (Fig. 12.12). While using any of the above instruments in the cervical os, give gentle traction on the tenaculum to ensure that the canal is properly aligned, so the cervical tract is more easily identified.

Step 4: Challenges sounding the uterine cavity (endocervical resistance)   Uterine sounds can be reusable and made of metal (available in 2 and 3 mm diameter sizes)

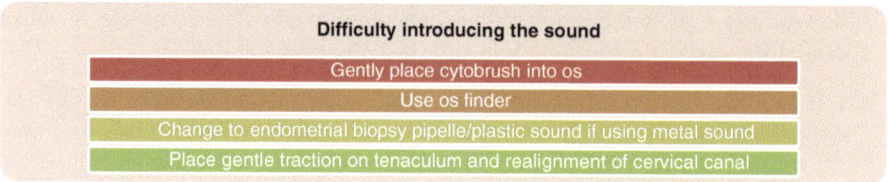

Fig. 12.7   Some steps the provider can take when faced with difficulty introducing a sound. (Source: Yoxthimer, Allen, Coles)

Fig. 12.8 Cytobrush. (Image source: Allen and Bickford (Women and Infants Hospital))

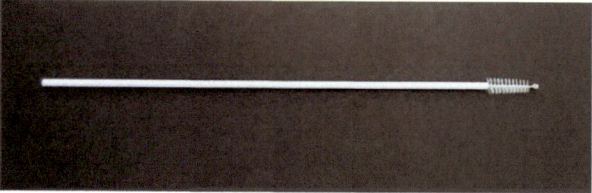

Fig. 12.9 Cervical os finder. (Image source: Allen and Bickford (Women and Infants Hospital))

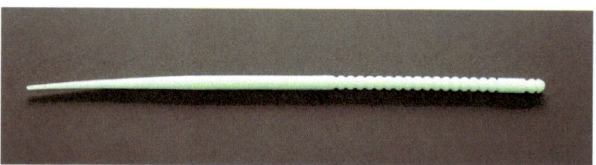

Fig. 12.10 Metal sound. (Image source: Allen and Bickford (Women and Infants Hospital))

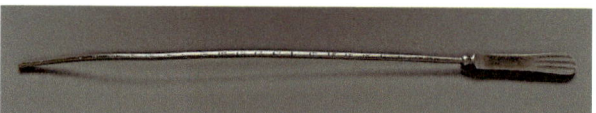

Fig. 12.11 Endometrial biopsy pipelle. (Image source: Allen and Bickford (Women and Infants Hospital))

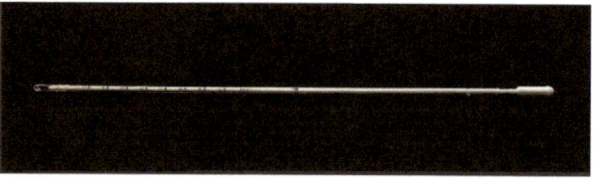

(Fig. 12.10) or disposable and made of plastic (available in 3 mm diameter size) (Fig. 12.12). Endometrial biopsy pipelles (3 mm) are also often used (Fig. 12.11) for uterine sounding. See Fig. 12.13 for an overview of steps to manage endocervical resistance. If the sound is easily introduced into the endocervical canal opening, but you are unable to pass through the canal, first, check the tenaculum location. You want to ensure that the teeth are not too deep and encroaching on the lumen of the endocervical canal, as this can cause constriction and resistance to sounding and placement. If the tenaculum is too deep or too close to the endocervical canal, then simply remove and replace the tenaculum on the cervix at either 11 and 1 o'clock or 5 and 7 o'clock positions on the anterior and posterior lip of cervix, respectively. The depth of the tenaculum bite should be approximately 0.5 cm, sufficient for stability but avoiding the endocervical canal. An alternative is to apply the tenaculum in the vertical position on the cervix, rather than horizontal.

If the tenaculum appears in normal position, then next try the endocervical canal realignment technique. Applying gentle traction, angle the tenaculum at various positions upward and downward and in lateral directions. With each endocervical canal realignment position, reattempt sounding until smooth passage of the instrument occurs. If realignment technique is not successful and you are using a standard metal sound, trial sounding using a different instrument, such as an endometrial biopsy pipelle or plastic uterine sound. With their small diameter and flexibility,

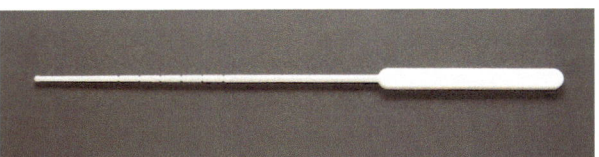

Fig. 12.12 Plastic sound. (Image source: Allen and Bickford (Women and Infants Hospital))

Step 4: Can you pass the sound through the endocervical canal?

Endocervical resistance	Obstruction	Large body habitus
Ensure tenaculum placement is not too close to endocervical canal	If visible canal obstruction –refer for removal prior to attempting placement	Lift pannus superiorly off of lower pelvic area
Realign cervical canal with tenaculum then resound		
Sound with endometrial biopsy pipelle or plastic sound (if using metal sound)		Place patient in McRoberts Position with legs fully flexed
Consider shorter speculum (e.g. Klopfer)		
Change tenaculum from anterior to posterior (or vice versa) then resound		

Fig. 12.13 An overview of steps to overcome endocervical resistance. (Source: Yoxthimer, Allen, Coles)

these devices can generally pass easily and can identify and move around contours that may be felt as resistance with a metal sound.

If you are still unable to pass a sound through the endocervical canal, then consider repositioning of the tenaculum to the opposite lip of the cervix (posterior or anterior). Begin sounding using the endometrial biopsy pipelle or plastic uterine sound. During sounding attempts, inspect the canal to ensure there is no prolapsing polyp/fibroid obstructing the canal. If there is an obvious obstruction from the polyp or fibroid, then removal of the benign tumor by an experienced provider will be indicated prior to IUD placement; this is unlikely to occur in AYAs. If endocervical resistance is thought to be secondary to large body habitus and pannus resistance, then trial the previously mentioned repositioning techniques including lifting the pannus of the patient off the pelvic area to midline position and/or McRoberts positioning. Managing endocervical resistance due to significant uterine flexion is addressed below.

Step 5: Challenges sounding the uterus due to uterine anteversion or retroversion (see Fig. 12.14) If you suspect significant anteversion or retroversion as a cause of endocervical resistance, we recommend positioning the patient low on the exam table so the buttocks are partially off of the table. This will allow for increased flexibility with speculum and tenaculum procedures. If the uterus is retroverted and retroflexed, also consider having the patient place their fists under their buttocks during the procedure to push the uterus forward. When there is difficulty sounding or placing the IUD device due to a severely anteverted and anteflexed uterus, body habitus permitting, a medical assistant can assist the provider with redirecting the position of the uterus from the bladder toward the midline:

- The medical assistant, positioned to the side of the patient at the level of the pelvis, will place their fingertips to a depth of 1 cm at the pubic bone.

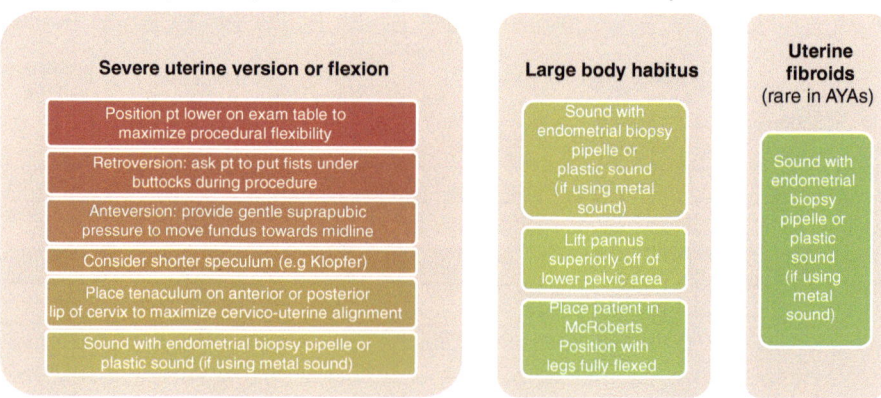

Fig. 12.14 An overview of steps to manage endocervical resistance due to anteverted or retroverted uteri. (Source: Yoxthimer, Allen, Coles)

- Then using steady fingertip pressure, the medical assistant will move their hands in a steady sweeping motion in the direction of the patient midline until reaching a level just above the suprapubic area.
- The steady sweep will try to lift and redirect the fundus more midline to reduce the angle between the cervix and uterine cavity.

If uterine flexion causes significant displacement of the cervix, place the tenaculum on the lip of the cervix that is best visualized. For a severely ante-verted/anteflexed uterus, placing the tenaculum on the anterior lip of the cervix may give the best traction. Similarly, for a severely retroverted/retroflexed uterus, placing the tenaculum on the posterior lip may provide best cavity alignment. If the sound does not pass further than 4–5 cm, it is likely still in the endocervical canal or at the uterine flexure. We recommend removing the sound, then trialing realignment of the uterine cavity by giving gentle traction in slightly different angling positions (back and slightly upward or downward), and again attempting resounding. If unsuccessful, trial sounding with a smaller sound (an endometrial biopsy pipelle or plastic uterine sound)—if not already using one. If still unsuccessful, consider changing the tenaculum to the opposite lip of the cervix to reattempt cavity alignment. A shorter speculum such as the Klopfer speculum (see Fig. 12.15) may also be warranted in these situations. The shorter speculum allows the angle between the cervix and uterus to be further straightened by the application of additional traction to the cervix without speculum blades impeding the descent of the cervix.

If sounding is challenging due to patient large body habitus, then we recommend utilizing the aforementioned strategies focused on body positioning, including lifting the pannus off the uterus and McRoberts positioning. If sounding is unsuccessful or equivocal (at lower limits of uterine sounding, e.g., 4–5 cm), then consider seeking ultrasound guidance assistance to ensure correct fundal placement.

Step 6: Challenges placing the IUD into the endometrial cavity Prior to placing the IUD, check to ensure it is loaded properly in the insertion tube and that the flange is set to the correct sounded uterine depth. When using the copper IUD inserter, ensure that the stabilizing rod is at the base of the IUD device inside the inserter tube. When using levonorgestrel (LNG) devices, ensure that the slider on the inserter handle is fully forward and that your thumb or finger is maintained on the slider in the forward most position. When introducing the IUD inserter tube into the vaginal vault, be cautious not to let the flange touch anything in the vaginal vault, including the speculum or walls of the vagina, as this could inadvertently change the flange setting and lead to errors in placement. When placing an LNG IUD, always remember to release the IUD arms 1.5–2 cm below the uterine fundus before advancing and deploying the IUD device at the fundus. These steps are outlined in Fig. 12.16 (below).

Fig. 12.15 The shorter, Klopfer speculum (top) as compared to Graves speculum (bottom). (Image source: Allen and Bickford (Women and Infants Hospital))

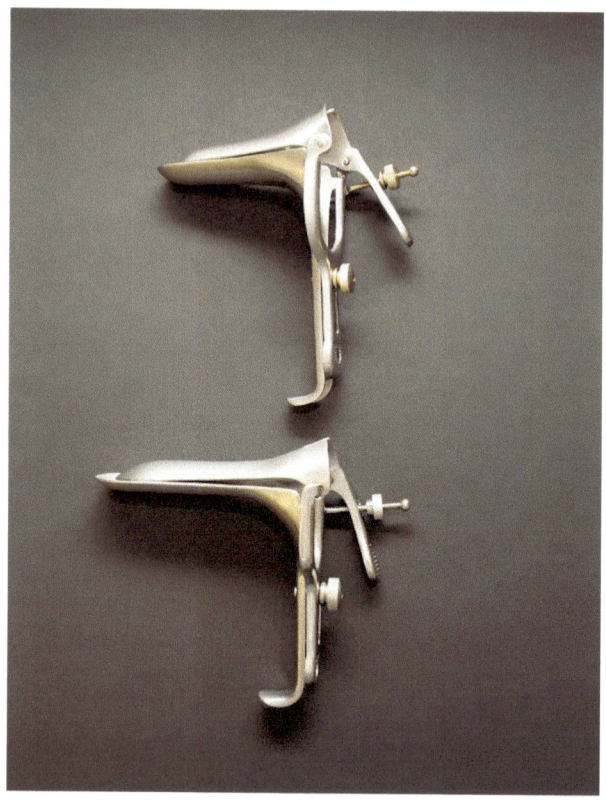

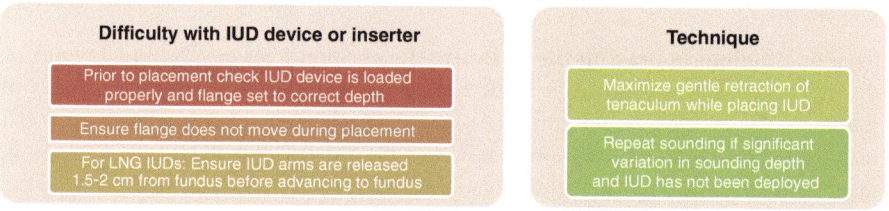

Step 6: Can you introduce the IUD inserter tube into the uterine cavity so that flange is flush with cervix (sounding depth)?

Difficulty with IUD device or inserter	Technique
Prior to placement check IUD device is loaded properly and flange set to correct depth	Maximize gentle retraction of tenaculum while placing IUD
Ensure flange does not move during placement	Repeat sounding if significant variation in sounding depth and IUD has not been deployed
For LNG IUDs: Ensure IUD arms are released 1.5-2 cm from fundus before advancing to fundus	

Fig. 12.16 Summary of difficulties with IUD device/inserter, along with some techniques to overcome these potential problems. (Source: Yoxthimer, Allen, Coles)

Here are some technique tips to address challenges placing the IUD within the endometrial cavity:

- Whenever in motion during IUD placement (e.g., sounding and IUD placement), maximize steady gentle tenaculum traction and angling positions as needed.
- Consider repositioning of the tenaculum if needed for best endocervical and cavity alignment.
- Take advantage of the curve in the LNG IUD applicators by turning them over (with curvature pointing toward the floor) for placement in a retroverted uterus.

- If the IUD applicator is not able to pass through the internal os of the cervix, further dilation may be required (see next section on cervical dilation).
- Ensure that the flange of the IUD inserter device is flushed with the cervix before deployment of the IUD at the fundus—this signifies correct fundal placement.
- If the flange is not flushed with the cervix and resistance is met, trial gentle traction upward or downward with the tenaculum, and reattempt to advance the IUD device gently.
- If unable to advance the IUD device further, and the flange is not flushed with the cervix, consider removal of the IUD inserter and resounding, possibly under ultrasound guidance.

Removing IUD inserter prior to deployment: If you are removing an IUD inserter from the uterine cavity *prior to IUD deployment* to attempt resounding, and you are using:

- An LNG IUD inserter, this can be removed with the loaded IUD device, and, after resounding, the same inserter can be used to place the same LNG IUD.
- A copper IUD inserted—removal will likely result in deployment of the IUD arms and device (the copper IUD unloading from the inserter tube into the uterus or vagina). If premature deployment of a copper IUD occurs, the IUD should be removed and discarded, and a new IUD should be used, due to vaginal contamination.

Case (continued)

After reassuring Anna that most IUDs are successfully and easily placed in AYAs, the provider prepares the instruments, including the os finder and endometrial biopsy pipelle. Because of Anna's elevated BMI, a condom was also added to the tray, in the event of vaginal wall prolapse. The patient has her mobile phone with her and plays some soft, calming music. On insertion of the speculum, the provider notes vaginal wall prolapse and places a condom cover over the speculum. Using the basic skills reviewed above, including endocervical canal realignment and repositioning of the tenaculum, the provider is unable to pass the sound or pipelle, and offers to use some further techniques for placement, which Anna accepts.

Advanced Skills for Challenging IUD Placements

For many experienced clinicians, advanced skills are rarely required for IUD insertion. In one retrospective study of 1177 AYAs undergoing IUD insertion at a clinic staffed mainly by advanced practice clinicians, the first attempt success rate was 96%, and insertion failures and IUD expulsions were not related to IUD type, age, or parity [8]. If IUD insertion is not successful with basic skills, it is reasonable to

Fig. 12.17 Examples of Pratt dilators. (Image source: Allen and Bickford (Women and Infants Hospital))

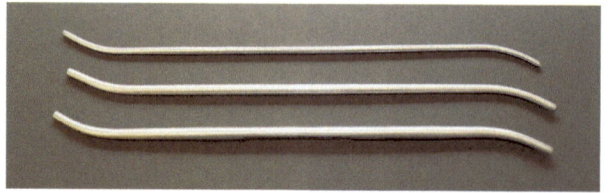

either refer the patient to a provider who can provide cervical dilation or offer the patient a repeat attempt after pretreatment with misoprostol. In the above study, 21 patients (1.8%) of the first attempt successes required ancillary measures, such as assistance from a second clinician, ultrasound, mechanical dilation, misoprostol, or paracervical block, which we discuss below.

Mechanical dilation If uterine sounding or insertion of the IUD applicator is unsuccessful despite the basic techniques described above, mechanical dilation with cervical dilators (see Fig. 12.17) may be required to insert the IUD. Pratt dilators are the most commonly used type of dilators, though Hegar and Hank dilators are also available. While the measurement system for dilators differs by type, all of these tapered rods allow cervical dilation to occur when gently inserted into the cervical canal. The amount of cervical dilation required depends both on the IUD applicator size and on the angle between the cervix and uterus. IUD inserters come in slightly different diameters: CuT380A IUD inserters are 4.0 mm, LNG 52 mg IUD inserters are 4.4 mm, and LNG 19.5 mg and 13.5 mg IUD inserters are 3.8 mm [24]. Due to their flexibility, plastic IUD applicators often need more room to navigate acute angles, compared to metal instruments (e.g., dilators or metal uterine sounds). In some instances, dilation above the insertion diameter and up to 7–7$^{2/3}$ mm (21 or 23 French Pratt dilator) may be required, especially if the uterus is particularly ante-flexed or retroflexed. A paracervical block can be considered for pain control with cervical dilation, as discussed in Chap. 9. In addition, some providers will use ultrasound guidance with more difficult cases requiring cervical dilation.

Pharmacologic dilation Misoprostol can also be used to assist with cervical dilation. Misoprostol is not recommended routinely for IUD insertion because it does not increase the rates of successful IUD insertion and can cause nausea and increased cramping before and during insertion [25, 26]. Nevertheless, there is some evidence that misoprostol can be helpful in those with a previously failed IUD insertion or with a prior difficult insertion due to known cervical stenosis [18, 27]. *Misoprostol regimens vary, but we recommend 400 mcg taken 2–3 hours before insertion, to be administered vaginally, buccally, or sublingually* [28, 29]. Buccal administration is generally preferred due to its convenience, with similar absorption to the vaginal route, and lower rates of gastrointestinal side effects compared to the sublingual route [30, 31].

Ultrasound guidance While ultrasound guidance is not required for IUD insertion or to confirm fundal placement, it can be helpful with very challenging insertions

[32]. The ultrasound can assist providers with navigating tortuous cervical canals or reassuring the provider that additional force can be applied safely under direct visualization. Ultrasound can also identify sharp uterine flexion (severely anteflexed or retroflexed), uterine anomalies, or obstructing uterine fibroids. In cases of *difficult insertion*, immediate post-procedure ultrasound can confirm fundal placement. Transabdominal ultrasound guidance does have limitations, especially in morbidly obese patients with empty bladders, where it may be more difficult to visualize the uterus.

Case (continued)

Due to the increased cervical resistance, the provider decided that cervical dilation would be the next appropriate step. Anna was offered a trial of gentle mechanical dilation, with or without local anesthesia. The patient opted for local anesthesia, and a paracervical block was used for pain control with cervical dilation. After dilation with a 21 Pratt dilator, the uterine sound was able to be passed and the IUD was placed successfully. Anna tolerated the procedure well.

Difficult IUD Removals

Case (continued after 3 years)

Anna has been using the CuT380A IUD happily for 3 years now. She presents to the health center after not being able to feel her IUD strings. She is having normal regular cycles and would like to continue to use her IUD for four more years. Upon performing a speculum exam, no strings are visualized.

Missing IUD strings Missing IUD strings are the primary reason for difficult IUD removals and occur in 5–15% of patients [33, 34]. In the vast majority of cases, the string has retracted into the cervical canal or uterine cavity with the IUD still in place. However, missing strings may also be a sign of an unnoticed IUD expulsion or, less likely, perforation into the abdominal cavity. In one large retrospective review of 14,935 patients using an IUD, 750 women (5%) presented with missing IUD strings [33]. Of these, the IUD was present in the uterus on ultrasound in 735 cases (98%), while nine women (1.2%) had expelled the device, and five women (0.7%) were found to have a perforation with the device in the pelvis.

If the IUD strings are not visualized on exam, an attempt can be made to sweep the strings out of the cervical canal with the cytobrush (Fig. 12.8) [35]. If IUD strings are still not visualized and the patient wishes to keep the device, then pregnancy should be ruled out and the patient should initiate backup contraception [36]. Next, an ultrasound should be done to attempt to locate the IUD. If no IUD is seen on ultrasound, we recommend an abdominal x-ray from the diaphragm to the pelvis be obtained. If the IUD is not seen on ultrasound or x-ray, it can be assumed that the patient had an unnoticed expulsion. If the device is documented to be located in the uterus, the patient can continue to rely on the device for contraception. If the strings continue to be missing at subsequent annual visits, some providers recommend repeat ultrasound confirmation that the IUD is still in situ, as expulsion can occur [33]. However, it is also reasonable to assess for changes in patients' bleeding or cramping patterns that may be concerning for an IUD expulsion and decide if ultrasound is clinically indicated using a shared decision-making model.

Case (continued)

Anna had an ultrasound that demonstrated an IUD correctly placed at the uterine fundus. It is now 7 years later, and she is ready to have her IUD removed and replaced. The strings are still not visualized, and Anna wants to know how her IUD will be removed.

IUD Removal with Missing Strings If the strings are not visible, and an individual desires IUD removal, an attempt can be made to locate the strings in the cervical canal with a cytobrush (as discussed above). If this is not successful, then you will need to

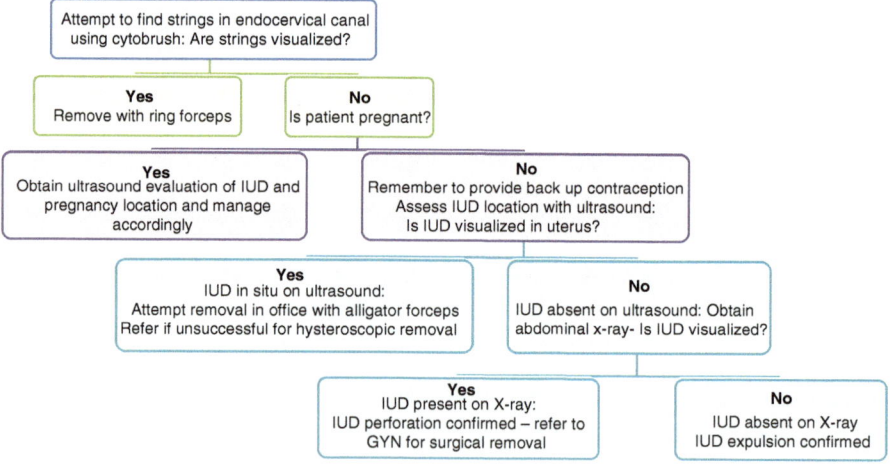

Fig. 12.18 Steps in IUD removal with missing strings. (Source: Yoxthimer, Allen, Coles)

Fig. 12.19 IUD thread retriever. (Image source: Allen and Bickford (Women and Infants Hospital))

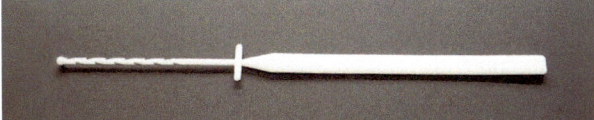

Fig. 12.20 Alligator forceps. (Image source: Allen and Bickford (Women and Infants Hospital))

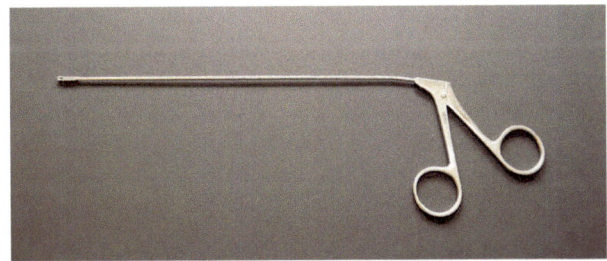

rule out pregnancy and confirm the presence of the IUD in the uterine cavity with ultrasound prior to instrumenting the uterine cavity. There are a variety of techniques that can be used to remove IUDs without visible strings in nonpregnant patients (see Fig. 12.18). IUD thread retrievers (Fig. 12.19) can be passed in into the uterine cavity with a clockwise twisting motion—both upon entry and exit—and assist in pulling the IUD strings down so that they are visible [35]. The IUD can then be removed in the routine fashion. IUD hooks (not pictured) are sometimes used but were originally designed to remove the loop and ring-shaped intrauterine devices, not the modern T-shaped IUDs. Therefore, most providers have abandoned the IUD hook in favor of alligator forceps (Fig. 12.20) [35]. These narrow devices can be inserted through the cervical canal and into the uterine cavity without cervical dilation. Using the alligator forceps with a tenaculum for cervical traction under ultrasound guidance is usually successful in removing the IUD in the office. Exploration of the uterine cavity with alligator forceps can be uncomfortable, so a paracervical block is advised. If alligator forceps are not available, a long curved Kelly clamp can be considered [37]. One final in-office technique (for providers trained in manual vacuum aspiration) is IUD removal using a manual vacuum aspirator with a 5 or 6 mm cannula. If removal fails with all of these techniques, hysteroscopic retrieval is the next step—either in the office, if available, or in a surgical setting by an obstetrician-gynecologist [38, 39].

Removal of IUDs in Pregnancy Use of IUDs decreases the overall risk of ectopic pregnancy, due to their incredibly high efficacy in preventing pregnancy [24]. Nevertheless, if an individual becomes pregnant with an IUD in place, ectopic pregnancy must be ruled out and the IUD must be located [36]. In one large study, approximately 27% of pregnancies with LNG IUDs and 15% of pregnancies with copper IUDs were ectopic in location [40]. Another study found that half of pregnancies with LNG IUDs were ectopic [41]. If the pregnancy is intrauterine and the IUD strings are visible, the IUD should be removed by the first provider who sees the patient, as the strings will soon migrate into the cervical canal and disappear from view with the enlarging uterus of pregnancy [42, 43]. While removal of the IUD is associated with a slightly increased risk for spontaneous abortion and premature delivery, leaving the device in situ will lead to an even further increased risk of spontaneous abortion, septic abortion, chorioamnionitis, and premature delivery [44]. Even if the patient plans pregnancy termination, IUD removal should not be deferred to the abortion provider. If the IUD strings are not visible, the cervical canal can be explored in pregnancy with the cytobrush and colposcopic magnification. However, intrauterine procedures are generally not advised [36]. Successful hysteroscopic or ultrasound-guided IUD removal in pregnancy has been reported; however, skilled surgeons are needed, and there is still a risk of adverse outcomes [42, 43, 45, 46]. Once the pregnancy has entered the second trimester, further attempts at removal without visible strings should be avoided.

Summary

Nulligravid and nulliparous AYAs have similar rates of successful IUD placement compared to older and multiparous individuals. Provider experience with IUD procedures is the most important factor contributing to successful provision of IUD services with patients of any age or parity. Most challenges that arise during IUD placement can be successfully resolved using strategies that *do not require advanced training*. When advanced skills are required, mechanical or pharmacologic dilation with or without ultrasound guidance will generally result in successful placement. Using algorithms to identify and overcome challenges that arise, such as those provided in this book, will improve success with IUD procedures.

Clinical Pearls
- AYAs and nulliparous individuals are not at higher risk of challenging IUD placements than other individuals.
- Understanding pelvic anatomy can help providers to problem solve challenges in IUD placement if they arise.
- Algorithms, such as those presented in this chapter, can help the majority of providers successfully place IUDs without advanced training.

References

1. McNicholas C, Madden T, Secura G, Peipert JF. The contraceptive CHOICE project round up: what we did and what we learned. Clin Obstet Gynecol. 2014;57:635–43.
2. Cohen R, Sheeder J, Kane M, Teal SB. Factors Associated With Contraceptive Method Choice and Initiation in Adolescents and Young Women. J Adolesc Health. 2017;61:454–60.
3. Colorado's success with long-acting reversible contraception (LARC). Department of Public Health and Environment [Internet]. [cited 3 Dec 2018]. Available: www.colorado.gov/pacific/cdphe/cfpi-report.

4. Daniels K, Daugherty J, Jones J, Mosher W. Current Contraceptive Use and Variation by Selected Characteristics Among Women Aged 15-44: United States, 2011-2013. Natl Health Stat Report. 2015;86:1–14.
5. Lindberg L, Santelli J, Desai S. Understanding the Decline in Adolescent Fertility in the United States, 2007-2012. J Adolesc Health. 2016;59:577–83.
6. Luchowski AT, Anderson BL, Power ML, Raglan GB, Espey E, Schulkin J. Obstetrician-gynecologists and contraception: practice and opinions about the use of IUDs in nulliparous women, adolescents and other patient populations. Contraception. 2014;89:572–7.
7. Harper CC, Blum M, de Bocanegra HT, Darney PD, Speidel JJ, Policar M, et al. Challenges in translating evidence to practice: the provision of intrauterine contraception. Obstet Gynecol. 2008;111:1359–69.
8. Teal SB, Romer SE, Goldthwaite LM, Peters MG, Kaplan DW, Sheeder J. Insertion characteristics of intrauterine devices in adolescents and young women: success, ancillary measures, and complications. Am J Obstet Gynecol. 2015;213:515.e1–5.
9. Marions L, Lövkvist L, Taube A, Johansson M, Dalvik H, Øverlie I. Use of the levonorgestrel releasing-intrauterine system in nulliparous women--a non-interventional study in Sweden. Eur J Contracept Reprod Health Care. 2011;16:126–34.
10. Bayer LL, Jensen JT, Li H, Nichols MD, Bednarek PH. Adolescent experience with intrauterine device insertion and use: a retrospective cohort study. Contraception. 2012;86:443–51.
11. Bahamondes MV, Hidalgo MM, Bahamondes L, Monteiro I. Ease of insertion and clinical performance of the levonorgestrel-releasing intrauterine system in nulligravidas. Contraception. 2011;84:e11–6.
12. Barnett C, Moehner S, Do Minh T, Heinemann K. Perforation risk and intra-uterine devices: results of the EURAS-IUD 5-year extension study. Eur J Contracept Reprod Health Care. 2017;22:424–8.
13. Jatlaoui TC, Riley HEM, Curtis KM. The safety of intrauterine devices among young women: a systematic review. Contraception. 2017;95:17–39.
14. Farmer M, Webb A. Intrauterine device insertion-related complications: can they be predicted? J Fam Plann Reprod Health Care. 2003;29:227–31.
15. Ireland LD, Allen RH. Pain Management for Gynecologic Procedures in the Office. Obstet Gynecol Surv. 2016;71:89–98.
16. Gemzell-Danielsson K, Mansour D, Fiala C, Kaunitz AM, Bahamondes L. Management of pain associated with the insertion of intrauterine contraceptives. Hum Reprod Update. 2013;19:419–27.
17. Bahamondes L, Mansour D, Fiala C, Kaunitz AM, Gemzell-Danielsson K. Practical advice for avoidance of pain associated with insertion of intrauterine contraceptives. J Fam Plann Reprod Health Care. 2014;40:54–60.
18. Christianson MS, Barker MA, Lindheim SR. Overcoming the challenging cervix: techniques to access the uterine cavity. J Low Genit Tract Dis. 2008;12:24–31.
19. Schorge J, Halvorson L, Schaffer J, Corton MM, Bradshaw K, Hoffman B. Williams Gynecology. 3rd ed: McGraw-Hill Education/Medical. Available at: www.accessmedicine.com; 2016.
20. Curtis KM, Tepper NK, Jatlaoui TC, Berry-Bibee E, Horton LG, Zapata LB, et al. U.S. Medical Eligibility Criteria for Contraceptive Use, 2016. MMWR Recomm Rep. 2016;65:1–103.
21. Higginbotham S, Society of Family Planning. Contraceptive considerations in obese women: release date 1 September 2009, SFP Guideline 20091. Contraception. 2009;80:583–90.
22. Nahum GG. Uterine anomalies. How common are they, and what is their distribution among subtypes? J Reprod Med. 1998;43:877–87.
23. Gottlieb AG, Galan HL. Shoulder dystocia: an update. Obstet Gynecol Clin N Am. 2007;34:501–31.. xii
24. ACOG Committee Opinion No. 735: Adolescents and Long-Acting Reversible Contraception: Implants and Intrauterine Devices. Obstet Gynecol. 2018;131:e130–9.
25. Zapata LB, Jatlaoui TC, Marchbanks PA, Curtis KM. Medications to ease intrauterine device insertion: a systematic review. Contraception. 2016;94:739–59.

26. Matthews LR, O'Dwyer L, O'Neill E. Intrauterine Device Insertion Failure After Misoprostol Administration: A Systematic Review. Obstet Gynecol. 2016;128:1084–91.
27. Bahamondes MV, Espejo-Arce X, Bahamondes L. Effect of vaginal administration of misoprostol before intrauterine contraceptive insertion following previous insertion failure: a double blind RCT. Hum Reprod. 2015;30:1861–6.
28. Espey E, Singh RH, Leeman L, Ogburn T, Fowler K, Greene H. Misoprostol for intrauterine device insertion in nulliparous women: a randomized controlled trial. Am J Obstet Gynecol. 2014;210:208.e1–5.
29. Fiala C, Gemzell-Danielsson K, Tang OS, von Hertzen H. Cervical priming with misoprostol prior to transcervical procedures. Int J Gynaecol Obstet. 2007;99(Suppl 2):S168–71.
30. Meckstroth KR, Whitaker AK, Bertisch S, Goldberg AB, Darney PD. Misoprostol administered by epithelial routes: Drug absorption and uterine response. Obstet Gynecol. 2006;108:582–90.
31. Chai J, Wong CYG, Ho PC. A randomized clinical trial comparing the short-term side effects of sublingual and buccal routes of misoprostol administration for medical abortions up to 63 days' gestation. Contraception. 2013;87:480–5.
32. Vickery Z, Madden T. Difficult intrauterine contraception insertion in a nulligravid patient. Obstet Gynecol. 2011;117:391–5.
33. Marchi NM, Castro S, Hidalgo MM, Hidalgo C, Monteiro-Dantas C, Villarroeal M, et al. Management of missing strings in users of intrauterine contraceptives. Contraception. 2012;86:354–8.
34. Tugrul S, Yavuzer B, Yildirim G, Kayahan A. The duration of use, causes of discontinuation, and problems during removal in women admitted for removal of IUD. Contraception. 2005;71:149–52.
35. Prabhakaran S, Chuang A. In-office retrieval of intrauterine contraceptive devices with missing strings. Contraception. 2011;83:102–6.
36. Curtis KM, Jatlaoui TC, Tepper NK, Zapata LB, Horton LG, Jamieson DJ, et al. U.S. Selected Practice Recommendations for Contraceptive Use, 2016. MMWR Recomm Rep. 2016;65:1–66.
37. Swenson C, Royer PA, Turok DK, Jacobson JC, Amaral G, Sanders JN. Removal of the LNG IUD when strings are not visible: a case series. Contraception. 2014;90:288–90.
38. Verma U, Astudillo-Dávalos FE, Gerkowicz SA. Safe and cost-effective ultrasound guided removal of retained intrauterine device: our experience. Contraception. 2015;92:77–80.
39. Turok DK, Gurtcheff SE, Gibson K, Handley E, Simonsen S, Murphy PA. Operative management of intrauterine device complications: a case series report. Contraception. 2010;82:354–7.
40. Heinemann K, Reed S, Moehner S, Minh TD. Comparative contraceptive effectiveness of levonorgestrel-releasing and copper intrauterine devices: the European Active Surveillance Study for Intrauterine Devices. Contraception. 2015;91:280–3.
41. Backman T, Rauramo I, Huhtala S, Koskenvuo M. Pregnancy during the use of levonorgestrel intrauterine system. Am J Obstet Gynecol. 2004;190:50–4.
42. Owen C, Sober S, Schreiber CA. Controversies in family planning: desired pregnancy, IUD in situ and no strings visible. Contraception. 2013;88:330–3.
43. Sanders AP, Fluker MR, Sanders BH. Saline Hysteroscopy for Removal of Retained Intrauterine Contraceptive Devices in Early Pregnancy. J Obstet Gynaecol Can. 2016;38:1114–9.
44. Brahmi D, Steenland MW, Renner R-M, Gaffield ME, Curtis KM. Pregnancy outcomes with an IUD in situ: a systematic review. Contraception. 2012;85:131–9.
45. McCarthy EA, Jagasia N, Maher P, Robinson M. Ultrasound-guided hysteroscopy to remove a levonorgestrel intrauterine system in early pregnancy. Contraception. 2012;86:587–90.
46. Schiesser M, Lapaire O, Tercanli S, Holzgreve W. Lost intrauterine devices during pregnancy: maternal and fetal outcome after ultrasound-guided extraction. An analysis of 82 cases. Ultrasound Obstet Gynecol. 2004;23:486–9.

Chapter 13
Adolescent and Young Adult IUD Delivery in Non-traditional Health Settings

Yasmin Z. Bahar, Mandy S. Coles, and Melanie A. Gold

Abbreviations

AYA   Adolescent and young adult
CDC   Centers for Disease Control and Prevention
ED   Emergency department
IUD   Intrauterine device
JJC   Juvenile justice center
LARC   Long-acting reversible contraception
LNG   Levonorgestrel
SBHC   School-based health center
STI   Sexually transmitted infections

Learning Objectives

Following completion of this chapter, you should be able to:

1. Describe how to effectively provide Intrauterine devices (IUDs) in non-traditional clinic settings.
2. Review the nuances of several non-traditional healthcare settings that may be barriers or facilitators to IUD delivery.
3. Anticipate planning and implementation needs when initiating or expanding provision of IUDs in non-traditional clinic settings.

Y. Z. Bahar (✉)
Department of Pediatrics, New York Presbyterian Columbia University Medical Center, New York, NY, USA
e-mail: yab9007@nyp.org

M. S. Coles
Department of Pediatrics, Boston University Medical Center, Boston, MA, USA

M. A. Gold
Department of Pediatrics, Division of Child and Adolescent Health, Columbia University Irving Medical Center/New York–Presbyterian Hospital, New York, NY, USA

© Springer Nature Switzerland AG 2019   169
M. S. Coles, A. Mays (eds.), *Optimizing IUD Delivery for Adolescents and Young Adults*, https://doi.org/10.1007/978-3-030-17816-1_13

Introduction

While traditional healthcare settings such as doctor's offices and clinics or health centers are the most common location for the receipt of medical care [1], they may present inadvertent barriers for Adolescent and young adults (AYAs), including issues with accessibility, transport, insurance coverage, and inability to pay [2]. Non-traditional health settings, such as School-based health centers (SBHCs), juvenile justice centers (JJCs), and Emergency departments (EDs) can help reduce some of the access issues faced by AYAs and can provide physically easier access to care [2]; IUD provision and management is one such service. In this chapter, we discuss options for providing IUDs to AYAs in non-traditional settings based on the literature and expert opinion (see Table 13.1).

Table 13.1 A summary of how to provide IUDs in non-traditional settings (Source: Modified from "Expanding Contraceptive Choice to the Underserved Through Delivery of Mobile Outreach Services.")

Making IUD services in non-traditional settings a reality [3]
1. Planning
(a) Needs assessment: Do we need outreach, and if so, where?
(i) Are there underserved populations in your program area, and if so, where are they located?
(ii) If yes, what are the main barriers to services for these populations?
(iii) Is IUD service provision in non-traditional settings an effective way to address these barriers and reach these populations?
(b) Identification of resources: What resources are available, and what resources do we need to find?
(i) Site selection and staffing
(ii) Guidelines and policies
(c) Cost analysis: Is this approach feasible from a cost perspective?
(d) Building partnership: Who are the key stakeholders, and how can we best plan and work together? *Remember to involve potential AYA patients, as well as youth-serving agencies*
(e) Development of an action plan: What are the key steps to starting and implementing the program? Who will be responsible for each step?
(i) Frequency of service delivery
(ii) Composition and training of health service delivery team
(iii) Promotion to the community
(iv) Follow-up and continuity of care activities
2. Implementation
(a) Main steps
(i) Schedule services
(ii) Prepare sites for service delivery
(iii) Inform client base
(iv) Create monitoring and ensure quality of care and follow-up for patients
(b) Main challenges and suggestions on how to address them
(i) Transportation issues
(ii) Financial and supply issues
(iii) Inadequate patient demands
3. Scale up
(a) Assess need for increasing service delivery

Case

Maria is a 15-year-old, cisgender female high school sophomore who wants to be a forensic scientist. She has been dating her boyfriend for a year, feels ready to have sex, and wants to make sure that she does not become pregnant. Maria discusses this with a peer educator in her school cafeteria, who shares information about her contraceptive options using a shared decision-making counseling framework. Later, in her health class, she hears a presentation on contraception from the school health educator. Maria tells the health educator that she is interested in the IUD and is referred to her SBHC. During this visit, Maria meets with the medical provider, who supplies her with more information about the different types of IUDs. Maria chooses to have a copper IUD placed that day. The SBHC medical assistant offers Maria support by holding her hand and helping her breathe during the procedure. After Maria has her IUD placed, she rests in the SBHC for 15 minutes and then returns to class. Several weeks later, Maria returns to her SBHC because she is worried about bleeding and cramping. She is seen immediately, is reassured about her IUD concerns, and is also offered testing for gonorrhea and chlamydia. Maria feels better by the end of her visit, and goes back to class. Over lunch, she shares her experience with her friend Stephanie, who also decides to schedule an appointment at the SBHC.

School-Based Health Centers (SBHCs)

While the provision of medical care in schools has existed for many years, the development of comprehensive—and primary care-focused—SBHCs began in earnest in the early 1970s [4, 5]. The 2016–2017 National School-Based Health Care Census identified 2584 SBHCs located in 48 states, the District of Columbia, and Puerto Rico (see Fig. 13.1). No SBHCs were identified in North Dakota and Wisconsin. Nearly half of the surveyed SBHCs provide care to communities in urban areas (46%), and more than one-third (36%) provide care to rural communities [6].

Strengths of SBHCs SBHCs provide direct contact with student patients, improve access to care [7], and allow providers to offer private and confidential reproductive healthcare visits consistent with state minor consent laws. SBHCs may receive grant funding for reproductive healthcare service delivery and can often provide care to patients regardless of insurance type or ability to pay. Among SBHCs that serve adolescents (defined in this survey as students in grades 6 and above), condoms were the contraceptive method most frequently available on site (41%), followed by oral contraceptive pills (30%) and emergency contraception (26%). Long-acting reversible contraception (LARC) methods (including IUDs and hormonal implants) were available at 21% of SBHCs serving adolescents [6].

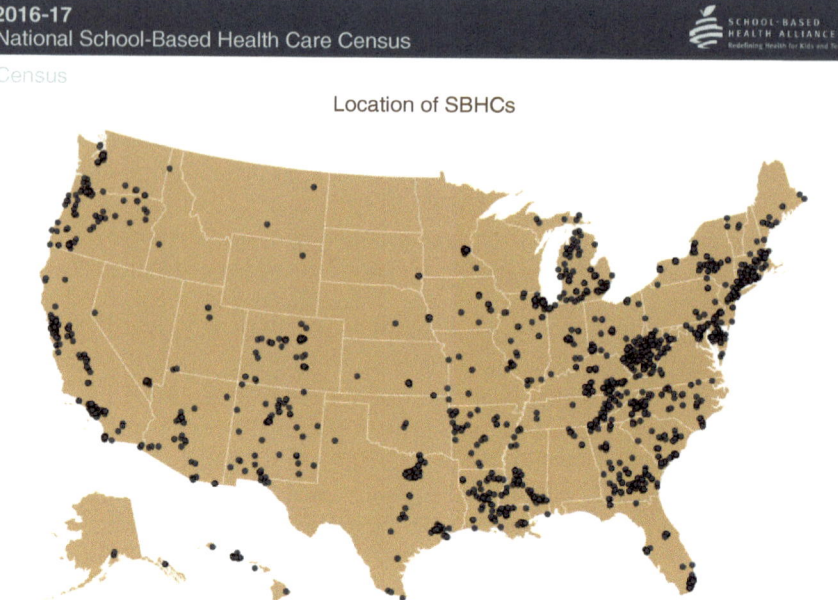

2016-17
National School-Based Health Care Census

Census

Location of SBHCs

SCHOOL-BASED
HEALTH ALLIANCE
Redefining Health for Kids and Teens

Fig. 13.1 A map representing numbers and density of SBHCs surveyed in the National School-Based Health Care Census (2016–2017) [6]

Multidisciplinary teams at SBHCs While medical providers supply much of the education around reproductive choice, students appreciate hearing information from a variety of different individuals at SBHCs [8]. Health educators (present at 12% of surveyed SBHCs) [9] can be instrumental by providing reproductive health education in both the classroom and within the SBHC. Health educators can conduct face-to-face sessions with patients as individuals or in groups. In New York City, the Office of School Health provides training for frontline staff members on reproductive health access and information; some SBHCs have opted to include mental and allied health staff in these training sessions. The goal of including multidisciplinary staff members is to ensure that everyone who interacts with students can deliver the same messages, ensure continuity, and provide accurate and evidence-based information.

Support partners in IUD provision at SBHCs The logistics of offering IUD services at SBHCs are unique and may require support from state departments of education or local school districts. Training school staff on what services SBHCs provide, as well as reviewing federal and state laws on minors' rights to reproductive healthcare, can be helpful in communicating with students and their parents/guardians.

Clinical pearls for IUD delivery in SBHCs:

• Use of health educators, when available, can be great resources for student health education, outreach, and connection to SBHCs. Advocating for health-educator positions as part of expanding services to include IUD provision can significantly increase clinical efficiency, device uptake, and student satisfaction with services.

- Multidisciplinary teams must be trained in the tenets of reproductive justice, the necessity of confidential care, and the full range of contraceptive services.

Case (continued)

Maria's friend Stephanie—a 16-year-old, cisgender female—does not have time to return to the SBHC for her IUD insertion before graduating from high school and contacts the health educator the next fall. She is now unstably housed and has no health insurance, so the health educator suggests services through a youth shelter or mobile van program. Before Stephanie is able to contact those two places, she goes to a JJC, where she is able to get her IUD placed.

Juvenile Justice Centers (JJCs)

AYAs in JJCs often represent some of the most vulnerable youth in a community and report higher rates of multiple sex partners, inconsistent condom use, early sexual debut, prior pregnancy, mental health issues (often co-occurring with substance abuse), housing instability, and food insecurity compared to other youth [10–14]. As the detention period may represent the only significant contact with the healthcare system for some AYAs in the juvenile justice system [11, 14], it can be a great opportunity to address multiple healthcare needs, including reproductive health. However, providers also need to be conscious of biases when extending care in these settings in order to avoid coercion. Youth are not able to move around freely, and others have authority over decisions regarding when and what they eat, when they can come and go in certain spaces, and when they wake and go to sleep [15]. Civil limitations such as these can subconsciously affect perception of choice around medical care. When counseling around IUDs for contraception, it is especially important to use shared decision-making counseling techniques (see Chap. 5) and ensure that AYAs in juvenile justice settings know they are free to choose the contraceptive method that is right for them without coercion [16].

Some of the advantages of providing IUD services at JJCs are that they are free to the patient, AYAs may be able to make frequent visits with the medical provider to talk about and follow up on their contraception, and often there are less time constraints for IUD counseling. Each JJC has standard requirements around how soon AYAs must see a medical provider after being detained. Most centers require that youth are seen within 24 hours, although some facilities have up to a 72-hour requirement. It is important to use the initial clinical visit as an opportunity to provide comprehensive medical care, including an overall health assessment that integrates sexual and reproductive health goals. As youth are both living and receiving their medical care in the JJC, AYAs who chose IUDs may be able to have frequent follow-up visits after the insertion and have any concerns addressed in a timely manner.

Clinical pearls for IUD delivery in JJCs:

- Communication and collaboration between the health center and the probation department (including staff) are important to ensure continuity across the JJC facility. Staff should also be educated on symptoms to expect after an IUD insertion and when it may be necessary to refer a patient for additional evaluation after IUD insertion.
- It is not only important to have policies in place to address follow-up after IUD insertion and management of post-insertion symptoms but also to ensure that probation staff members are aware of follow-up and symptom management plans.
- Employing shared decision-making counseling principles [17] (see Chap. 5) is key when discussing contraception with JJC youth to ensure patient reproductive autonomy.

Emergency Department

While EDs are busy clinical settings where patients present for both emergent and urgent concerns [18], they also represent a potential site for the provision of IUDs and contraceptive implants. Some AYAs come to EDs with concerns of pregnancy or Sexually transmitted infections (STIs) [19, 20], while others may be at risk for pregnancy or presenting for non-related concerns. We know that AYAs are less likely to attend preventive health visits; thus, education on reproductive health is important at any clinical encounter [21, 22]. Many ED providers refer to patients interested in contraception to family planning clinics, adolescent clinics, or primary care providers. However, delay in providing contraception is a missed opportunity, and places the patient at risk for an unintended pregnancy [23, 24].

There is a paucity of literature on IUD insertions in the ED. One article discussed consideration of obtaining a gynecology consult for insertion of the copper IUD as emergency contraception after sexual assault [25]. Personal communications with a provider who researched placing IUDs in ED settings (A. Koyama, personal communication, May 14, 2018) found that patients reported more interest in using the contraceptive pill or implant than in the IUD. Providers in this setting were also resistant to performing procedures that they did not view as emergent and felt they would not be placing enough devices to maintain proficiency. In weighing the cost of the devices, combined with evidence that lack of experience in inserting IUDs increases the possibility of expulsion [26, 27], Dr. Koyama successfully worked with the hospital's adolescent and family planning clinics to improve same-day access to IUD insertions for AYAs referred from the ED (A. Koyama, personal communication, May 14, 2018). Along with same-day referral from the emergency room, additional data suggest that AYAs are also interested in receiving LARC while in the ED [24].

Although the aforementioned institution was not able to provide IUD insertions in the ED, Dr. Koyama did share some important information to help advance this practice for others in the future. Billing for IUD insertions and devices was raised as a potential challenge, as many EDs are reimbursed at flat rates based on diagnosis and not by visit complexity. Dr. Koyama was able to negotiate this challenge by using grant-funded devices which did not have to be billed for. Providers were also concerned that follow-up would be an issue for patients receiving IUDs in an ED setting. However, this issue has been managed at other non-traditional and mobile care sites as discussed below by providing information on community-based clinics. It is important to address the potential for contraceptive coercion when considering future efforts to provide contraception in the ED, as AYAs may feel like they need to agree to a certain contraceptive option in order to receive the emergent or urgent clinical care that they need. Additionally, it is helpful to have an IUD champion in the ED to involve stakeholders early to address issues with billing and reimbursement, identify opportunities for provider training, and increase patient education and interest.

Clinical Pearls for IUD insertion in EDs

- Assess patient interest in IUD insertion in ED settings prior to programmatic development.
- Identify an IUD provider champion in the ED to increase success.
- Involve stakeholders early to help address potential billing challenges, which are important to the success of IUD delivery in ED settings.
- In the event that the ED does not have the capacity to provide IUDs within the department, create a same-day LARC referral partnership with an AYA clinic or family planning site to help improve access.

Healthcare Programs for Homeless and Unstably Housed AYAs

As defined by Dorsen, vulnerability in homeless AYAs is defined as "the constellation of past, present and future risk, perceived or real, because of the common human experience of risk, the increased vulnerability of the adolescent period, the consequences of family disruption, and the increased risks of life on the street [28]." Lack of access to health-promoting resources, including regular medical care, is one of the many identified factors that can impact this vulnerability. Healthcare programs for homeless and unstably housed AYAs, such as those located at drop-in and shelter-based clinics, seek to provide stability for these AYAs and may be more commonly used than other medical services [29]. As rates of pregnancy are substantially higher among homeless than stably housed youth [30], these sites are also ideal locations for the delivery of the full spectrum of contraceptive options, including IUDs.

Medical services targeted toward unstably housed AYAs may often exist as programs of a larger satellite community clinics or federally qualified health centers. These larger health centers often have grant funding or an existing capacity to support the up-front costs of IUD services. Devices and equipment for IUD insertions may be provided by the health center, and disposable instruments are often useful in these settings (see Chap. 8 for more information). If there is only one medical provider on-site, it is important that they are able to provide the full range of contraceptive options, including IUDs. One advantage of providing IUDs in shelter settings is that AYAs often live in the same location where they are receiving healthcare. As a result, medical providers have the opportunity to follow up with and assess how patients are doing after their IUD insertion. Vulnerable youth who are not living in shelters often use these medical services too, as youth shelters are designed as safe spaces where AYAs can access trusted services. AYAs may be referred by providers at other youth-serving agencies or local health departments. Despite AYAs' generally positive reactions to health services within shelters, some identified barriers to use of services include perceived restrictive rules and concerns about confidentiality and mandated reporting [29].

One survey of facilities that provided IUD placement services to unstably housed AYAs reported a number of barriers to providing these services to AYAs. These included lack of provider training, lack of insurance, insufficient funding to provide contraceptive services, high no-show rates for IUD insertions after initial appointments for labs (not in line with evidence-based guidelines [31]), concern for lack of follow-up if complications were to develop, and competing complex medical, mental health, and substances abuse issues [32]. Many of these concerns are not unique to programs serving unstably housed AYAs and have been discussed throughout this text, while others are unique to programs serving this population. As it has been well documented that requiring two visits for an IUD insertion is a barrier to AYAs [33, 34], it is important that providers are comfortable with same-day insertion and have the necessary devices and insertion supplies on hand.

Clinical pearls for IUD insertion in healthcare programs for homeless or unstably housed AYAs

- It is important to reduce barriers to access by offering same-day IUD insertions to AYAs in medical services targeted at unstably housed youth.
- AYA housing status or social vulnerability is not a contraindication to IUD use or suggestive of risk of complication; providers should focus on evidence-based guidelines to determine eligibility and safety for IUD use.

Inpatient Settings

There is a scarcity of literature about providing IUDs to AYAs who are not postpartum within inpatient settings. However, in some medical centers, adolescent medicine providers are already offering IUDs on an outpatient basis and are also taking care of many AYAs in the inpatient setting. As these providers are already discussing sexual and reproductive health as part of their social history taking with inpatient AYAs—and also have the skills to offer a full spectrum of contraceptive options for those who are interested—offering this service on an inpatient basis may be both reasonable and doable.

Providers from an adolescent medicine program at the University of Rochester Medical Center began offering IUDs as an option to inpatient AYAs in 2012. It was the experience of one of these providers that patients who were admitted for eating disorders, intentional ingestion, or suicidality were often also interested in discussing contraception prior to discharge (K. Greenberg, personal communication, May 24, 2018). Supplies for IUD insertion were available in the adolescent medicine clinic, which had sterilized equipment for IUD insertions ("IUD trays") set up and easy for providers to move from the adjoining building (clinic) to the inpatient unit. The physical environment on inpatient units can be a particular challenge, Dr. Greenberg noted; inpatient facilities were not set up for gynecologic procedures, and staff members were sometimes needed to facilitate patient positioning and easy access to supplies.

Challenges to inpatient provision of IUD services Payment for devices and procedures can also be a significant barrier to provision of IUD services in an inpatient setting. Dr. Greenberg noted that providers were initially reimbursed for the devices themselves, but not for the insertion procedure. More recently, the division stopped receiving reimbursement for the devices themselves and had to stop inserting IUDs in the inpatient setting (K. Greenberg, personal communication, May 24, 2018). Partnering with family planning programs who may have access to grant funding for devices, or directly working with insurance companies to advocate for payment for devices and procedures—such as the unbundling of family planning codes and reimbursement from the global labor and delivery package to decrease barriers to immediate postpartum LARC methods—are a few options that can help to improve access. As an alternative, Dr. Greenberg shared that providers give patients an appointment in the adolescent medicine clinic on the same day as their discharge, so they can have their IUD placed as soon as they leave the inpatient unit, but before leaving the medical center and going home. Additional concerted and strategic efforts to provide IUDs in inpatient settings could continue to expand service delivery and improve AYA access.

Clinical pearls for IUD insertion in inpatient settings

- Consider facility and room design when planning for new or updated inpatient units to allow options for gynecologic procedures, such as IUD insertions, to be performed.
- Monitor reimbursement for IUD insertion procedures and devices closely, in order to guarantee payment for services and allow for opportunities for advocacy with insurance companies as needed.

Mobile Health Programs

Mobile health clinics, created to reach underserved or medically disenfranchised communities, can be ideal for AYAs who have difficulty engaging with more traditional healthcare services. These programs can provide health education and patient navigation services [35], as well as direct medical care, and are a cost-effective way to bring services to highly underserved populations [29, 36]. Mobile health programs can go to where AYAs are in the community—health fairs, parks, or other areas where unstably housed youth are known to gather—and are often affiliated with a clinic, youth-serving agency, or medical institution.

As previously discussed, rates of pregnancy are substantially higher among unstably housed and vulnerable AYAs [30]. While most mobile health programs are not currently offering IUD services to clients, these sites provide an opportunity to bring the full spectrum of contraceptive options to those who may be most in need. Provision of services can be communicated via social media, through flyers inside the mobile clinic or at other sites (shelters, food pantries, and drop-in centers) frequented by youth, or via outreach workers from youth-serving agencies, including social service agencies.

Challenges to IUD provision in mobile health programs While mobile health clinics clearly allow providers to reach AYAs who might otherwise not engage in healthcare, there are also challenges to providing IUDs in these settings. Little has been published on the development of these programs in the USA, though there are many successful examples internationally [37–39]. Guidelines for expanding contraceptive choice through mobile outreach do exist, as outlined in Table 13.1 [3]. Mobile healthcare programs usually have limited space and may have only one private exam room. Another unique challenge of providing IUD insertions in mobile vans is that they may not have a space for rest or respite after the procedure. Some programs have addressed this by creating a private respite site adjacent the mobile van, using a chair where the patient can rest after the procedure (A. Mays, personal communication, May 16, 2018). As unstably housed AYAs often move around over time, having regular follow-up appointments may be challenging. It is important that AYAs know when the mobile van will return to different locations. AYAs should also have information on where to get care if they have any urgent concerns after IUD placement. Alternate ways of communicating with patients after IUD provision include via text messaging, apps, social media posts, mobile phones, or communication with providers at youth-serving agencies. In the event of positive STI tests results, local health departments can assist in finding and treating patients.

Clinical Pearls for IUD insertion in mobile healthcare programs

- It is important to be fluid in the process of IUD delivery in a mobile health program. Consideration of private space and places for respite after insertion is an integral part of this care.

- Partnering with youth-serving agencies, local health departments, and community AYA clinics can help to strengthen IUD delivery in mobile health programs.

Considerations in Providing IUDs at Non-traditional Clinical Sites

While some of the challenges to providing IUDs in non-traditional settings are unique to the site of care (as discussed above), there are many similarities across care sites. The start-up cost of an IUD program may be high, especially given the cost of the individual devices. In clinics with no support from a sponsor organization, the clinic may have to find funds for the up-front cost of buying the supplies involved in IUD insertion. Please see the "Additional Resources" section at the back of this text for additional information. Providers must also consider whether they want to use sterilizable equipment or disposable equipment, as each has its overall benefits and challenges (see Chap. 8). More information on these kits is also available in the "Additional Resources" section of this textbook. Limited staffing can also present an issue, as the medical assistant may need to perform a time out prior to the procedure, assist the medical provider during the IUD insertion, or support the patient during the procedure. The entire medical team, including community partners and organizational members, should be comfortable with IUDs being provided on site and aware of the tenets of reproductive justice and the importance of patient confidentiality.

Conclusion

Non-traditional health settings have the ability to respond to gaps in reproductive healthcare by addressing access barriers that AYAs may face in traditional health settings, particularly among highly vulnerable youth. While all of the sites discussed in this chapter have the ability to offer same-day IUD placements and meet AYAs in their communities, programs may not currently exist. For most non-traditional sites, a one-size-fits-all policy approach regarding IUD placement for AYAs is impractical. It is important to be thoughtful and tailored in planning and implementing IUD provision in non-traditional settings while following existing guidelines and building community partnerships. The Centers for Disease Control and Prevention (CDC) Quality Family Planning Guidelines [40] provide an evidence-based roadmap on how to implement these services. Lastly, maintaining patient confidentiality and preventing contraceptive coercion, especially with AYAs who are underserved or medically disenfranchised, is of utmost importance.

Overall Clinical Pearls

- Involve stakeholders early on, as most of the challenges may be around billing and reimbursement. Make a business plan beforehand, and determine how to fund the start-up costs of launching an IUD service in a non-traditional setting.
- Educate clinical and nonclinical staff members. It is critical that all team members understand that, although it is a non-traditional setting, IUDs are a safe and viable option for AYAs seeking healthcare in these settings.
- Tailor IUD service delivery (including protocols, instrument type, and space determination) to the specific needs and resources of the clinical site.
- Ensure staff are comfortable with same-day IUD insertion. Quickstart guidelines will help to optimize IUD delivery in non-traditional settings.
- Consult existing guidelines (see Table 13.1 above) for expanding contraceptive choice to non-traditional sites. These guidelines include performing a needs assessment, identifying resources, determining feasibility from a cost perspective, building partnerships, developing and implementing an action plan, and addressing challenges.

References

1. National Center for Health Statistics. Summary health statistics for U.S. children: national health interview survey. Bethesda: National Center for Health Statistics; 2017.
2. Decker M, Berglas N, Brindis C. A call to action: developing and strengthening new strategies to promote adolescent sexual health. Societies. 2015;5:686–712.
3. Expanding contraceptive choice to the underserved through delivery of mobile outreach services: a handbook for program planners [Internet]. [cited 3 Dec 2018]. Available: https://www.k4health.org/sites/default/files/expanding_contraceptive_choice.pdf.
4. Edwards LE, Steinman ME, Hakanson EY. An experimental comprehensive high school clinic. Am J Public Health. 1977;67:765–6.
5. Kirby D. Comprehensive school-based health clinics: a growing movement to improve adolescent health and reduce teen-age pregnancy. J Sch Health. 1986;56:289–91.
6. Love H, Soleimanpour S, Panchal N, Schlitt J, Behr C, Even M. 2016–17 national school-based health care census report. Washington, D.C: School-Based Health Alliance; 2018.
7. School-based health centers: improving health, well-being and educational success. In: American Public Health Association [Internet]. [cited 3 Dec 2018]. Available: https://www.apha.org/-/media/files/pdf/sbhc/well_being_in_schools.
8. Sangraula M, Garbers S, Garth J, Shakibnia EB, Timmons S, Gold MA. Integrating long-acting reversible contraception services into New York City school-based health centers: quality improvement to ensure provision of youth-friendly services. J Pediatr Adolesc Gynecol. 2017;30:376–82.
9. 2013-14 census of school-based health centers: methodology, key report data details, and acknowledgements. In: School-based health alliance [Internet]. [cited 3 Dec 2018]. Available: http://www.sbh4all.org/wp-content/uploads/2015/02/2013-14-Census-Data-and-Methods.pdf.
10. Golzari M, Hunt SJ, Anoshiravani A. The health status of youth in juvenile detention facilities. J Adolesc Health. 2006;38:776–82.
11. Feinstein RA, Lampkin A, Lorish CD, Klerman LV, Maisiak R, Oh MK. Medical status of adolescents at time of admission to a juvenile detention center. J Adolesc Health Care. 1998;22:190–6.

12. Griel LC III, Loeb SJ. Health issues faced by adolescents incarcerated in the juvenile justice system. J Forensic Nurs. 2009;5:162–79.
13. Feldmann JM. Caring for incarcerated youth. Curr Opin Pediatr. 2008;20:398–402.
14. Committee on Adolescence. Health care for youth in the juvenile justice system. Pediatrics. 2011;128:1219–35.
15. Mendel RA. Maltreatment of youth in U.S. juvenile corrections facilities: an update. In: The Annie E. Casey foundation [Internet]. [cited 3 Dec 2018]. Available: https://www.aecf.org/m/resourcedoc/aecf-maltreatmentyouthuscorrections-2015.pdf.
16. Sufrin C, Baird S, Clarke J, Feldman E. Family planning services for incarcerated women: models for filling an unmet need. Int J Prison Health. 2017;13:10–8.
17. Dehlendorf C, Grumbach K, Schmittdiel JA, Steinauer J. Shared decision making in contraceptive counseling. Contraception. 2017;95:452–5.
18. Coster JE, Turner JK, Bradbury D, Cantrell A. Why do people choose emergency and urgent care services? A rapid review utilizing a systematic literature search and narrative synthesis. Acad Emerg Med. 2017;24:1137–49.
19. Cox S, Dean T, Posner SF, Jamieson DJ, Curtis KM, Johnson CH, et al. Disparities in reproductive health-related visits to the emergency department in Maryland by age and race, 1999–2005. J Women's Health. 2011;20:1833–8.
20. Curtis KM, Hillis SD, Jr Kieke BA, Brett KM, Marchbanks PA, Peterson HB. Visits to emergency departments for gynecologic disorders in the United States, 1992–1994. Obstet Gynecol. 1998;91:1007–12.
21. Jr Irwin CE, Adams SH, Park MJ, Newacheck PW. Preventive care for adolescents: few get visits and fewer get services. Pediatrics. 2009;123:e565–72.
22. Chung PJ, Lee TC, Morrison JL, Schuster MA. Preventive care for children in the United States: quality and barriers. Annu Rev Public Health. 2006;27:491–515.
23. Miller MK, Randell KA, Barral R, Sherman AK, Miller E. Factors associated with interest in same-day contraception initiation among females in the pediatric emergency department. J Adolesc Health. 2016;58:154–9.
24. Hoehn EF, Hoefgen H, Chernick LS, Dyas J, Krantz L, Zhang N, et al. A pediatric emergency department intervention to increase contraception initiation among adolescents. Acad Emerg Med. 2018; https://doi.org/10.1111/acem.13565.
25. Larsen J, Patty Cason FNP. IUDs in the ED - emergency physicians monthly. In: Emergency physicians monthly [Internet]. 16 Jan 2014 [cited 3 Dec 2018]. Available: http://epmonthly.com/article/iuds-in-the-ed/.
26. Andersson K, Ryde-Blomqvist E, Lindell K, Odlind V, Milsom I. Perforations with intrauterine devices. Report from a Swedish survey. Contraception. 1998;57:251–5.
27. Caliskan E, Oztürk N, Dilbaz BO, Dilbaz S. Analysis of risk factors associated with uterine perforation by intrauterine devices. Eur J Contracept Reprod Health Care. 2003;8:150–5.
28. Dorsen C. Vulnerability in homeless adolescents: concept analysis. J Adv Nurs. 2010;66:2819–27.
29. De Rosa CJ, Montgomery SB, Kipke MD, Iverson E, Ma JL, Unger JB. Service utilization among homeless and runaway youth in Los Angeles, California: rates and reasons. J Adolesc Health. 1999;24:190–200.
30. Greene JM, Ringwalt CL. Pregnancy among three national samples of runaway and homeless youth. J Adolesc Health. 1998;23:370–7.
31. Curtis KM, Jatlaoui TC, Tepper NK, Zapata LB, Horton LG, Jamieson DJ, et al. U.S. selected practice recommendations for contraceptive use, 2016. MMWR Recomm Rep. 2016;65:1–66.
32. Saver BG, Weinreb L, Gelberg L, Zerger S. Provision of contraceptive services to homeless women: results of a survey of health care for the homeless providers. Women Health. 2012;52:151–61.
33. Pritt NM, Norris AH, Berlan ED. Barriers and facilitators to adolescents' use of long-acting reversible contraceptives. J Pediatr Adolesc Gynecol. 2017;30:18–22.
34. Bergin A, Tristan S, Terplan M, Gilliam ML, Whitaker AK. A missed opportunity for care: two-visit IUD insertion protocols inhibit placement. Contraception. 2012;86:694–7.

35. Hill C, Zurakowski D, Bennet J, Walker-White R, Osman JL, Quarles A, et al. Knowledgeable neighbors: a mobile clinic model for disease prevention and screening in underserved communities. Am J Public Health. 2012;102:406–10.
36. Oriol NE, Cote PJ, Vavasis AP, Bennet J, Delorenzo D, Blanc P, et al. Calculating the return on investment of mobile healthcare. BMC Med. 2009;7:27.
37. Hubacher D, Akora V, Masaba R, Chen M, Veena V. Introduction of the levonorgestrel intrauterine system in Kenya through mobile outreach: review of service statistics and provider perspectives. Glob Health Sci Pract. 2014;2:47–54.
38. Cleland J, Ali M, Benova L, Daniele M. The promotion of intrauterine contraception in low- and middle-income countries: a narrative review. Contraception. 2017;95:519–28.
39. Azmat SK, Hameed W, Mustafa G, Hussain W, Ahmed A, Bilgrami M. IUD discontinuation rates, switching behavior, and user satisfaction: findings from a retrospective analysis of a mobile outreach service program in Pakistan. Int J Women's Health. 2013;5:19–27.
40. Gavin L, Pazol K, Ahrens K. Update: providing quality family planning services - recommendations from CDC and the U.S. office of population affairs, 2017. MMWR Morb Mortal Wkly Rep. 2017;66:1383–5.

Appendix: Additional Resources

Chapter 1: The Intrauterine Device and Adolescents: History and Present

- Roberts D. *Killing the Black Body: Race, Reproduction, and the Meaning of Liberty.* Vintage: 2014.
- Further information on reproductive justice available at Sister Song: Women of Color Reproductive Justice Collective—https://www.sistersong.net/reproductive-justice/

Chapter 2: Making Your Office Accessible for Adolescent and Young Adult IUD Services

Adolescent-Friendly Health Services (presentation). Adolescent Sexual and Reproductive Health Education Project (ARSHEP), part of Physicians for Reproductive Choice. Available for download at—https://prh.org/arshep-ppts/

Information on state's minor consent laws

- American Civil Liberties Union—www.aclu.org
- Guttmacher Institute—https://www.guttmacher.org/state-policy/laws-policies

Emergency Contraception Birth Control that Works After Sex (educational materials/chart). Available in Spanish and English at—https://beyondthepill.ucsf.edu/educational-materials

Evidence-Based Sexual Health Information Apps and websites—

- Bedsider Birth Control Support Network—Bedsider.org
- The Reproductive Health Access Project (RHAP)—Reproductiveaccess.org

© Springer Nature Switzerland AG 2019
M. S. Coles, A. Mays (eds.), *Optimizing IUD Delivery for Adolescents and Young Adults*, https://doi.org/10.1007/978-3-030-17816-1

- TeenSource: Teen Health Resources and Information—Teensouce.org
- Planned Parenthood Federation of America—Plannedparenthood.org
- As well as myriad period-tracking apps.

Drawing a Picture: Adolescent Centered Medical Homes (video). Adolescent Health Initiative—https://www.youtube.com/watch?v=vAu5ad827I8

Birth Control Across the Gender Spectrum (also printed at the end of this chapter). Reproductive Health Access Project—https://www.reproductiveaccess.org/wpcontent/uploads/2018/06/bc-across-gender-spectrum.pdf

Best Practices for Youth-Friendly Clinical Services Advocates for Youth—

- Website—https://advocatesforyouth.org/resources/health-information/bp-youth-friendly-services/
- PDF version—https://advocatesforyouth.org/wp-content/uploads/storage//advfy/documents/bp-youth-friendly-services.pdf

Your First Pelvic Exam Center for Young Women's Health—https://youngwomenshealth.org/2013/08/22/pelvic-exam/

Characteristics of Youth-Friendly Health Care Desiderio, G. Healthy Teen Network. October 8, 2014—http://www.healthyteennetwork.org/blog/characteristics-youth-friendly-health-care-services/

EC4U Toolkit K4Health—
https://www.k4health.org/toolkits/emergency-contraception

Achieving Quality Health Services for Adolescents *Pediatrics*. June 2016; 138 (2). AAP News and Journals Gateway—http://pediatrics.aappublications.org/content/138/2/e20161347

Adolescent Friendly Services: Key Criteria and Assessment Tool. Serrano J, Shafii T, UW School of Med. (Adapted from WHO 2009)— http://www.k12.wa.us/HIVSexualhealth/pubdocs/AdolescentFriendlyServices_OSPI.pdf

Society for Adolescent Health and Medicine (SAHM) Resources

- Routine Sexual and Reproductive Health Resources— https://www.adolescenthealth.org/Resources/Clinical-Care-Resources/Sexual-Reproductive-Health/Resources/Routine-Sexual-Reproductive-Healthcare.aspx#R-Services
- Sexual and Reproductive Health Care: A Position Paper of the Society for Adolescent Health and Medicine. *Journal of Adolescent Health* 2014; 54(4):491-6.
- Improving Knowledge About, Access to, and Utilization of Long-Acting Reversible Contraception Among Adolescents and Young Adults. *J Adolesc Health* 2017; 60(4):472-474.

Adolescent and Youth Friendly Resource Guide Vermont Department of Health—http://www.amchp.org/programsandtopics/AdolescentHealth/Lists/Resources/DispForm.aspx?ID=13

Youth Centered Care Toolkit National Adolescent and Young Adult Health Information Center—http://nahic.ucsf.edu/resource_center/toolkit-youth-centered-care/

WHO Global Standards for Quality Youth-Centered Care Volumes 1 and 2 (Strategies and Implementation Guide). 2015—http://apps.who.int/iris/bitstream/handle/10665/183935/9789241549332_vol1_eng.pdf?sequence=1

LARC Quick Coding Guide The American College of Obstetrics and Gynecology (also printed at the end of this chapter)—https://www.acog.org/-/media/Departments/LARC/Coding-Guide-2018FINAL.pdf

Chapter 3: Types of IUDs and Mechanism of Action

Method-specific information sheets available at:

- Bedsider Birth Control Support Network—www.bedsider.org
- The Reproductive Health Access Project (RHAP)—www.reproductiveaccess.org

Facts Are Important: Emergency Contraception (EC) and Intrauterine Devices (IUDs) Are Not Abortifacients Handout. June 2014. The American College of Obstetricians and Gynecologists (also printed at the end of this chapter)— https://www.acog.org/-/media/Departments/Government-Relations-and-Outreach/FactsAreImportantEC.pdf

Chapter 4: Addressing IUD Efficacy, Eligibility, Myths, and Satisfaction with Adolescents and Young Adults

CDC Medical Eligibility Criteria for Contraceptive Use Centers for Disease Control and Prevention (CDC). Direct links are available (on the website, or as printed at the end of this chapter)—https://www.cdc.gov/reproductivehealth/contraception/mmwr/mec/summary.html

- The USA MEC and USA SPR apps.
- Print version of the Medical Eligibility Criteria for Contraceptive Use, 2016—https://www.cdc.gov/reproductivehealth/contraception/mmwr/mec/summary.html

- MEC Summary Chart (1 page, double sided)—https://www.cdc.gov/reproductivehealth/contraception/pdf/summary-chart-us-medical-eligibility-criteria_508tagged.pdf
- Effectiveness of Contraceptive Methods (1 page, also printed at the end of this chapter)—https://www.cdc.gov/reproductivehealth/contraception/unintendedpregnancy/pdf/Contraceptive_methods_508.pdf

CDC USA Selected Practice Recommendations (USA SPR) for Contraceptive Use Centers for Disease Control and Prevention (CDC). Direct links are available (on the website, or as listed below)—https://www.cdc.gov/reproductivehealth/contraception/mmwr/spr/summary.html

- The USA MEC and USA SPR apps.
- Print version of the MMWR USA Selected Practice Recommendations for Contraceptive Use—https://www.cdc.gov/mmwr/volumes/65/rr/rr6504a1.htm?s_cid=rr6504a1_w
- When to Start Using Specific Contraceptive Methods (1 page)—https://www.cdc.gov/reproductivehealth/contraception/pdf/When-To-Start_508Tagged.pdf
- Recommended Actions After Late or Missed Combined Oral Contraceptives (1 page, double sided)—https://www.cdc.gov/reproductivehealth/contraception/pdf/Recommended-Actions-Late-Missed_508Tagged.pdf
- Management of Women with Bleeding Irregularities While Using Contraception (2 pages)—https://www.cdc.gov/reproductivehealth/contraception/pdf/Management-During-Contraception_508Tagged.pdf

Five Myths About the IUD, Busted. M. Rodrigues. September 12, 2017. Bedsider — https://www.bedsider.org/features/243-5-myths-about-the-iud-busted

Facts Are Important: Emergency Contraception (EC) and Intrauterine Devices (IUDs) Are Not Abortifacients Handout. June 2014. The American College of Obstetricians and Gynecologists (also printed at the end of this chapter)— https://www.acog.org/-/media/Departments/Government-Relations-and-Outreach/FactsAreImportantEC.pdf

Chapter 5: IUD Counseling: What's Choice Got to Do With It?

Long-Acting Reversible Contraception Statement of Principles Sister Song: Women of Color Reproductive Justice Collective and National Women's Health Network (also printed at the end of this chapter)—https://www.nwhn.org/wp-content/uploads/2017/02/LARCStatementofPrinciples.pdf

Supporting AYA Sexual Empowerment, Sexual Readiness, and Sexual Consent Rights, Respect, Responsibility: Don't Have Sex Without Them A Lesson Plan from Rights, Respect, Responsibility: A K-12 Curriculum. [cited

18 Jan 2019]. Advocates for Youth—https://advocatesforyouth.org/wp-content/uploads/3rscurric/documents/10-Lesson-1-3Rs-RightsRespectResponsibility.pdf

Hanging Out or Hooking Up: A Train the Trainers Curriculum on Responding to Adolescent Relationship Abuse February 2, 2015. Futures Without Violence—https://www.futureswithoutviolence.org/hanging-hooking-train-trainers-curriculum-responding-adolescent-relationship-abuse/

Chapter 6: Just Do It: The When and How of IUD Insertion

CDC USA Selected Practice Recommendations (USA SPR) for Contraceptive Use Centers for Disease Control and Prevention (CDC)—https://www.cdc.gov/reproductivehealth/contraception/mmwr/spr/summary.html

QuickStart Algorithm The Reproductive Health Access Project (RHAP) (also printed at the end of this chapter)—https://www.reproductiveaccess.org/wp-content/uploads/2014/12/QuickstartAlgorithm.pdf

USA Medical Eligibility Criteria for Contraceptive Use Centers for Disease Control and Prevention (also printed at the end of this chapter)—https://www.cdc.gov/reproductivehealth/contraception/pdf/summary-chart-us-medical-eligibility-criteria_508tagged.pdf

LARC Insertion: Immediate Postpartum Period Innovating Education and Reproductive Health—http://innovating-education.org/2018/04/larc-insertion-immediate-postpartum-period/

Chapter 7: Consenting and Pre-procedural Counseling for IUD Insertion: What to Expect and What to Talk About

Minor Consent Laws Information available at the Guttmacher Institute—www.guttmacher.org/state-policy/explore/minors-access-contraceptive-services

Chapter 8: Integrating IUD Provision into Your Practice: Site Preparedness, Staff Training, and Procedural Steps

RHAP Patient Handouts The Reproductive Health Access Project (RHAP)—

- Copper IUD User Guide (also printed at the end of this chapter)—https://www.reproductiveaccess.org/resource/copper-iud-user-guide/
- Progestin IUD User Guide (also printed at the end of this chapter)—https://www.reproductiveaccess.org/resource/progestin-iud-user-guide/
- IUD Fact Sheet—https://www.reproductiveaccess.org/resource/iud-facts/
- RHAP Aftercare Handout—https://www.reproductiveaccess.org/resource/iud-aftercare-instructions/

RHAP LARC Readiness Checklist The Reproductive Health Access Project (RHAP) (available as a Word document download, also printed at the end of this chapter)—
https://www.reproductiveaccess.org/programs/hartcenter/getting-started/

RHAP IUD Consent Form The Reproductive Health Access Project (RHAP)—
https://www.reproductiveaccess.org/resource/iud-consent-form/

RHAP Procedure Note Templates The Reproductive Health Access Project (RHAP)

- IUD insertion (from the EPIC system). This template can be adapted for other EHR systems—https://www.reproductiveaccess.org/resource/iud-insertion-note/
- IUD removal (from the EPIC system). This template can be adapted for other EHR systems—https://www.reproductiveaccess.org/resource/iud-removal-note/

RHAP Clinical IUD Policy and Procedure The Reproductive Health Access Project—https://www.reproductiveaccess.org/resource/iud-policy-procedure/

RHAP Supply List Contains equipment and supplies needed for IUD insertion and removal. The Reproductive Health Access Project (RHAP) (also printed at the end of this chapter)—https://www.reproductiveaccess.org/resource/iud-insertion-removal-supplies-list/

Clinic and Provider Tools UCSF Beyond the Pill—https://beyondthepill.ucsf.edu/clinic-tools

Innovating Education and Reproductive Health: LARC Insertion and Removal Series Bixby Center for Global and Reproductive Health—http://innovating-education.org/course/larc-insertion-series/

Birth Control That Really Works Contraception video, 8.5 minutes. UCSF Bixby Center for Global Reproductive Health—https://vimeo.com/123257511

No Touch Technique for Copper IUD Innovating Education in Reproductive Health—https://innovating-education.org/2018/10/this-is-how-i-teach-no-touch-technique-for-cooper-iud/

Training Centers and Opportunities Various organizations can help with logistical assistance and proctoring support—

- RHAP Hands-on Reproductive Health Training Center contains information on setting up hands-on training and getting started with LARC in your health center. The Reproductive Health Access Project—https://www.reproductiveaccess.org/programs/hartcenter/
- Providing Quality Contraceptive Counseling and Education: not IUD specific, but a good resource for broader staff training. CARDEA—http://www.cardeaservices.org/resourcecenter/providing-quality-contraceptive-counseling-education-a-toolkit-for-training-staff
- Approach. Upstream USA—https://www.upstream.org/approach/
- Beyond the Pill (UCSF)—https://beyondthepill.ucsf.edu/site-training
- LARC Clinical Training Opportunities. American College of Obstetrics and Gynecology (also printed at the end of this chapter)—https://www.acog.org/-/media/Departments/LARC/LARC-Clinical-Training-Opportunities-Replaceable.pdf

Papaya Workshop Information

- The Papaya Workshop teaches manual vacuum aspiration, IUD placement, and other gynecologic skills, using papayas as uterine models. The Papaya Workshop: Innovating Education in Reproductive Health—https://papayaworkshop.org/
- Training in MVA using Papayas. The Reproductive Health Access Project—https://www.reproductiveaccess.org/wp-content/uploads/2014/12/mva_training_using_papayas.pdf

IUD Competency Checklists

- IUD Competency Checklist. Beyond the Pill and UCSF—https://beyondthepill.ucsf.edu/sites/beyondthepill.ucsf.edu/files/Beyond%20the%20Pill%20IUD%20Competency%20Checklists.pdf
- IUD Competency Checklist. Upstream—http://www.upstream.org/wp-content/uploads/2015/11/IUD-Competency-Checklist.pdf

IUD Reimbursement and Revenue

LARC Quick Coding Guides

- The American College of Obstetrics and Gynecology (also printed at the end of this chapter)—https://www.acog.org/-/media/Departments/LARC/Coding-Guide-2018FINAL.pdf
- Beyond the Pill and UCSF—https://beyondthepill.ucsf.edu/sites/beyondthepill.ucsf.edu/files/LARC%20Quick%20Coding%20Guide%20Supplement_6.29.17.pdf

LARC Modeling Tool. CAI's resource is intended to support healthcare service providers to examine assumptions about the affordability of long-acting reversible contraception (LARC) methods. CAI—https://www.caiglobal.org/caistage/index.php?option=com_content&view=article&id=692&Itemid=1246

Information on 340B Pricing. Health Resources and Services Administration—https://www.hrsa.gov/opa/

IUD Manufacturers Patient Assistance Programs

- Liletta Patient Savings Program—https://www.lilettahcp.com/access-reimbursement/liletta-patient-savings-program
- Mirena and Skyla IUD Patient Assistance Program (ARCH Foundation)—http://www.archfoundation.com/about.htm
- Paragard IUD Patient Assistance Program—http://www.patientassistance.com/profile/duramedpharmaceticalsinc-426/

Chapter 10: Nonpharmacologic Approaches to Pain Management with IUD Insertion

Pain After IUD Insertion: Use Acupressure on Spleen 6 Educational handout on Spleen 6 for SBHC patients. L Warren, RC Passmore. 2018—(Printed at the end of this chapter).

Chapter 12: Challenging IUD Procedures

Algorithms for Steps to Manage Difficult IUD Insertions and for How to Remove an IUD with Missing Strings Located in the text of Chapter 12, and printed at the end of this chapter.

Patient Requests IUD Removal, Strings Are not Visible Reproductive Health Access Project—https://www.reproductiveaccess.org/wp-content/uploads/2017/12/2017-11-27-IUD-removal-no-strings-algorithm.pdf

Chapter 13: Adolescent and Young Adult IUD Delivery in Non-traditional Health Settings

Expanding Contraceptive Choice to the Underserved Through Delivery of Mobile Outreach Services: A Handbook for Program Planners [Internet]. [cited 3 Dec 2018]. K4Health—https://www.k4health.org/sites/default/files/expanding_contraceptive_choice.pdf

Sample Onsite IUD Protocol Reproductive Health Access Project (also printed at the end of this chapter)—http://reproductiveaccess.org/wp-content/uploads/2015/01/Sample-Onsite-IUD-Protocol.doc

National School-Based Health Care Census Report School-Based Health Alliance. Washington, D.C.—https://www.sbh4all.org/school-health-care/national-census-of-school-based-health-centers/

BIRTH CONTROL ACROSS THE GENDER SPECTRUM

CAN YOU GET PREGNANT?

If you have a uterus and ovaries, you can get pregnant. This is true even if you take testosterone. Although it may stop your monthly bleeding, testosterone does not keep you from getting pregnant.

CAN YOU GET SOMEONE PREGNANT?

If you have a penis and testes, you can get someone pregnant. This is true even if you take estrogen. Estrogen may lower your sperm count, but it does not keep you from getting someone pregnant.

BIRTH CONTROL FOR PEOPLE TAKING TESTOSTERONE

There are several birth control options for people who have a uterus and ovaries and who take testosterone. The progestin pill, implant, IUD, and shot may help decrease monthly bleeding. Some people use one of these methods just to control bleeding, even if they don't need birth control. Progestin does not interact with testosterone. The copper IUD prevents pregnancy and contains no hormones. Condoms prevent pregnancy and sexually transmitted infections (STIs).

BIRTH CONTROL FOR PEOPLE TAKING ESTROGEN

People who have a penis and testes and who take estrogen can choose any birth control method.

PERMANENT OPTIONS

Permanent methods are great for people who don't ever want to get pregnant. These include tubal ligation, Essure, hysterectomy, orchiectomy, and vasectomy.

DON'T FORGET ABOUT SEXUALLY TRANSMITTED INFECTIONS!

Condoms can prevent human immunodeficiency virus (HIV) and other STIs. There are two types of condoms, internal and external. Both types help to prevent pregnancy and infections.

• •

BIRTH CONTROL CHOICES ACROSS THE GENDER SPECTRUM

Method	How well does it work?	How to Use	Pros	Cons
The Implant Nexplanon®	> 99%	A health care provider places it under the skin of the upper arm. It must be removed by a health care provider.	It may last up to 5 years. It often decreases cramps. After 1 year, you may have no monthly bleeding at all. It may lower the risk of uterine lining cancer, ovarian cancer, and polycystic ovary syndrome (PCOS).	May cause spotting. It may cause mood changes.
Progestin IUD Liletta®, Mirena®, Skyla®, and others	> 99%	A health care provider places it in the uterus. It is usually removed by a health care provider.	It works for 3 to 7 years, depending on which IUD you choose. It may improve monthly bleeding and cramps. After 1 year, you may have no monthly bleeding at all. It may lower the risk of uterine lining cancer, ovarian cancer, and polycystic ovary syndrome (PCOS).	May cause spotting.
Copper IUD ParaGard®	> 99%	A health care provider places it in the uterus. It is usually removed by a health care provider.	May be left in place for up to 12 years	May cause spotting (if you are taking testosterone, this may not be an issue).

over ➡

• •

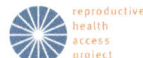

reproductive health access project

BIRTH CONTROL ACROSS THE GENDER SPECTRUM

Method	How well does it work?	How to Use	Pros	Cons
The Shot Depo-Provera	94%	Get a shot every 3 months. You can get the shot at a health care office, or you can give yourself the shot.	Each shot works for 12 weeks. It usually decreases monthly bleeding. After 1 year, you may have no monthly bleeding at all. It may lower the risk of uterine lining cancer, ovarian cancer, and polycystic ovary syndrome (PCOS).	It may cause spotting, weight gain, depression, hair or skin changes, or change in sex drive. It may cause delay in getting pregnant after you stop the shots. Side effects may last up to 6 months after you stop the shots.
Progestin-Only Pills Camila, Nor-QD® Micronor	91%	You must take the pill at the same time daily.	It's easy to use. It may lower the risk of uterine lining cancer, ovarian cancer, and polycystic ovary syndrome (PCOS).	It often causes spotting, which may last for many months. It may cause depression, hair or skin changes, or change in sex drive.
External Condom	82%	Use a new condom each time you have sex. Use a polyurethane condom if allergic to latex	Can buy at many stores. Can put on as part of sex play/foreplay. Can help prevent early ejaculation. Can be used for oral, vaginal, and anal sex	Can decrease sensation. Can cause loss of erection. Can break or slip off
Internal Condom	79%	Use a new condom each time you have sex. Use lubrication as needed	Can put in as part of sex play/foreplay. Can be used for anal and vaginal sex. May increase pleasure when used for anal and vaginal sex. Good for people with latex allergy	Can decrease sensation. May be noisy. May be hard to insert. May slip out of place during sex. Requires a prescription from your health care provider
Withdrawal Pull-out	78%	Pull penis out of vagina before ejaculation (that is, before coming)	Costs nothing	Less pleasure for some. Does not work if penis is not pulled out in time. Must interrupt sex
Diaphragm Caya® and Milex®	88%	Must be used each time you have sex. Must be used with spermicide	Can last several years. Costs very little to use. May protect against some infections, but not HIV	Using spermicide may raise the risk of getting HIV. Should not be used with vaginal bleeding or infection. Raises risk of bladder infection
Spermicide Cream, gel, sponge, foam, inserts, film	72%	Insert spermicide each time you have sex	Can buy at many stores. Can insert as part of sex play/foreplay. Comes in many forms: cream, gel, sponge, foam, inserts, film	May raise the risk of getting HIV. May irritate vagina, penis. Cream, gel, and foam can be messy
Emergency Contraception Pills Progestin EC (Plan B One-Step® and others) and ulipristal acetate (ella®)	58-94% Ulipristal acetate EC works better than progestin EC if you are overweight. Ulipristal acetate EC works better than progestin EC in the 2-5 days after sex	Works best the sooner you take it after unprotected sex. You can take EC up to 5 days after unprotected sex. If pack contains 2 pills, take both together	Available at pharmacies, health centers, or health care providers: call ahead to see if they have it. People of any age can get progestin EC without a prescription, and it doesn't interact with testosterone.	May cause stomach upset or nausea. Your next monthly bleeding may come early or late. May cause spotting. Ulipristal acetate EC requires a prescription, and we don't know whether or not it interacts with testosterone. May cost a lot

Remember, these methods do not protect against human immunodeficiency virus (HIV) or other sexually transmitted infections (STIs). Always use condoms to protect yourself!

· ·

August 2018 / www.reproductiveaccess.org

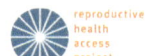 reproductive health access project

LARC Quick Coding Guide

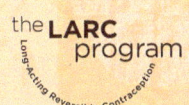

2018 UPDATE

Coding for the Contraceptive Implant and IUDs

CORRECT CODING can result in more appropriate compensation for services and devices. To help practices receive appropriate payment for providing the contraceptive implant and intrauterine devices (IUDs), the American College of Obstetricians and Gynecologists' Long-Acting Reversible Contraception (LARC) Program, in collaboration with the ACOG Coding Department, has prepared this updated quick reference guide to coding for LARC methods. The information included in this guide is current as of May 9, 2018. For more information about the LARC Program and coding for LARC methods, go to **http://www.acog.org/larc.**

Basic Contraceptive Implant Coding

The diagnostic coding will vary, but usually will be selected from the Z30.01- (encounter for initial prescription of contraceptives) and Z30.4- (encounter for surveillance of contraceptives) series in ICD-10-CM. These codes are:

Z30.017 Encounter for initial prescription of implantable subdermal contraceptive

This code is reported for the initial prescription, counseling, advice, and insertion of the implant, even when the insertion is performed at a separate encounter

Z30.46 Encounter for surveillance of implantable subdermal contraceptive

This code is reported for checking, reinsertion, or removal of the implant

The contraceptive implant is a single-rod etonogestrel-releasing contraceptive device inserted under the skin of the upper arm. The insertion and/or removal of the implant are reported using one of the following CPT (Current Procedural Terminology) codes:

11981 Insertion, non-biodegradable drug delivery implant

11982 Removal, non-biodegradable drug delivery implant

11983 Removal with reinsertion, non-biodegradable drug delivery implant

CPT procedure codes do not include the cost of the supply. Report the supply separately using a HCPCS (Healthcare Procedural Coding System) code:

J7307 Etonogestrel (contraceptive) implant system, including implant and supplies

Basic IUD Coding

Most IUD services will be linked to a diagnosis code from the Z30.01- (encounter for initial prescription of contraceptives) and Z30.43- (encounter for surveillance of intrauterine contraceptive device) series.

Z30.014 Encounter for initial prescription of intrauterine contraceptive device

This code includes the initial prescription of the IUD, counseling, and advice, but excludes the IUD insertion

Z30.430 Encounter for insertion of intrauterine contraceptive device

Z30.431 Encounter for routine checking of intrauterine contraceptive device

Z30.432 Encounter for removal of intrauterine contraceptive device

Z30.433 Encounter for removal and reinsertion of intrauterine contraceptive device

Intrauterine devices include the copper IUD and the hormonal IUDs. The insertion and/or removal of IUDs are reported using one of the following CPT codes:

58300 Insertion of IUD

58301 Removal of IUD

CPT procedure codes do not include the cost of the supply. Report the supply separately using a HCPCS code:

J7296 Levonorgestrel-releasing intrauterine contraceptive system (Kyleena®), 19.5 mg (5 year duration)

J7297 Levonorgestrel-releasing intrauterine contraceptive system (Liletta®), 52 mg (4 year duration)

J7298 Levonorgestrel-releasing intrauterine contraceptive system (Mirena®), 52 mg (5 year duration)

J7300 Intrauterine copper contraceptive (Paragard®) (10 year duration)

J7301 Levonorgestrel-releasing intrauterine contraceptive system (Skyla®), 13.5 mg (3 year duration)

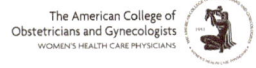

The American College of
Obstetricians and Gynecologists
WOMEN'S HEALTH CARE PHYSICIANS

Reporting Contraceptive Services with Other Services

Under some circumstances, an Evaluation and Management (E/M) services code, a procedure code, and a HCPCS code may all be reported.

ACOG Fellows and their staff can submit specific coding questions to the ACOG Department of Health Economics' coding ticket database at **acogcoding.freshdesk.com** or by fax to 202-484-7480. Questions are answered in the order received, usually within 1–3 weeks. There is no charge for this service, but no more than 3 questions per practice are to be submitted each month.

E/M Services Code Only

If a patient comes in to discuss contraception options but no procedure is provided at that visit:

- If the discussion takes place during an annual preventive visit (99381–99387 or 99391–99397), it is included in the Preventive Medicine code. The discussion is not reported separately.

- If the discussion takes place during an E/M office or outpatient visit (99201–99215), an E/M services code may be reported if an E/M service (including history, physical examination, or medical decision making or time spent counseling) is documented. Link the E/M code to ICD-10-CM diagnosis code Z30.014 (encounter for initial prescription of intrauterine contraceptive device) or Z30.017 (encounter for initial prescription of implantable subdermal contraceptive) when applicable.

E/M Services Code and Procedure Code

If discussion of contraceptive options takes place during the same encounter as a procedure, such as insertion of a contraceptive implant or IUD, it may or may not be appropriate to report both an E/M services code and the procedure code:

- If the clinician and patient discuss a number of contraceptive options, decide on a method, and then an implant or IUD is inserted during the visit, an E/M service may be reported, depending on the documentation.

- If the patient comes into the office and states, "I want an IUD," followed by a brief discussion of the benefits and risks and the insertion, an E/M service is not reported since the E/M services are minimal.

- If the patient comes in for another reason and, during the same visit, a procedure is performed, then both the E/M services code and procedure may be reported.

If reporting both an E/M service and a procedure, the documentation must indicate a significant, separately identifiable E/M service. The documentation must indicate either the key components (history, physical examination, and medical decision making) or time spent counseling. Counseling must be documented as more than 50% of the time spent face-to-face with the patient. Note the "typical times" listed in outpatient E/M services codes 99201–99215. For example, if an established patient is seen for 25 minutes, including 15 minutes spent counseling, report code 99214 — this code lists a "typical time" of 25 minutes. The level of history, physical examination, and medical decision making do not matter in selecting this code. Providers should consult third-party payers before instituting this coding practice to ensure compliance with specific plan guidelines.

A modifier 25 (significant, separately identifiable E/M service on the same day as a procedure or other service) is added to the E/M code to indicate that this service was significant and separately identifiable from the insertion. This indicates that two distinct services were provided: an E/M service and a procedure.

Contraceptive Implant Coding: Specific Clinical Scenarios

E/M Service and Implant Insertion

The following table illustrates coding when an implant insertion and an office visit occur at the same encounter. Under certain circumstances and when supported by documentation, it may be appropriate to report a CPT procedure code, an E/M code, and a HCPCS supply code for the one visit. Diagnostic codes are reported based on services provided, such as outpatient or preventive services, as appropriate.

▶ **Coding for Implant Insertion and E/M Service**

CPT PROCEDURES AND SERVICES	MODIFIER	DIAGNOSIS(ES)
11981 Insertion, non-biodegradable drug delivery implant		Z30.017 Encounter for initial prescription of implantable subdermal contraceptive
992XX E/M based either on the key components or time spent counseling	25	Z30.017 Encounter for initial prescription of implantable subdermal contraceptive
HCPCS SUPPLY CODES		
J7307 Etonogestrel (contraceptive) implant system, including implant and supplies		Z30.017 Encounter for initial prescription of implantable subdermal contraceptive

OR

CPT PROCEDURES AND SERVICES	MODIFIER	DIAGNOSIS(ES)
11981 Insertion, non-biodegradable drug delivery implant		Z30.017 Encounter for initial prescription of implantable subdermal contraceptive
9939X or 9938X Preventive E/M service based on age and whether a new or established patient	25	Z01.41- Routine gynecological examination (series) Z01.411 with abnormal findings Z01.419 without abnormal findings Z30.017 Encounter for initial prescription of implantable subdermal contraceptive
HCPCS SUPPLY CODES		
J7307 Etonogestrel (contraceptive) implant system, including implant and supplies		Z30.017 Encounter for initial prescription of implantable subdermal contraceptive

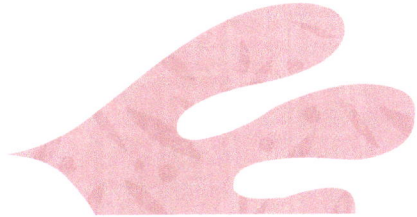

Implant Reassessment

ICD-10-CM code Z30.46 (encounter for surveillance of implantable subdermal contraceptive) is assigned for a follow-up visit in the office to check, reinsert, or remove the implant. If the patient has symptoms, report these as secondary diagnoses. For example, code S40.021 (contusion of right upper arm) or other physical symptoms such as code R11.0 (nausea)

Same Day Implant Removal and Reinsertion

The following chart shows coding when an implant is removed and a new one inserted during an office visit. When appropriate and supported by documentation, a CPT procedure code, an E/M code, and a HCPCS supply code are reported for the one visit.

► **Coding for Same Day Removal and Reinsertion of Implant with an E/M Service**

CPT PROCEDURES AND SERVICES	MODIFIER	DIAGNOSIS(ES)
11983 Removal with reinsertion, non-biodegradable drug delivery implant		Z30.46 Encounter for surveillance of implantable subdermal contraceptive
992XX E/M based either on the key components or time spent counseling	25	Z30.46 Encounter for surveillance of implantable subdermal contraceptive
HCPCS SUPPLY CODES		
J7307 Etonogestrel (contraceptive) implant system, including implant and supplies		Z30.46 Encounter for surveillance of implantable subdermal contraceptive

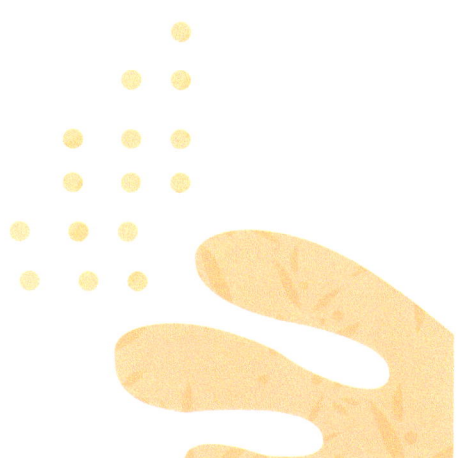

IUD Coding: Specific Clinical Scenarios

E/M Service and IUD Insertion

The following table illustrates coding when an IUD insertion and an office visit occur at the same encounter. Under certain circumstances and when supported by documentation, it may be appropriate to report a CPT procedure code, an E/M code, and a HCPCS supply code for the one visit. Diagnostic codes are reported based on services provided, such as outpatient or preventive services, as appropriate.

▶ **Coding for IUD Insertion and E/M Service**

CPT PROCEDURES AND SERVICES	MODIFIER	DIAGNOSIS(ES)
58300 Insertion of IUD		Z30.430 Encounter for insertion of intrauterine contraceptive device
992XX E/M based either on the key components or time spent counseling	25	Z30.014 Encounter for initial prescription of intrauterine contraceptive device
HCPCS SUPPLY CODES		
J7296 Levonorgestrel-releasing intrauterine contraceptive system (Kyleena®), 19.5 mg (5 year duration) J7297 Levonorgestrel-releasing intrauterine contraceptive system (Liletta®), 52 mg (4 year duration) J7298 Levonorgestrel-releasing intrauterine contraceptive system (Mirena®), 52 mg (5 year duration) J7300 Intrauterine copper contraceptive (Paragard®) (10 year duration) J7301 Levonorgestrel-releasing intrauterine contraceptive system (Skyla®), 13.5 mg (3 year duration)		Z30.430 Encounter for insertion of intrauterine contraceptive device

OR (continued next page)

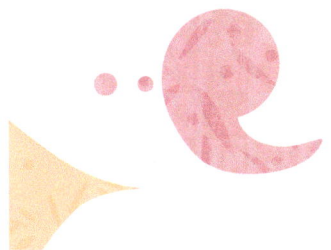

CPT PROCEDURES AND SERVICES	MODIFIER	DIAGNOSIS(ES)
58300 Insertion of IUD		Z30.430 Encounter for insertion of intrauterine contraceptive device
9939X or 9938X Preventive E/M service based on age and whether a new or established patient	25	Z01.41- Routine gynecological examination (series) Z01.411 with abnormal findings Z01.419 without abnormal findings Z30.014 Encounter for initial prescription of intrauterine contraceptive device

HCPCS SUPPLY CODES		
J7296 Levonorgestrel-releasing intrauterine contraceptive system (Kyleena®), 19.5 mg (5 year duration) J7297 Levonorgestrel-releasing intrauterine contraceptive system (Liletta®), 52 mg (4 year duration) J7298 Levonorgestrel-releasing intrauterine contraceptive system (Mirena®), 52 mg (5 year duration) J7300 Intrauterine copper contraceptive (Paragard®) (10 year duration) J7301 Levonorgestrel-releasing intrauterine contraceptive system (Skyla®), 13.5 mg (3 year duration)		Z30.430 Encounter for insertion of intrauterine contraceptive device

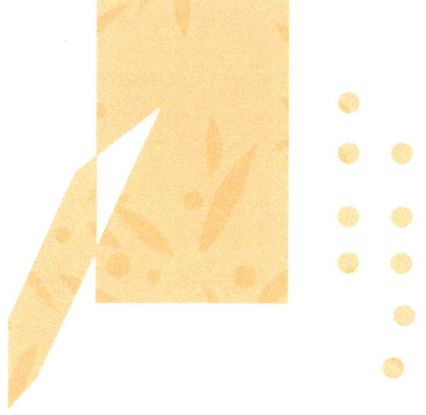

Use of Ultrasound

The performance of an ultrasound to check IUD placement is not bundled into the IUD insertion (code 58300), and it is not common practice to use ultrasound to confirm placement. Therefore, this should not be routinely billed. However, ultrasonography may be used to confirm the location of the IUD when the qualified clinicician incurs a difficult IUD placement (e.g., severe pain, uterine perforation, etc.). If ultrasound is used, one of the following codes is added:

- Code 76857   Ultrasound, pelvic [nonobstetric], real time with image documentation; limited or follow-up, or
- Code 76830   Ultrasound, transvaginal

Occasionally, ultrasound is needed to guide IUD insertion. If ultrasound is used, add code 76998 (ultrasonic guidance, intraoperative).

IUD Reassessment

ICD-10-CM code Z30.431 (encounter for routine checking of intrauterine contraceptive device) is assigned for a follow-up visit in the office to check the proper placement of the IUD.

Difficult Insertions

The 22 modifier can be reported if the work required to insert an IUD is substantially greater than usual. The 22 modifier can also be reported in the case of an unsuccessful insertion followed by a successful insertion during the same surgical session. A modifier 22 is added to code 58300 (insertion of IUD) (i.e., 58300-22).

Documentation must support the substantial additional work and the reason for the additional work, such as: increased intensity or time, increased technical difficulty of performing the procedure, severity of patient's condition, increased physical and mental effort required. The qualified clinician should specifically document the total time of the procedure and how it compares with the typical duration of the procedure.

Discontinued IUD Insertion

On occasion, a clinician may elect to discontinue the IUD insertion due to extenuating circumstances or a threat to the patient's well-being. A modifier 53 (discontinued procedure) is added to code 58300 (insertion of IUD) (i.e., 58300-53). This modifier is used when a procedure is started but discontinued and no other procedure is performed during the visit.

Modifier 53 provides a way to receive partial payment for work performed before the procedure is discontinued. It is not necessary to reduce the fee. The payer will determine the fee for the service. The payer may require documentation showing how much work was actually performed. This modifier is also useful because it tells the payer that the procedure was unsuccessful. If the procedure is performed successfully at a later date, the payer will be more likely to recognize that the first claim (reported with a modifier 53) and the second one are not duplicates.

Same Day IUD Removal and Reinsertion

The following chart shows coding when an IUD is removed and a new one inserted during an office visit. When appropriate and supported by documentation, two CPT procedure codes, an E/M code, and a HCPCS supply code are reported for the one visit. A modifier 51 (multiple procedures) is added to code 58300.

▶ **Coding for Same Day Removal and Reinsertion of IUD with an E/M Service**

CPT PROCEDURES AND SERVICES	MODIFIER	DIAGNOSIS(ES)
58301 Removal of IUD		
58300 Insertion of IUD	51	Z30.433 Encounter for removal and reinsertion of intrauterine contraceptive device
992XX E/M based either on the key components or time spent counseling	25	
HCPCS SUPPLY CODES		
J7296 Levonorgestrel-releasing intrauterine contraceptive system (Kyleena®), 19.5 mg (5 year duration)		
J7297 Levonorgestrel-releasing intrauterine contraceptive system (Liletta®), 52 mg (4 year duration)		
J7298 Levonorgestrel-releasing intrauterine contraceptive system (Mirena®), 52 mg (5 year duration)		Z30.433 Encounter for removal and reinsertion of intrauterine contraceptive device
J7300 Intrauterine copper contraceptive (Paragard®) (10 year duration)		
J7301 Levonorgestrel-releasing intrauterine contraceptive system (Skyla®), 13.5 mg (3 year duration)		

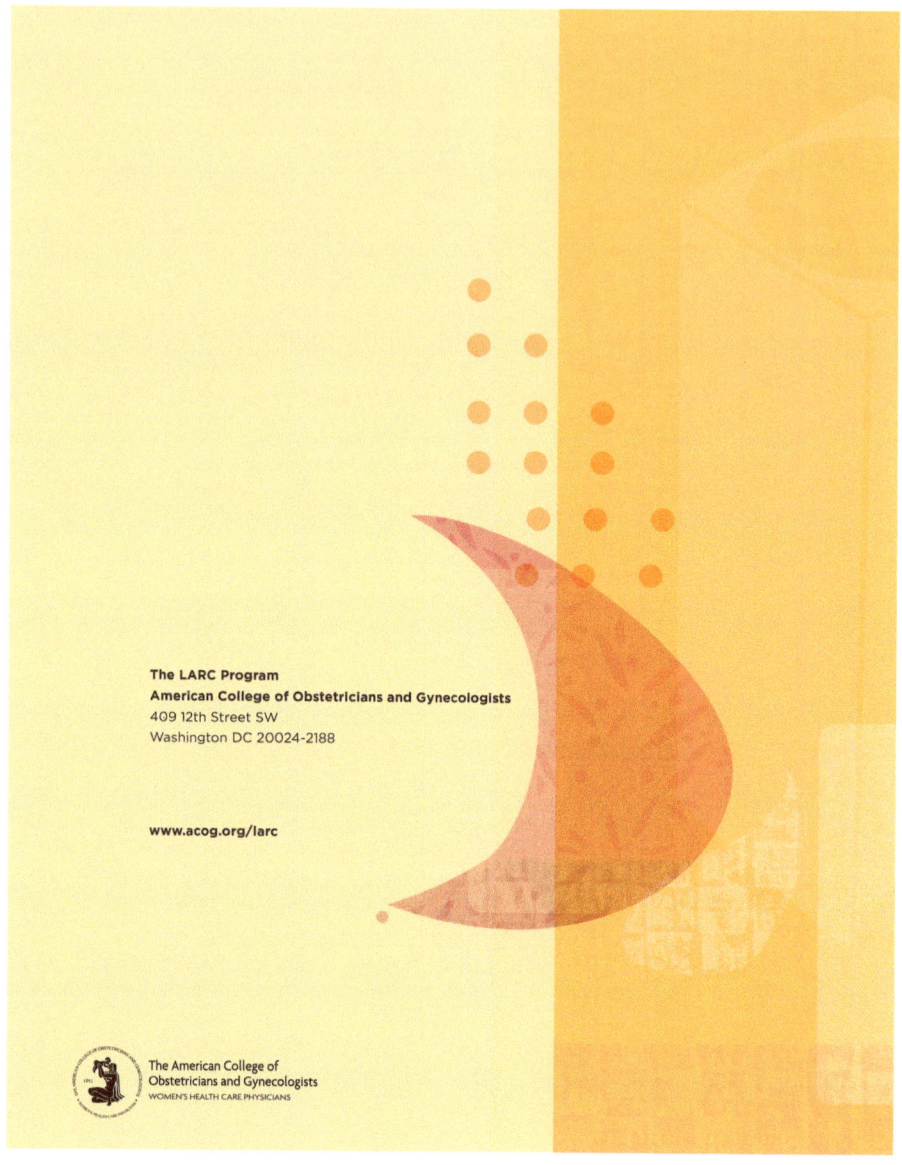

The LARC Program
American College of Obstetricians and Gynecologists
409 12th Street SW
Washington DC 20024-2188

www.acog.org/larc

The American College of
Obstetricians and Gynecologists
WOMEN'S HEALTH CARE PHYSICIANS

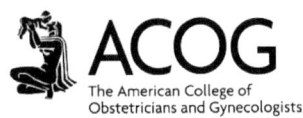

June 2014

The American College of
Obstetricians and Gynecologists

Facts Are Important
Emergency Contraception (EC) and
Intrauterine Devices (IUDs) are Not Abortifacients

Facts are very important, especially when discussing the health of the American public. Contrary to assertions made by some, emergency contraception and IUDs do not cause abortions, and therefore are not abortifacients. Here are the scientific facts.

Emergency contraception (EC) does not cause medical abortions. A woman can take mifepristone to cause a medical abortion, terminating an early existing pregnancy. EC however only works <u>before</u> a pregnancy is established. Review of the scientific evidence suggests that EC cannot prevent implantation of a fertilized egg. EC is not effective after implantation; it <u>cannot end a pregnancy</u> and is <u>not an abortifacient</u>.

Contraceptives v. Abortifacients
Understanding the difference between a contraceptive and an abortifacient requires an understanding of the biological processes leading to pregnancy and how various forms of contraception work to prevent pregnancy.

Fertilization: Occurs when a viable egg fuses with viable sperm. Because sperm can remain viable in the female reproductive tract for approximately five days and an egg for up to one day, sexual intercourse can result in fertilization from five days before ovulation up to one day after.

Implantation: Following fertilization, the blastocyst (the fertilized egg) may implant into the lining of the uterus (the endometrium), which typically occurs over the course of several days – between 5-9 days following fertilization.[i,ii]

Pregnancy: Is established only at the conclusion of implantation of a fertilized egg.[iii,iv] This scientific definition of pregnancy is also the legal definition of pregnancy, accepted by governmental agencies and all major U.S. medical organizations.[v]

Contraceptive: An agent which prevents fertilization of an egg or prevents implantation of a fertilized egg, preventing a pregnancy from taking place.[1]

Emergency contraception: A drug or device used after intercourse has occurred, but before pregnancy is established, to prevent pregnancy. EC works much like traditional contraceptives, but provides protection after-the-fact in the event of contraception failure (i.e. a broken condom) or unprotected sex, including sexual assault.[vi,vii] Plan B and ella are two FDA-approved emergency contraceptives.

Abortifacient: An agent that disturbs an embryo already implanted in the uterine lining, after a pregnancy has been established.[viii]

ECs are Not Abortifacients
There is no scientific evidence that FDA-approved emergency contraceptives affect an existing pregnancy; no EC is classified as an abortifacient.

There are two types of EC pills available in the U.S.: those containing levonorgestrel (LNG) and those containing ulipristal acetate (UPA). Plan B, Plan B One-Step, Next Choice One Dose and others are hormonal pills containing 1.5 mg LNG.

---

[1] Not all blastocysts implant. The limited data available suggests that even under optimal conditions and timing, no more than 40% of blastocysts eventually implant in the endometrium. *See* Diedrich, *et al.*, *The role of the endometrium and embryo in human implantation*, 13 HUM. REPROD. UPDATE 365 (2007)

LNG, which has long been approved at lower dosage levels for use in ordinary contraceptives, has been approved as EC since 1999 and is the most commonly used form of EC. Ella, which came on the market in 2010, contains 30 mg UPA and acts on human progesterone receptors.

LNG and UPA function primarily, if not exclusively, by inhibiting ovulation, thereby preventing fertilization from occurring. LNG and UPA do not affect implantation of a fertilized egg or harm or end an established pregnancy.[ix] UPA works later in the pre-ovulatory cycle, when LNG is no longer effective. The fact that UPA EC works when taken later than LNG EC does not mean that UPA EC prevents implantation. **There is no scientific evidence that UPA EC affects implantation. LNG EC has been widely studied, and current scientific evidence shows that it works by preventing or disrupting ovulation, but is not effective after ovulation has already occurred.**[x]

Opponents of EC frequently cite the FDA-approved product label for LNG products, which states that "it may inhibit implantation (by altering the endometrium)."[xi] This product label has not been updated since the product was approved in 1999 and does not reflect current research, including recent studies showing that LNG does not cause changes to the endometrium (uterine lining) that would hamper implantation.[xii,xiii]

Another form of contraception approved by the FDA – the copper Intrauterine Device CuT380A (Cu-IUD) – is effective as an EC when inserted up to five days following intercourse. Copper ions released from the IUD create an environment that is toxic to sperm, preventing fertilization.[xiv] Copper can also alter the endometrial lining, but studies show that this alteration can prevent implantation, but not disrupt implantation. **Because Cu-IUDs prevent rather than disrupt pregnancy, they too are properly classified as contraceptives, not abortifacients.**[xv]

The American Congress of Obstetricians and Gynecologists (ACOG), representing nearly 58,000 ob-gyns and partners in women's health, supports robust, factual debates on issues of importance to the American people. We urge you to call on us for expert understanding of issues related to women's health.

---

[i] Wilcox et al., *Timing of Sexual Intercourse in Relation to Ovulation. Effects on Probability of Conception*, 333 NEW ENG. J.MED. 1517 (1995)
[ii] Dunson et al., *Day-Specific Probabilities of Clinical Pregnancy Based on Two Studies With Imperfect Measures of Ovulation*, 14 HUM. REPROD. 1835 (1999)
[iii] OBSTETRIC-GYNECOLOGIC TERMINOLOGY: WITH SECTION ON NEONATOLOGY AND GLOSSARY OF CONGENITAL ABNORMALITIES 299, 327 (E.G. Hughes, ed., F.A. Davis Co. 1972)
[iv] *Statement on Contraceptive Methods* (Am. Coll. of Obstetricians & Gynecologists, Wash., D.C., Jul. 1998)
[v] *See, e.g.*, 45 C.F.R § 46.202 (recognizing pregnancy as "the period of time from implantation to delivery")
[vi] Gemzell-Danielsson et al., *Emergency Contraception—Mechanisms of Action*, 87 CONTRACEPTION 300, 300 (2013) ("emergency contraception (EC) is defined as the use of any drug or device after an unprotected intercourse to prevent an unintended pregnancy")
[vii] Croxatto et al., *Mechanism of Action of Hormonal Preparations Used for Emergency Contraception: A Review of the Literature*, 63 CONTRACEPTION 111, 112 (2001) ("emergency contraception is used after coitus but before pregnancy has become established.")
[viii] *See* COCHRANE LIBRARY, http://www.thecochranelibrary.com/view/0/index.html (search"Abortifacient Agents").
[ix] Gemzell-Danielsson et al. at 305; *Access to Emergency Contraception*, ACOG Comm. Op. 542, 120 OBSTET GYNECOL 1250 (2012)
[x] Noe et al.; Novikova et al., *Effectiveness of Levonorgestrel Emergency Contraception Given Before or After Ovulation – A Pilot Study*, 75 CONTRACEPTION 112 (2007)
[xi] FDA, LABELING FOR PLAN B ONE STEP, *available at* http://www.accessdata.fda.gov/drugsatfda_docs/label/2009/021998lbl.pdf
[xii] Durand et al., *On the Mechanisms of Action of Short-Term Levonorgestrel Administration in Emergency Contraception*, 64 CONTRACEPTION 227, 233 (2001)
[xiii] Noe et al. at 486-492
[xiv] Gemzell-Danielsson et al. at 305
[xv] FDA, BIRTH CONTROL GUIDE, *available at* http://www.fda.gov/downloads/ForConsumers/ByAudience/ForWomen/FreePublications/UCM282014.pdf

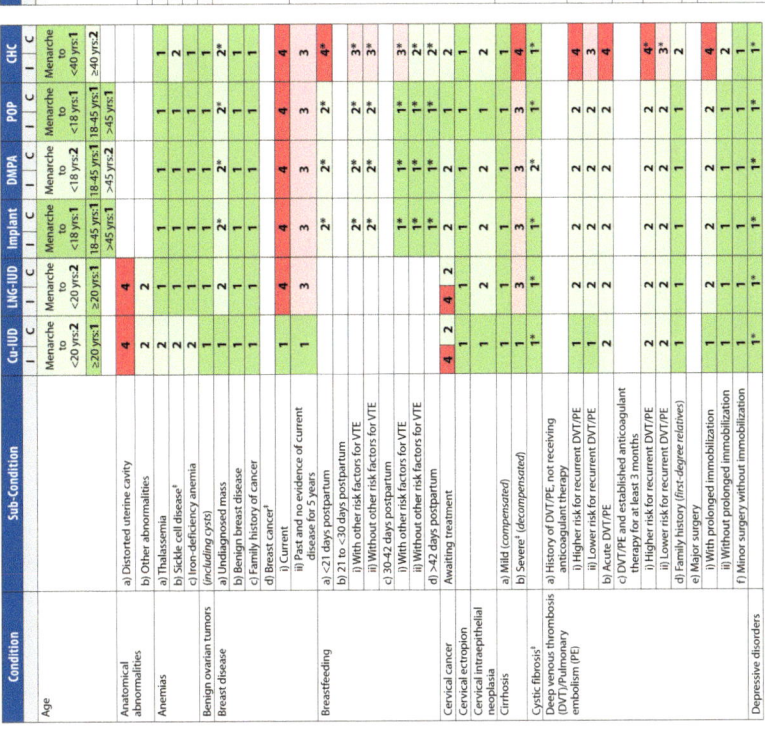

Summary Chart of U.S. Medical Eligibility Criteria for Contraceptive Use

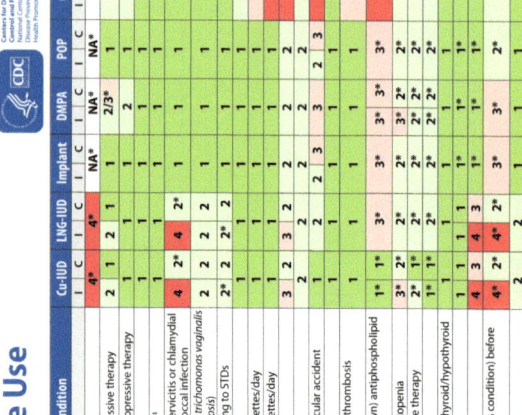

Centers for Disease Control and Prevention
National Center for Chronic Disease Prevention and Health Promotion

Condition	Sub-Condition	Cu-IUD I	Cu-IUD C	LNG-IUD I	LNG-IUD C	Implant I	Implant C	DMPA I	DMPA C	POP I	POP C	CHC I	CHC C
Hypertension	a) Adequately controlled hypertension	1*		1*		1*		2*		1*		3*	
	b) Elevated blood pressure levels (properly taken measurements)												
	i) Systolic 140–159 or diastolic 90-99	1*		1*		1*		2*		1*		3*	
	ii) Systolic ≥160 or diastolic ≥100²	1*		2*		2*		3*		2*		4*	
	c) Vascular disease	1*		2*		2*		3*		2*		4*	
Inflammatory bowel disease (Ulcerative colitis, Crohn's disease)		1		1		1		2		2		2/3*	
Ischemic heart disease³	Current and history of	1		2	3	2	3	3		2	3	4	
Known thrombogenic mutations³		1*		2*		2*		2*		2*		4*	
Liver tumors	a) Benign												
	i) Focal nodular hyperplasia	1		2		2		2		2		2	
	ii) Hepatocellular adenoma³	1		3		3		3		3		4	
	b) Malignant (hepatoma)	1		3		3		3		3		4	
Malaria		1		1		1		1		1		1	
Multiple risk factors for atherosclerotic cardiovascular disease	(e.g., older age, smoking, diabetes, hypertension, low HDL, high LDL, or high triglyceride levels)	1		2		2*		3*		2*		3/4*	
Multiple sclerosis	a) With prolonged immobility	1		1		1		2		1		3	
	b) Without prolonged immobility	1		1		1		1		1		1	
Obesity	a) Body mass index (BMI) ≥30 kg/m²	1		1		1		1		1		2	
	b) Menarche to <18 years and BMI ≥ 30 kg/m²	1		1		1		2		1		2	
Ovarian cancer³		1		1		1		1		1		1	
Parity	a) Nulliparous	2		2		1		1		1		1	
	b) Parous	1		1		1		1		1		1	
Past ectopic pregnancy		1		1		1		1		2		1	
Pelvic inflammatory disease	a) Past												
	i) With subsequent pregnancy	1	1	1	1	1		1		1		1	
	ii) Without subsequent pregnancy	2	2	2	2	1		1		1		1	
	b) Current	4	2*	4	2*	1		1		1		1	
Peripartum cardiomyopathy³	a) Normal or mildly impaired cardiac function												
	i) <6 months	2		2		1		1		1		4	
	ii) ≥6 months	2		2		1		1		1		3	
	b) Moderately or severely impaired cardiac function	2		2		2		2		2		4	
Postabortion	a) First trimester	1*		1*		1*		1*		1*		1*	
	b) Second trimester	2*		2*		1*		1*		1*		1*	
	c) Immediate postseptic abortion	4		4		1*		1*		1*		1*	
Postpartum (nonbreastfeeding women)	a) <21 days												
	b) 21 days to 42 days												
	i) With other risk factors for VTE												3*
	ii) Without other risk factors for VTE												2
	c) >42 days												1
Postpartum (in breastfeeding or non-breastfeeding women, including cesarean delivery)	a) <10 minutes after delivery of the placenta												
	i) Breastfeeding	1*		2*									
	ii) Nonbreastfeeding	1*		1*									
	b) 10 minutes after delivery of the placenta to <4 weeks	2*		2*									
	c) ≥4 weeks	1*		1*									
	d) Postpartum sepsis	4		4									

Condition	Sub-Condition	Cu-IUD I	Cu-IUD C	LNG-IUD I	LNG-IUD C	Implant I	Implant C	DMPA I	DMPA C	POP I	POP C	CHC I	CHC C
Pregnancy		4*		4*		NA*		NA*		NA*		NA*	
Rheumatoid arthritis	a) On immunosuppressive therapy	2	1	2	1	1		2/3*		1		2	
	b) Not on immunosuppressive therapy	1		1		1		1		1		1	
Schistosomiasis	a) Uncomplicated	1		1		1		1		1		1	
	b) Fibrosis of the liver³	1		1		1		1		1		1	
Sexually transmitted diseases (STDs)	a) Current purulent cervicitis or chlamydial infection or gonococcal infection	4	2*	4	2*	1		1		1		1	
	b) Vaginitis (including trichomonas vaginalis and bacterial vaginosis)	2	2	2	2	1		1		1		1	
	c) Other factors relating to STDs	2*	2	2*	2	1		1		1		1	
Smoking	a) Age <35	1		1		1		1		1		2	
	b) Age ≥35, <15 cigarettes/day	1		1		1		1		1		3	
	c) Age ≥35, ≥15 cigarettes/day	1		1		1		1		1		4	
Solid organ transplantation³	a) Complicated	3	2	3	2	2		2		2		4	
	b) Uncomplicated	2		2		2		2		2		2*	
Stroke³	History of cerebrovascular accident	1		2		2	3	3		2	3	4	
Superficial venous disorders	a) Varicose veins	1		1		1		1		1		1	
	b) Superficial venous thrombosis (acute or history)	1		1		1		1		1		3*	
Systemic lupus erythematosus³	a) Positive (or unknown) antiphospholipid antibodies	1*	1*	3*		3*		3*	3*	3*		4*	
	b) Severe thrombocytopenia	3*	2*	2*		2*		3*	2*	2*		2*	
	c) Immunosuppressive therapy	2*	1*	2*		2*		2*	2*	2*		2*	
	d) None of the above	1*	1*	2*		2*		2*	2*	2*		2*	
Thyroid disorders	Simple goiter/ hyperthyroid/hypothyroid	1		1		1		1		1		1	
Tuberculosis³ (see also Drug Interactions)	a) Nonpelvic	1		1		1		1		1		1*	
	b) Pelvic	4	3	4*	3	1*		1*		1*		1*	
Unexplained vaginal bleeding	(suspicious for serious condition) before evaluation	4*	2*	4*	2*	3*		3*		2*		2*	
Uterine fibroids		2		2		1		1		1		1	
Valvular heart disease	a) Uncomplicated	1		1		1		1		1		2	
	b) Complicated³	1		1		1		1		1		4	
Vaginal bleeding patterns	a) Irregular pattern without heavy bleeding	1		1	1	2		2		2		1	
	b) Heavy or prolonged bleeding	2*		1*	2*	2*		2*		2*		1*	
Viral hepatitis	a) Acute or flare	1		1		1		1		1		3/4*	2
	b) Carrier/Chronic	1		1		1		1		1		1	
Drug Interactions													
Antiretroviral therapy	All other ARV's are 1 or 2 for all methods. Fosamprenavir (FPV)	1/2*		1/2*	1*	2*		2*		2*		3*	
Anticonvulsant therapy	a) Certain anticonvulsants (phenytoin, carbamazepine, barbiturates, primidone, topiramate, oxcarbazepine)	1		1		2*		1*		3*		3*	
	b) Lamotrigine	1		1		1		1		1		3*	
Antimicrobial therapy	a) Broad spectrum antibiotics	1		1		1		1		1		1	
	b) Antifungals	1		1		1		1		1		1	
	c) Antiparasitics	1		1		1		1		1		1	
	d) Rifampin or rifabutin therapy	1		1		2*		1*		3*		3*	
SSRIs		1		1		1		1		1		1	
St. John's wort		1		1		2		1		2		2	

Updated in 2017. This summary sheet only contains a subset of the recommendations from the U.S. MEC. For complete guidance, see: http://www.cdc.gov/reproductivehealth/unintendedpregnancy/USMEC.htm. Most contraceptive methods do not protect against sexually transmitted diseases (STDs). Consistent and correct use of the male latex condom reduces the risk of STDs and HIV.

CS266008-A

Effectiveness of Family Planning Methods

Most Effective	Reversible			Permanent		How to make your method most effective
	Implant	Intrauterine Device (IUD)	Male Sterilization (Vasectomy)	Female Sterilization (Abdominal, Laparoscopic, Hysteroscopic)		After procedure, little or nothing to do or remember.
Less than 1 pregnancy per 100 women in a year	0.05 %*	LNG - 0.2 % Copper T - 0.8 %	0.15 %	0.5 %		**Vasectomy and hysteroscopic sterilization:** Use another method for first 3 months.

	Injectable	Pill	Patch	Ring	Diaphragm	**Injectable:** Get repeat injections on time.
6-12 pregnancies per 100 women in a year	6 %	9 %	9 %	9 %	12 %	**Pills:** Take a pill each day. **Patch, Ring:** Keep in place, change on time. **Diaphragm:** Use correctly every time you have sex.

	Male Condom	Female Condom	Withdrawal	Sponge		Condoms, sponge, withdrawal, spermicides: Use correctly every time you have sex.
18 or more pregnancies per 100 women in a year	18 %	21 %	22 %	24 % parous women 12 % nulliparous women		**Fertility awareness-based methods:** Abstain or use condoms on fertile days. Newest methods (Standard Days Method and TwoDay Method) may be the easiest to use and consequently more effective.

	Fertility-Awareness Based Methods	Spermicide
Least Effective	24 %	28 %

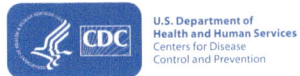

* The percentages indicate the number out of every 100 women who experienced an unintended pregnancy within the first year of typical use of each contraceptive method.

CS 242797

CONDOMS SHOULD ALWAYS BE USED TO REDUCE THE RISK OF SEXUALLY TRANSMITTED INFECTIONS.

Other Methods of Contraception

Lactational Amenorrhea Method: LAM is a highly effective, temporary method of contraception.

Emergency Contraception: Emergency contraceptive pills or a copper IUD after unprotected intercourse substantially reduces risk of pregnancy.

U.S. Department of Health and Human Services
Centers for Disease Control and Prevention

Adapted from World Health Organization (WHO) Department of Reproductive Health and Research, Johns Hopkins Bloomberg School of Public Health/Center for Communication Programs (CCP). Knowledge for health project. Family planning: a global handbook for providers (2011 update). Baltimore, MD; Geneva, Switzerland: CCP and WHO; 2011; and Trussell J. Contraceptive failure in the United States. Contraception 2011;83:397–404.

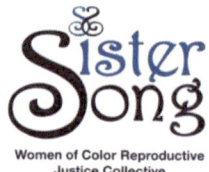
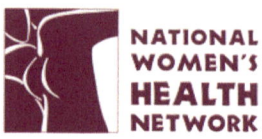

Long-Acting Reversible Contraception
Statement of Principles

We believe that people can and do make good decisions about the risks and benefits of drugs and medical devices when they have good information and supportive health care. We strongly support the inclusion of long-acting reversible contraceptive methods (LARCs) as part of a well-balanced mix of options, including barrier methods, oral contraceptives, and other alternatives. We reject efforts to direct women[1] toward any particular method and caution providers and public health officials against making assumptions based on race, ethnicity, age, ability, economic status, sexual orientation, or gender identity and expression. People should be given complete information and be supported in making the best decision for their health and other unique circumstances.

We call on the reproductive health, rights, and justice communities, including clinicians, professional associations, service providers, public health agencies, private funders and others to endorse the following principles.

We acknowledge the complex history of the provision of LARCs and seek to ensure that counseling is provided in a consistent and respectful manner that neither denies access nor coerces anyone into using a specific method.

- Many of the same communities now aggressively targeted by public health officials for LARCs have also been subjected to a long history of sterilization abuse, particularly people of color, low-income and uninsured women, Indigenous women, immigrant women, women with disabilities, and people whose sexual expression was not respected.

We commit to ensuring that people are provided comprehensive, scientifically accurate information about the full range of contraceptive options in a medically ethical and culturally competent manner in order to ensure that each person is supported in identifying the method that best meets their needs.

- A one-size-fits-all focus on LARCs at the exclusion of a full discussion of other methods ignores the needs of each individual and the benefits that other contraceptive methods provide. A woman seeking care who is preemptively directed to a LARC may be better

---

[1] While we use "woman" and "women" throughout this statement, we recognize that these terms do not encompass the full range of people who utilize contraception and who may be impacted by coercive practices. We also use the gender-inclusive "their" and "them" as singular pronouns.

served by a barrier method that reduces the spread of HIV and other sexually transmitted infections (STIs); a pill, patch, or ring that allows her to control her menstrual cycle; or any method that she can choose to stop using on her own without the approval of clinician.

- Women—particularly young women, elderly women, women of color, LGBTQ individuals, and low-income women—frequently report that clinicians talk down to them, do not take their questions seriously, and treat them as though they do not have the basic human right to determine what happens with their bodies. Only affordable coverage of all options and a comprehensive, medically accurate, and culturally competent discussion of them will ensure treatment of the whole human being and truly meet the health and life needs of every woman.

Advocates and the medical community must balance efforts to emphasize contraception as part of a healthy sex life beyond the fear of unintended pregnancy with appropriate counseling and support for people who seek contraception for other health reasons.

- The current focus on straight, cisgender women limits the health information given to people whose primary need may not be for preventing pregnancy, but for treating endometriosis, ovarian cysts, heavy or painful menstrual cycles, and more. This current focus also reinforces a limited set of public health outcomes that have been historically problematic, rather than respecting the bodily autonomy and rights of all women.

- Health care providers need good information to effectively consult with their patients. We seek to ensure access to training and up-to-date information on the benefits and possible drawbacks or limitations of any given option so that health professionals and clinic staff are able to provide the highest quality counseling for each and every patient.

The decision to obtain a LARC should be made by each person on the basis of quality counseling that helps them identify what will work best for them. No one should be pressured into using a certain method or denied access based on limitations in health insurance for the insertion or removal of LARC devices.

- Too often, providers receive biased promotional information from funders and pharmaceutical companies. It is critical that providers receive information that doesn't privilege LARC over other methods.

- Governments, foundations, and providers should reject explicit and implicit targets or goals for total numbers of LARCs inserted, which inappropriately bias the conversation between women and clinicians and can lead to coercion.

- Governments, foundations, and providers should reject incentives that limit patient choice, such as vouchers that can only be redeemed for LARCs.

The decision to cease using a long-acting method should be made by each individual with support from their health professional without judgment or obstacles.

- A woman who wants her LARC removed should have her decision respected and her LARC promptly removed, even if her clinician believes that she might ultimately be happy with the device if she were to wait.

- Removal of a LARC can be more demanding than insertion, but many women face significant obstacles when they want their LARC removed. Every clinic that offers a LARC should also have clinicians trained and able to remove LARCs and should offer appointments for removal at that same site. Likewise, providers should make clear that if women are not insured at the time they want their LARC removed, they may have to pay for removal out of pocket.

- When programs are implemented to increase access to LARCs, they should clearly address issues of removal, particularly how the needs of patients will be met if and when a program ends.

The current enthusiasm for LARCs should not distract from the ongoing need to support other policies and programs that address the full scope of healthy sexuality.

- Comprehensive sexuality education must be fully funded and supported.

- LARCs are an important addition to the range of options, but they are not the only option. The medical community must not only ensure access to and information about the full range of current methods, but also support continued research to develop new options to continue to improve quality of care and support women and families.

Women should have the right and the ability to control their own fertility whether planning, preventing or terminating a pregnancy. Marginalized communities, and particularly women of color, have experienced many forms of reproductive oppression, from forced sterilization to restrictions on abortion access to coercive limits on their ability to have children, and they continue to face high rates of maternal mortality.

We believe articulating these principles is necessary to protect the bodily autonomy and to respect the agency, health and dignity of marginalized women so that those who have historically been oppressed or harmed feel safe when making reproductive decisions. This is a critical step forward. This is what reproductive justice looks like.

Quick Start Algorithm — Patient requests a new birth control method:

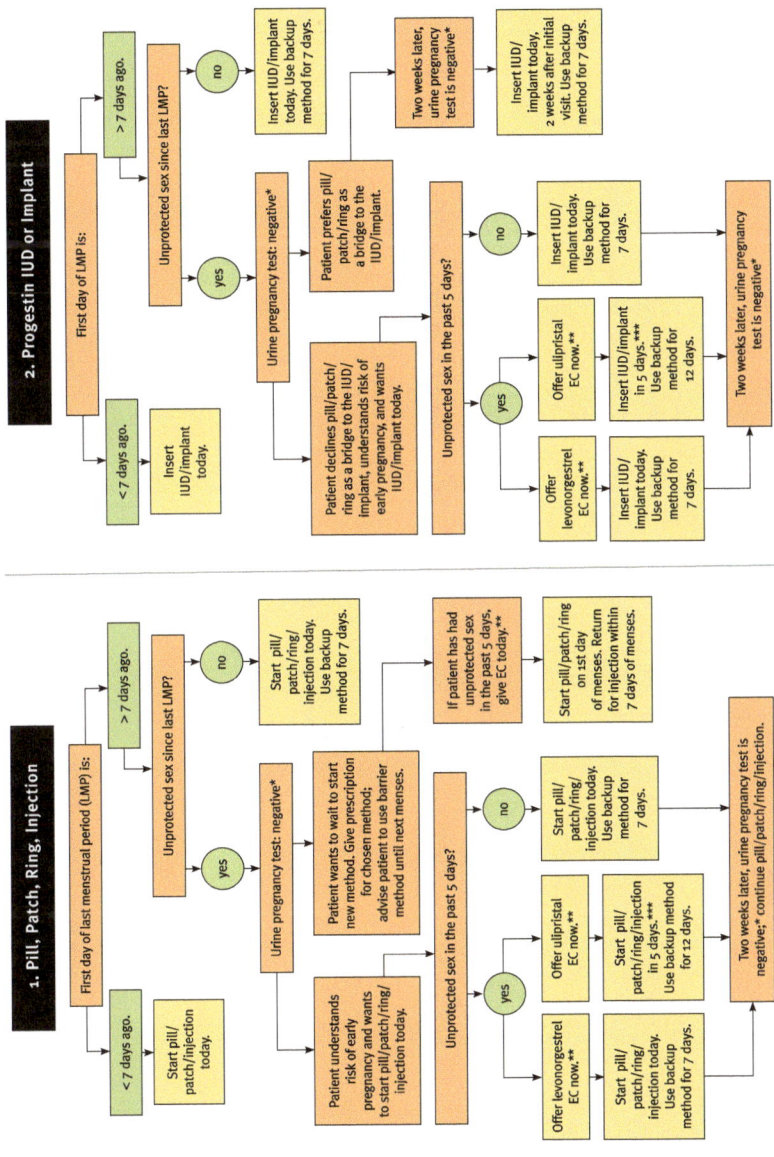

* If pregnancy test is positive, provide options counseling.
** For patients with body mass index over 25, levonorgestrel EC works no better than placebo. For those who had unprotected sex 3-5 days ago, ulipristal EC has higher efficacy than levonorgestrel EC.
*** Because ulipristal EC may interact with hormonal contraceptives, the new method should be started no sooner than 5 days after ulipristal EC. Consider starting injection/IUD/implant sooner if benefit outweighs risk.

Quick Start Algorithm — Patient requests a new birth control method:

3. Copper IUD

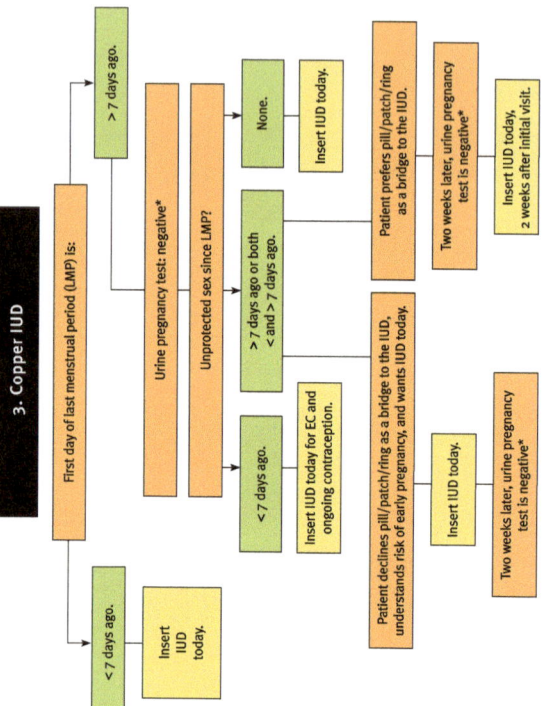

First day of last menstrual period (LMP) is:

- < 7 days ago. → Insert IUD today.

- > 7 days ago. → Urine pregnancy test: negative*
  - Unprotected sex since LMP?
    - None. → Insert IUD today.
    - > 7 days ago or both < and > 7 days ago.
      - Patient prefers pill/patch/ring as a bridge to the IUD. → Two weeks later, urine pregnancy test is negative* → Insert IUD today, 2 weeks after initial visit.
      - Patient declines pill/patch/ring as a bridge to the IUD, understands risk of early pregnancy, and wants IUD today.
        - Insert IUD today.
        - Two weeks later, urine pregnancy test is negative*
    - < 7 days ago. → Insert IUD today for EC and ongoing contraception.

* If pregnancy test is positive, provide options counseling.

Citation: Curtis KM, Jattaoui TC, Tepper NK, et al. U.S. Selected Practice Recommendations for Contraceptive Use, 2016. MMWR Recomm Rep 2016;65(No. RR-4):1–66. DOI: http://dx.doi.org/10.15585/mmwr.rr6504a1.

FACT SHEET : COPPER IUD

Remember, the copper IUD **does not protect you from Sexually Transmitted Infections or HIV.** Always use condoms to protect yourself!

HOW DOES THE COPPER IUD WORK?

- The copper IUD is a T-shaped plastic rod that stays in your uterus. It releases small amounts of copper. Copper kills sperm. Without live sperm, you cannot get pregnant.
- No method of birth control is 100% effective. The copper IUD is over 99% effective.

AFTER THE COPPER IUD IS INSERTED, WHEN CAN I HAVE SEX?

- You must wait 24 hours after the IUD is placed before you can use tampons or have sex.

WHEN DOES THE COPPER IUD START WORKING?

- The copper IUD works right after it is placed in you. It may be inserted up to 5 days after unprotected sex to prevent pregnancy.

HOW LONG DOES THE COPPER IUD LAST?

- The copper IUD works for 10-12 years.

WHAT DO I NEED TO DO AFTER I HAVE THE IUD INSERTED?

- Some women like to check their IUD's string after each period. To check, insert a finger into your vagina and feel for the cervix. (It feels like the tip of your nose.) You should feel the string near your cervix. **Do not** pull on the string.

WHAT DO I DO IF AND WHEN I DECIDE TO GET PREGNANT?

- When you are ready, your health care provider will remove your IUD. Most women get pregnant soon after removal.

HOW DOES THE COPPER IUD HELP ME?

- You do not need to think about birth control before or during sex.
- You do not need refills (as you do for the pill).
- You can use the copper IUD while breastfeeding.
- The copper IUD costs less than most types of birth control.

HOW WILL I FEEL HAVING THE IUD IN ME?
HOW WILL MY BODY CHANGE?

- You will not feel the IUD in you.
- You may have cramps and heavy periods. Ibuprofen can help. You can take up to 4 pills (800 mg) of Ibuprofen every 8 hours with food. To prevent cramps, take Ibuprofen when your period starts and keep taking it every 8 hours for the first 2-3 days of your period. You can also put a hot water bottle on your belly if you have bad cramps.

DOES THE COPPER IUD HAVE RISKS?

- The copper IUD is very safe. Serious problems are rare. If you have the following symptoms **within the first 3 weeks** after the IUD is inserted, see your health care provider:
  - Fever (>101ºF)
  - Chills
  - Strong pain in your belly
- If you have the following symptoms **at any time** while you have an IUD in you, see your health care provider:
  - Feeling pregnant (breast tenderness, nausea, vomiting)
  - Positive home pregnancy test

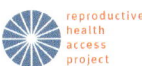

reproductive
health
access
project

June 2015 / www.reproductiveaccess.org

FACT SHEET :

PROGESTIN IUD –
MIRENA®, LILETTA®, SKYLA®, and others

Remember, the progestin IUD **does not protect you from Sexually Transmitted Infections or HIV.** Always use condoms to protect yourself!

HOW DOES THE PROGESTIN IUD WORK?
- The progestin IUD is a T-shaped plastic rod that stays in your uterus. It contains a hormone (progestin) like the ones your body makes. The hormone blocks sperm from reaching the egg and stops the release of eggs. If sperm cannot reach an egg, you cannot get pregnant.
- No method of birth control is 100% effective. The progestin IUD is over 99% effective.

AFTER THE PROGESTIN IUD IS INSERTED, WHEN CAN I HAVE SEX?
- You must wait 24 hours after the IUD is placed before you can use tampons or have sex.

WHEN DOES THE PROGESTIN IUD START WORKING?
- The progestin IUD starts to work 7 days after it is inserted. For 7 days after your IUD is inserted, **use condoms or continue your pills/patch/ring as back-up**.

HOW LONG DOES THE PROGESTIN IUD LAST?
- The progestin IUD works for 3 to 7 years, depending on which IUD you choose.

IS THERE ANYTHING I NEED TO DO AFTER HAVING THE IUD INSERTED?
- Some people like to check their IUD's string after each period. To check, insert a finger into your vagina and feel for the cervix. (It feels like the tip of your nose.) You should feel the string near your cervix. **Do not** pull on the string.

WHAT DO I DO IF AND WHEN I DECIDE TO GET PREGNANT?
- When you are ready, your health care provider will remove your IUD. Most people get pregnant soon after removal.

HOW DOES THE PROGESTIN IUD HELP ME?
- You do not need to think about birth control before or during sex.
- You do not need refills (as you do for the pill).
- You can use the progestin IUD while breastfeeding.
- You may have less cramping and bleeding with periods.
- The progestin IUD costs less than most types of birth control.

HOW WILL I FEEL HAVING THE PROGESTIN IUD IN ME?
HOW WILL MY BODY CHANGE?
- You will not feel the IUD in you.
- You may have cramps and spotty periods for the first few months. Ibuprofen can help. You can take up to 4 pills (800 mg) of Ibuprofen every 8 hours with food. To prevent cramps, take Ibuprofen when your period starts and keep taking it every 8 hours for the first 2-3 days of your period. You can also put a hot water bottle on your belly if you have bad cramps.
- You may stop having periods after 1-2 years with the progestin IUD. This is normal.
- You may have spotting, bloating, nausea, headaches, or breast tenderness.

DOES THE PROGESTIN IUD HAVE RISKS?
- The progestin IUD is very safe. Serious problems are rare. If you have the following symptoms **within the first 3 weeks** after getting an IUD, see your health care provider:
    - Fever (>101ºF)
    - Chills
    - Strong or sharp pain in your stomach or belly
- If you have the following symptoms **at any time** while you have an IUD in you, see your health care provider:
    - Feeling pregnant (breast tenderness, nausea, vomiting)
    - Positive home pregnancy test

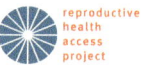

reproductive
health
access
project

March 2017 / www.reproductiveaccess.org

Intra-Uterine Device (IUD) Insertion Equipment List

IUD (Paragard, Liletta, Mirena, or Skyla)

Sterile Instruments:
Small speculum
Tenaculum
Scissors
Ringed forceps
Needle extender
Metal cup
4 x 4's

Also:
- Uterine Sound-Dilator
- **OR** Os finders- disposable (size I, II, and III) and disposable uterine sound
- **One** 10 mL syringe of combined: **OR**   **One** 10 mL syringe of combined:
    - 2.5 mL of 1 % Lidocaine   2.5 mL of 0.25%
      Marcaine
    - 2.5 mL of 0.9% Bacteriostatic NaCl   2.5 mL of 0.9%
      Bacteriostatic NaCl
    - 0.5 mL of 8.4% Sodium Bicarbonate
- 18 g needle to draw up medication
- 22 g 1 ½ to attach to syringe

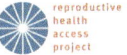

Intra-Uterine Device (IUD) Removal Equipment List

IUD Removal (simple)
- Small speculum (plastic)
- Ringed forceps
- Large OB swabs (large cotton swabs)
- Contraceptive options handout if desired

IUD Removal Complex (sterile)
- Small sterile speculum
- Tenaculum
- Ringed forceps
- Sterile 4 x 4's
- Alligator forceps and IUD hook
- 10 mL syringe of combined: **OR**   10 mL syringe of
  combined:
  - 5 mL of 1 % Lidocaine   5 mL of 0.25%
    Marcaine
  - 5 mL of 0.9% Bacteriostatic NaCl   5 mL of 0.9%
    Bacteriostatic NaCl
  - 0.5 mL 8.4% Sodium Bicarbonate
- 18 g needle to draw up medication
- 22g 1 ½ to attach to syringe

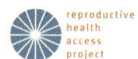

LARC Readiness Checklist
Site:
Date:
Completed by:

Issue/Requirement	Status/Notes
Facility Considerations	
1. Adequate, private exam room with exam table	
2. Appropriate IUD/implant insertion and removal supplies resource: http://www.reproductiveaccess.org/wp-content/uploads/2015/01/IUD-Insertion-Set-up-Supplies.pdf	
3. Space for storing IUD/implant devices	
4. Space for storing sterile and non-sterile equipment.	
5. Sterilization of equipment ☐ Onsite ☐ Transport from offsite facility	
Administrative Considerations	
1. Chart note template for IUD insertion/removal visit resource: http://www.reproductiveaccess.org/resources/?rsearch=epic&rtopic%5B%5D=46	
2. Chart note template for implant insertion/removal visit resource: http://www.reproductiveaccess.org/resources/?rsearch=epic&rtopic%5B%5D=45	

LARC Readiness Checklist
Site:
Date:
Completed by:

3. Billing and coding codes up to date resources: http://www.reproductiveaccess.org/resource s/?rsearch=epic&rtopic%5B%5D=45 http://www.reproductiveaccess.org/resource s/?rsearch=Coding&rtopic%5B%5D=45	
5. System for appointment scheduling	
6. System for ordering/tracking supplies	
Clinical Considerations	
1. IUD and implant protocols in place. resources: http://www.reproductiveaccess.org/resource /depo-provera-policy-procedures/ http://www.reproductiveaccess.org/resource /iud-policy-procedure/	
2. Procedure for sterilizing equipment in place.	
3. IUD and implant consent forms available. resources: http://www.reproductiveaccess.org/resource /iud-consent-form/ http://www.reproductiveaccess.org/resource /progestin-implant-consent-form/	
4. Patient education materials available. resources: http://www.reproductiveaccess.org/resource s/?rsearch=&rtopic%5B%5D=46&rtype%5B%5D =61 http://www.reproductiveaccess.org/resource s/?rsearch=&rtopic%5B%5D=45&rtype%5B%5D =61	

LARC Readiness Checklist
Site:
Date:
Completed by:

5. Patient after care information available. resources: http://www.reproductiveaccess.org/resources/?rsearch=&rtopic%5B%5D=45&rtype%5B%5D=62 http://www.reproductiveaccess.org/resources/?rsearch=&rtopic%5B%5D=46&rtype%5B%5D=62	
6. QA systems in place	
7. Malpractice coverage (verify for pediatricians)	

LARC Clinical Training Opportunities

Method-Specific Training Opportunities

- **Kyleena® (levonorgestrel-releasing intrauterine system) 19.5mg: | Bayer HealthCare Pharmaceuticals**
  - To watch an insertion and removal video: https://hcp.kyleena-us.com/#insertionandremoval
  - To request a training: 1-888-84-BAYER (1-888-842-2937)
  - For more information: https://hcp.kyleena-us.com/

- **Liletta® (levonorgestrel-releasing intrauterine system) 52mg | Medicines360**
  - To watch an insertion and removal video: https://www.lilettahcp.com/resources/placement
  - To request a training: https://www.lilettahcp.com/request-a-rep or 1-800-678-1605
  - For more information: https://www.lilettahcp.com

- **Mirena® (levonorgestrel-releasing intrauterine system) 52mg | Bayer HealthCare Pharmaceuticals**
  - To watch an insertion and removal video: http://hcp.mirena-us.com/mirena-insertion-removal-video/
  - To request a training: 1-888-84-BAYER (1-888-842-2937)
  - For more information: http://hcp.mirena-us.com/

- **Nexplanon® (etonogestrel implant) 68mg | Merck & Co., Inc.**
  - To request a training: https://www.nexplanontraining.com/request-clinical-training/in-person-training/
  - For more information: https://www.merckconnect.com/nexplanon/overview.html

- **ParaGard® (intrauterine copper contraceptive) | CooperSurgical, Inc.**
  - To watch an insertion and removal video: http://hcp.paragard.com/Resources/Videos.aspx
  - To request a training: 1-877-PARAGARD (1-877-727-2427)
  - For more information: http://hcp.paragard.com/

- **Skyla® (levonorgestrel-releasing intrauterine system) 13.5mg | Bayer HealthCare Pharmaceuticals**
  - To watch an insertion and removal video: http://hcp.skyla-us.com/insertion-and-removal/
  - To request a training: 1-888-84-BAYER (1-888-842-2937)
  - For more information: http://hcp.skyla-us.com/

Brand Name	Description	FDA-Approved Duration of Use	Researched Extended Use	Size (horizonal x vertical)	Inserter Tube Diameter	Typical Use Failure Rate
Kyleena®	19.5mg LNG IUD	5 years	N/A	28mm x 30mm	3.8mm	0.20%*
Liletta®	52mg LNG IUD	4 years	Up to 5 years	32mm x 32mm	4.4mm	0.20%*
Mirena®	52mg LNG IUD	5 years	Up to 7 years	32mm x 32mm	4.4mm	0.20%*
Nexplanon®	68mg ENG implant	3 years	Up to 5 years	40mm x 2mm	N/A	0.05%
Paragard®	Copper IUD	10 years	Up to 12 years	32mm x 36mm	4.01mm	0.80%
Skyla®	13.5mg LNG IUD	3 years	N/A	28mm x 30mm	3.8mm	0.20%*

Table information from device prescribing information and ACOG Practice Bulletin No. 186.   *for all LNG IUDs

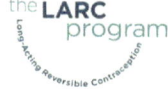
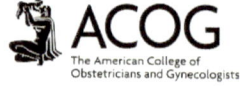

General Training Opportunities

- **Beyond the Pill**

  The Beyond the Pill program from the Bixby Center for Global Reproductive Health at the University of California, San Francisco (UCSF) partners with health care providers, researchers, and educators to improve women's access to effective contraception and reproductive health care. This training program is designed to increase provider knowledge and skills for IUDs and implants, and improve women's access to these methods of birth control.
  - For free online training: http://beyondthepill.ucsf.edu/online-training
  - For on-site training information: http://beyondthepill.ucsf.edu/site-training
  - To request an on-site training: Jennifer Grand at Jennifer.Grand@ucsf.edu or 1-415-502-0331

- **Contraceptive Technology**

  Contraceptive Technology hosts conferences that cover advances in women's health and contraception and topics including new and future methods of contraception, sexuality, recurrent vaginitis, adolescent health, and STD treatment. The conferences include interactive sessions and hands-on workshops.
  - For information on upcoming training sessions:
    http://www.contraceptivetechnology.org/conferences/upcoming-ct-conferences/

- **Essential Access Health**

  Essential Access Health's Learning Exchange is a resource for information about best practices in the provision of quality, patient-centered sexual and reproductive health care in diverse settings. Training formats include hands-on clinical practica in IUD and implant placement, Family Planning Health Worker Certification trainings, live webinars, online courses, in-person trainings, and an annual conference. The Learning Exchange also offers custom trainings and is a certified provider of continuing education credits.
  - For a list of training opportunities: http://www.essentialaccesshealth.org
  - To request an on-site training: Jasmine Hutchinson at jhutchinson@essentialaccess.org

- **National Clinical Training Center for Family Planning**

  The National Clinical Training Center for Family Planning (NCTCFP) provides training for family planning Nurse Practitioners, Certified Nurse Midwives, Physicians and Physician Assistants. NCTCFP offers a national family planning training symposium, reproductive health conference, and clinical webinars.
  - For a list of training opportunities: http://www.ctcfp.org/larc
  - For more information: Kimberly Carlson at 1-866-91-CTCFP (1-866-912-8237) or carlsonkim@umkc.edu

- **Upstream USA**

  Upstream USA provides on-site, comprehensive consulting and technical training to health centers so that they can provide the full range of contraceptive methods, same day, including IUDs and implants. This training includes CME/CE-accredited content for clinicians, such as LARC placement skills, and offers counseling tips for health educators, counselors, and medical assistants and in-depth revenue cycle management assistance and/or coding review for billing and financial staff.
  - For on-site training information: http://www.upstream.org/our-training/
  - To request an on-site training: Peter Belden at peter@upstream.org

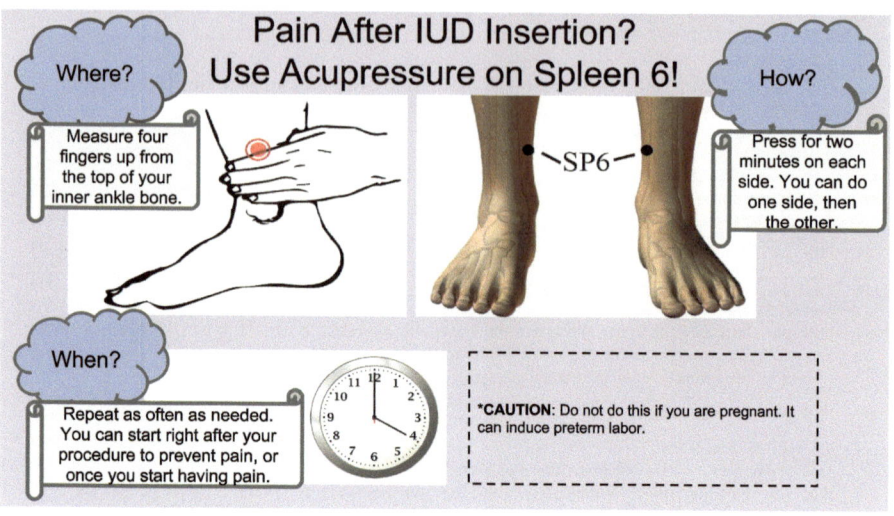

Step 1: Does patient have anxiety before or during IUD placement?

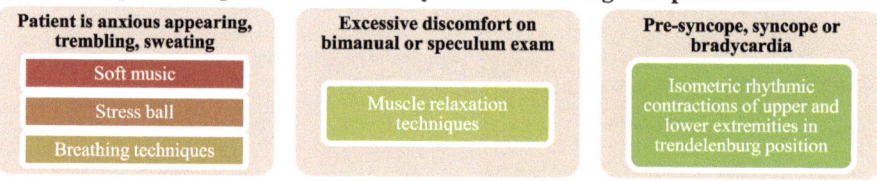

Step 2: Do you have complete visualization of the cervix?

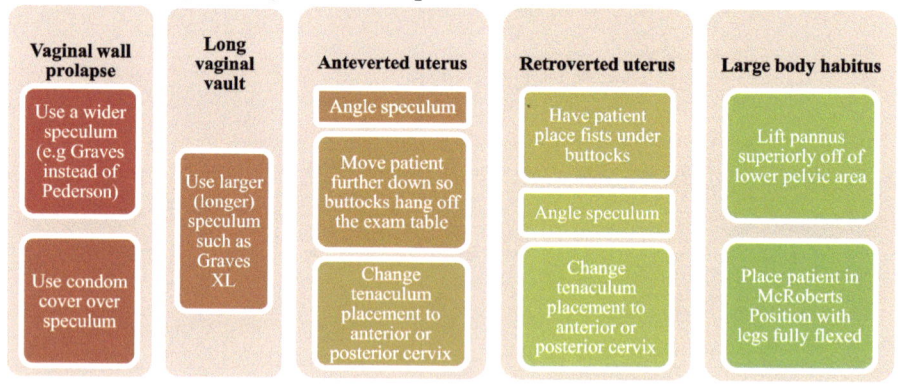

Step 3: Can you introduce a sound into the cervical os?

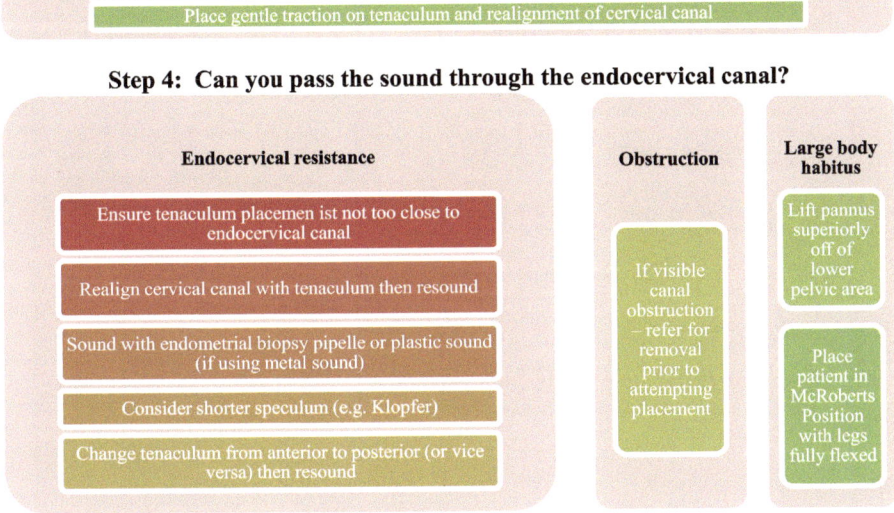

Difficulty introducing the sound

Gently place cytobrush into os

Use os finder

Change to endometrial biopsy pipelle/plastic sound if using metal sound

Place gentle traction on tenaculum and realignment of cervical canal

Step 4: Can you pass the sound through the endocervical canal?

Endocervical resistance

Ensure tenaculum placemen ist not too close to endocervical canal

Realign cervical canal with tenaculum then resound

Sound with endometrial biopsy pipelle or plastic sound (if using metal sound)

Consider shorter speculum (e.g. Klopfer)

Change tenaculum from anterior to posterior (or vice versa) then resound

Obstruction

If visible canal obstruction – refer for removal prior to attempting placement

Large body habitus

Lift pannus superiorly off of lower pelvic area

Place patient in McRoberts Position with legs fully flexed

Step 5: Can you successfully sound the uterus to > 5 cm depth?

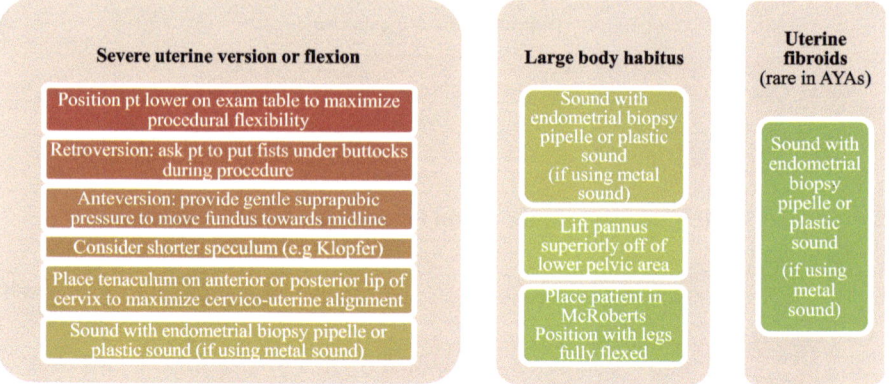

Step 6: Can you introduce the IUD inserter tube into the uterine cavity so that flange is flush with cervix (sounding depth)?

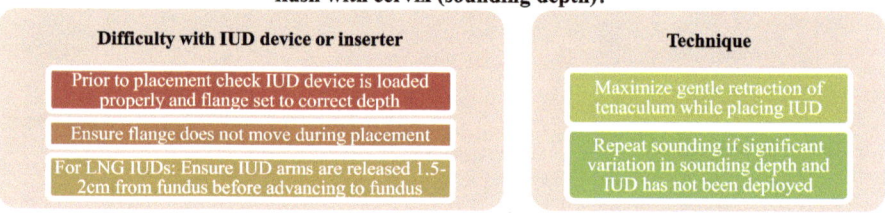

Algorithm 2: IUD Removal with Missing Strings

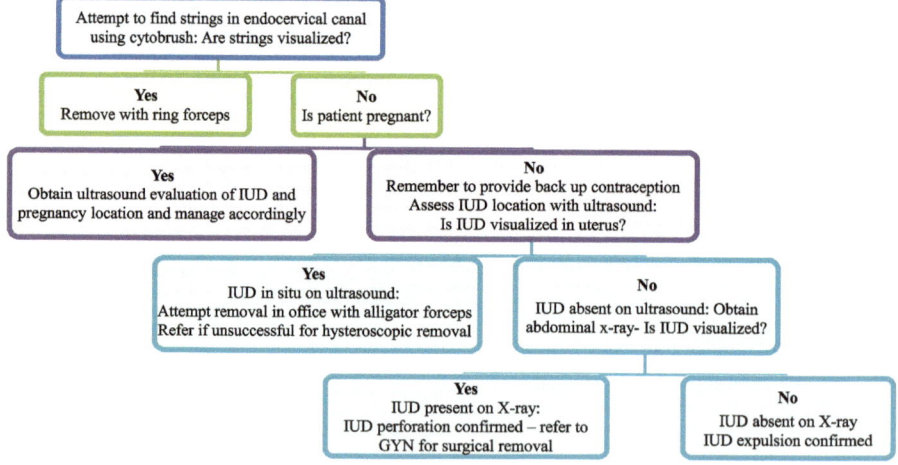

Sample Onsite IUD Protocol

1. Provider Training and Credentialing Processes

    a. Group trainings: Develop and convene general trainings for all SBHC staff. Topics should include IUD overview, values clarification relating to IUDs and adolescents, patient flow, IUD follow-up care, and customer service.

    b. Preceptorships: Preceptorships will be the mainstay of provider training, either on-site at the sponsoring institution (SI)'s high volume procedure session or, on-site at the provider's school-based health center under supervision of an trained preceptor:

        i. Providers will be observed at least twice for each of the two IUDs (Mirena and Paragard) respectively, or until competence with the procedure is established. This can be done either at the SI high volume procedure session or under supervision by a trained preceptor at the school-based health center site. Providers can be scheduled to go to the SI procedure session during school holidays and summer sessions.

        ii. An observational form will be used for each insertion (at SI and at the school-based health center). The form will assess competency in four domains (medical knowledge, interpersonal and communication skills, patient care/skills IUD insertion general, and patient care/skills IUD insertion specific to Mirena and/or Paragard). There is no need to identify the patient's name and medical record number on the observational form, and that a paper copy of the form is sufficient.

        iii. Once the provider has been deemed competent, the program's medical director will be notified by the supervising physician to make a formal request to the respective Departmental Chairperson for adding this procedure to the list of credentialed procedures. Credentialing for each of the IUD products should be done separately. The complete observation form (with all fields indicating a competent level) will go into the provider's personnel file.

        iv. Medically Trained Personnel (LPN, RN, PCA, PCT) Trainings: Prior to assisting the school- health provider at the school- health site, the staff person will spend one-half day session at the SI or at another SBHC already inserting IUDs in order to observe IUD insertion procedures, along with the SI's designated Patient Care Technician who is assigned to the reproductive health sessions. LPNs can be scheduled to go to the SI during school holidays and summer sessions.

4/12/2019

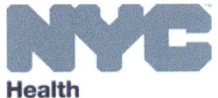

2. Site Phase-Ins: One provider at each SBHC in a High School/Campus will be designated for training as an IUD inserter.

    a. Step One - Initial Site. Supervising physician will initiate program on [start date]. Allow time during the pilot phase to address issues with the procedures and protocols before expansion to other sites.

    b. Step Two - Implement program to remaining sites one at a time with trained and credentialed IUD inserters.

3. Clinical Care Protocol

    a. Appointments for IUD insertion will be scheduled in a 30-minute appointment slot. Appointments for IUD removal will be scheduled in a 15-minute appointment slot.

    b. Two to three appointments per morning will be scheduled for IUD insertion. Initially, appointments will only be scheduled once a week during initial phase-in of the protocol. Adjustments will be made based on demand and capacity, in consultation with supervising physicians. No appointments will be scheduled when supervising physician is not available on-site until SBHC provider has been signed off.

    c. Site Back Up System: During working hours, providers will contact supervising physician directly for clinical back up. A back-up for the supervising physician must be designated. During off-hours, patients will be instructed (verbally and in writing on the "Post-Insertion Instruction sheet") to call the on-call provider telephone number. Back-up for the on-call provider must be designated and a telephone number assigned.

    d. Parent Communication Protocol: a specific protocol will be created to train all SBHC staff about how to respond to a parent/guardian who inadvertently learns about an otherwise confidential IUD insertion procedure. The protocol will be contextualized in the overall procedures around confidentiality for any form of contraception, and will include discussion of avoiding parent/guarding disclosure as part of overall contraception counseling. The protocol will include instructions to contact the Medical Director immediately in the case of inadvertent parent/guardian disclosure; the medical director will contact the supervising physician and director of the sponsoring institution.

4/12/2019

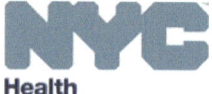
Health

4. Supplies

    a. A required equipment list must be created for each site's needs (see sample attached).

    b. Determine how IUD devices will be ordered and articulate in this section of the protocol.

5. Infection Control

    a. All sites, prior to initiation of the IUD Insertion Protocol, will be visited from a representative from the Infection Control Division.

    b. All sites will follow standard procedures for infection control, by first soaking the items in an approved cidal agent as per SI Infection Control Division in the designated "dirty area," and then decontaminating in the Autoclave.

    c. When autoclaves are available onsite, develop and articulate procedures in this section of the protocol.

6. Evaluation/Continuous Quality Improvement

    a. All appointments and actual insertions will be documented using a standard time out procedure and observation form/EMR template.

    b. Create a plan that includes an assessment strategy, time frame, and specific measures of interest. Examples of outcome indicators can include:

        i. % of IUD appointments with completed IUD insertions

        ii. % of sexually active females (within 90 days) with IUD insertions

        iii. % of sexually active females on contraception who have had a IUD insertion

        iv. % increase of IUD insertions from baseline of protocol initiation

        v. % of IUDs removed

4/12/2019

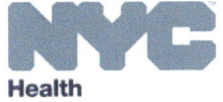

Checklist for onsite IUD Readiness

- ☐ IUD credentialing on file

- ☐ Allied staff training completed

- ☐ Infection control signed off

- ☐ Supplies onsite

- ☐ Tool cleansing protocol in place

- ☐ Appointment system in place

- ☐ Adverse event protocol in place

- ☐ Phone call and back-up plan delineated

- ☐ Supervision plan for onsite IUD in place

- ☐ Plan for initial IUD insertions in place
    - will supervisor be onsite?
    - who will oversee clinical issues as they arise?

- ☐ Physical environment meets criteria

4/12/2019

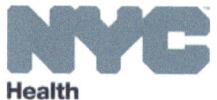

Index

A
Abortifacients, 48
Acupuncture, 114, 123, 128, 130
Adolescent-friendly services, 12
American Academy of Pediatrics (AAP), 7–8, 42
American College of Obstetricians and
        Gynecologists (ACOG), 7, 8, 37,
        42, 47, 56, 76, 77
Atmosphere and materials, 14–16
Awareness and misconceptions, 6

B
Best practices and real-world applications, 13
Bleeding patterns, 66
Breastfeeding, 77

C
Call center/scheduling staff tips and scripts, 20
CHOICE Project, 50
Clinic-wide training, 96
Consent process
    duration of action, 85
    ectopic pregnancy, 87
    expulsion, 86
    infection, 86
    informed consent, 84, 85
    insertion, 88
    menstrual bleeding and cramping patterns,
        85, 86
    patients expectation, 89
    pelvic exam counseling, 87, 88
    perforation, 87
    pre-procedural counseling, 87

    standardized procedural informed consent
        templates, 87
    uterine anatomy, 88
Consumerist counseling, 59
Contemporary, 4, 5, 7, 8
Contraception abuse, 58, 59
Contraceptive counseling, 61, 62
    bleeding patterns, 66 (*see also* Consent
        process)
    consumerist counseling, 59
    contraception abuse and reproductive
        coercion, 58, 59
    directive counseling, 59, 60
    effectiveness, 56, 64, 65
    first-line method, 56
    IUD removal, 65
    perfect contraceptive use, 56
    placement, continuation, and removal, 56
    SDM, 60–64
    sexual readiness, 57, 58
Contraindications, 49
Copper intrauterine devices (IUDs), 4, 13,
        36–38, 48, 75
Cramping patterns, 85, 86
CuT380A IUD, 36

D
Dalkon shield, 2–4, 86
Diagnosis Related Group (DRG) code, 77
Directive counseling, 59, 60

E
Ectopic pregnancy, 47

© Springer Nature Switzerland AG 2019
M. Coles, A. Mays (eds.), *Optimizing IUD Delivery for Adolescents and Young
Adults*, https://doi.org/10.1007/978-3-030-17816-1